The Kidney

Editors

KIM ZUBER
JANE S. DAVIS

PHYSICIAN ASSISTANT CLINICS

www.physicianassistant.theclinics.com

Consulting Editor
JAMES A. VAN RHEE

April 2022 • Volume 7 • Number 2

ELSEVIER

1600 John F. Kennedy Boulevard • Suite 1800 • Philadelphia, Pennsylvania, 19103-2899

http://www.theclinics.com

PHYSICIAN ASSISTANT CLINICS Volume 7, Number 2
April 2022 ISSN 2405-7991, ISBN-13: 978-0-323-89734-1

Editor: Katerina Heidhausen
Developmental Editor: Axell Ivan Jade Purificacion

Physician Assistant Clinics (ISSN: 2405–7991) is published quarterly by Elsevier Inc., 360 Park Avenue South, New York, NY 10010-1710. Months of issue are January, April, July, and October. Periodicals postage paid at New York, NY and additional mailing offices. Subscription prices are $150.00 per year (US individuals), $305.00 (US institutions), $100.00 (US students), $150.00 (Canadian individuals), $320.00 (Canadian institutions), $100.00 (Canadian students), $150.00 (international individuals), $320.00 (international institutions), and $100.00 (international students). Foreign air speed delivery is included in all *Clinics* subscription prices. All prices are subject to change without notice. POSTMASTER: Send address changes to *Physician Assistant Clinics*, Elsevier Periodicals Customer Service, 11830 Westline Industrial Drive, St. Louis, MO 63146. Customer Service Health Sciences Division, Subscription Customer Service, 3251 Riverport Lane, Maryland Heights, MO 63043. **Customer Service: 1-800-654-2452 (U.S. and Canada); 314-447-8871 (outside U.S. and Canada). Fax: 314-447-8029. E-mail: journalscustomerservice-usa@elsevier.com (for print support); journalsonlinesupport-usa@elsevier.com (for online support).**

Reprints. For copies of 100 or more, of articles in this publication, please contact the Commercial Reprints Department, Elsevier Inc., 360 Park Avenue South, New York, NY 10010-1710. Tel. 212-633-3874; Fax: 212-633-3820; E-mail: reprints@elsevier.com.

Physician Assistant Clinics is covered in *EMBASE/Excerpta Medica and ESCI.*

PROGRAM OBJECTIVE
The goal of the Physician Assistant Clinics is to keep practicing physician assistants up to date with current clinical practice by providing timely articles reviewing the state of the art in patient care.

TARGET AUDIENCE
Physician Assistants and other healthcare professionals

LEARNING OBJECTIVES
Upon completion of this activity, participants will be able to:
1. Review the pathology, clinical presentation, risk factors, classification systems, comorbidities, and complications of kidney disease to facilitate in appropriate diagnosis and staging.
2. Discuss:
    a. treatment and management of kidney disease with the appropriate use of clinical practice guide-lines, diagnostic studies, treatment therapies including pharmacotherapy, hemodialysis, lifestyle modifications, and kidney replacement.
    b. Relationship with vital organs
    c. Ethical considerations of end-of-life care
    d. Risk and impact of kidney disease in special populations
3. Recognize the relevance of the U.S. military and its role in the development of the role of the physician assistant and its advocacy effects in recognizing nephrology as a specialty and treatment of kidney disease.

ACCREDITATION
The Elsevier Office of Continuing Medical Education (EOCME) is accredited by the Accreditation Council for Continuing Medical Education (ACCME) to provide continuing medical education for physicians.

The EOCME designates this journal-based CME activity for a maximum of 17 *AMA PRA Category 1 Credit*(s)™. Physicians should claim only the credit commensurate with the extent of their participation in the activity.

All other health care professionals requesting continuing education credit for this enduring material will be issued a certificate of participation.

DISCLOSURE OF CONFLICTS OF INTEREST
The EOCME assesses conflict of interest with its instructors, faculty, planners, and other individuals who are in a position to control the content of CME activities. All relevant conflicts of interest that are identified are thoroughly vetted by EOCME for fair balance, scientific objectivity, and patient care recommendations. EOCME is committed to providing its learners with CME activities that promote improvements or quality in healthcare and not a specific proprietary business or a commercial interest.

The planning committee, staff, authors, and editors listed below have identified no financial relationships or relationships to products or devices they or their spouse/life partner have with commercial interest related to the content of this CME activity:
Molly E. Band, MHS, PA-C; Samantha Gwyn Collins, PA-C; Jyothi Digambaranath, PhD, PA-S; Harvey A. Feldman, MD, FACP, FASN; Kimberly Gadulka, MA, CCC-SLP, PA-S; Dale Marie Gomez, PA-C; Rebecca Grillo, PA-C, RD, LD/N; Brittany Heady, PA-C; Rodney Ho, PhD, MPH, PA-C, Psychiatry-CAQ; Caroline Jackson, PharmD candidate; Pradeep Kuttysankaran; Claretha Lyas, MD; Rebecca Maxson, PharmD, BCPS; Megan McKay, PA-S; Ciara Mitchell, MA, RD, LD; Amy Mosman, MMS, PA-C; Becky Ness, PA-C, MPAS, DFAAPA, FNKF; Nguyen H. Park, MS, PA-C, DFAAPA; Lindsay Paige Penninger, PA-C; Flor A. Rangel, DMD, PA-S; Michaela Rekow, PA-C; Dawn E. Rosenbaum, MHS, PA-C; Marlene Shaw-Gallagher, MS, PA-C; Faraaz Siddiqui, PA-S; Melanie T. Stapleton, MS-PAS, PA-C; Kelly A. Sweeney, PA-S; Doreen Thomas-Payne, MSN, BSN, RN, PMHNP-BC; Kendra A. Thomsen, MPAS, PA-C; Julie C. Utley, MPAS, PA-C; Kara-Ann Valentine, MMS, PA-C; Troy Zimmerman, BA; Kim Zuber, PAC, MS

The planning committee, staff, authors and editors listed below have identified financial relationships or relationships to products or devices they or their spouse/life partner have with commercial interest related to the content of this CME activity:
Jane S. Davis, DNP: *Speakers Bureau*: Amgen, Bayer

UNAPPROVED/OFF-LABEL USE DISCLOSURE
The EOCME requires CME faculty to disclose to the participants:

1. When products or procedures being discussed are off-label, unlabelled, experimental, and/or investigational (not US Food and Drug Administration [FDA] approved); and
2. Any limitations on the information presented, such as data that are preliminary or that represent ongoing research, interim analyses, and/or unsupported opinions. Faculty may discuss information about pharmaceutical agents that is outside of FDA-approved labelling. This information is intended solely for CME and is not intended to promote off-label use of these medications. If you have any questions, contact the medical affairs department of the manufacturer for the most recent prescribing information.

TO ENROLL
The CME program is available to all Physician Assistant Clinics subscribers at no additional fee. To subscribe to the Physician Assistant Clinics, call customer service at 1-800-654-2452 or sign up online at www.physicianassistant.theclinics.com.

METHOD OF PARTICIPATION
In order to claim credit, participants must complete the following:
1. Complete enrolment as indicated above
2. Read the activity
3. Complete the CME Test and Evaluation. Participants must achieve a score of 70% on the test. All CME Tests and Evaluations must be completed online

CME INQUIRIES/SPECIAL NEEDS
For all CME inquiries or special needs, please contact elsevierCME@elsevier.com.

Contributors

CONSULTING EDITOR

JAMES A. VAN RHEE, MS, PA-C
Associate Professor, Program Director, Yale School of Medicine, Yale Physician Assistant Online Program, New Haven, Connecticut

EDITORS

KIM ZUBER, PAC, MS
Executive Director, American Academy of Nephrology PAs, St Petersburg, Florida

JANE S. DAVIS, DNP
Division of Nephrology, University of Alabama at Birmingham, Birmingham, Alabama

AUTHORS

MOLLY E. BAND, MHS, PA-C
Pediatric Urology, Yale New Haven Hospital, New Haven, Connecticut

SAMANTHA GWYN COLLINS, PA-C
Carolina Kidney Associates, Greensboro, North Carolina

JANE S. DAVIS, DNP
Division of Nephrology, University of Alabama at Birmingham, Birmingham, Alabama

JYOTHI DIGAMBARANATH, PhD, PA-S
University of Detroit Mercy, Detroit, Michigan

HARVEY A. FELDMAN, MD, FACP, FASN
Physician Assistant Program, Nova Southeastern University, Ft Lauderdale, Florida

KIMBERLY GADULKA, MA, CCC-SLP, PA-S
University of Detroit Mercy, Detroit, Michigan

DALE MARIE GOMEZ, PA-C
Physician Assistant, Mid Atlantic Nephrology Associates, Baltimore, Maryland

REBECCA GRILLO, PA-C, RD, LD/N
Renal Hypertension Center, Hudson, Florida

BRITTANY HEADY, PA-C
St. Louis Kidney Consultants, St Louis, Missouri

RODNEY HO, PhD, MPH, PA-C, Psychiatry-CAQ
Adjunct Instructor, University of West Florida, JBSA–Lackland

CAROLINE JACKSON, PharmD candidate
Auburn University Harrison School of Pharmacy, Auburn, Alabama

CLARETHA LYAS, MD
Assistant Professor, Division of Nephrology, Chronic Kidney Disease Clinic, Director, University of Alabama at Birmingham, Birmingham, Alabama

REBECCA MAXSON, PharmD, BCPS
Associate Clinical Professor, Auburn University Harrison School of Pharmacy, Auburn, Alabama

MEGAN MCKAY, PA-S
University of Detroit Mercy, Detroit, Michigan

CIARA MITCHELL, MA, RD, LD
University of Alabama at Birmingham, Trussville, Alabama

AMY MOSMAN, MMS, PA-C
Division of Nephrology, Saint Louis University, St Louis, Missouri

BECKY NESS, PA-C, MPAS, DFAAPA, FNKF
Instructor of Medicine, Mayo College of Medicine, Mayo Clinic Health System – SW Region, Mankato, Minnesota

NGUYEN H. PARK, MS, PA-C, DFAAPA
National Institutes of Health/NHGRI/ACMG, Genomic Medicine Program Management Fellow, Bethesda, Maryland

LINDSAY PAIGE PENNINGER, PA-C
Carolina Kidney Associates, Greensboro, North Carolina

FLOR A. RANGEL, DMD, PA-S
University of Detroit Mercy, Detroit, Michigan

MICHAELA REKOW, PA-C
Nephrology Department, Medical College of Wisconsin, Wauwatosa, Wisconsin

DAWN E. ROSENBAUM, MHS, PA-C
Geisinger Medical Group, Danville, Pennsylvania

MARLENE SHAW-GALLAGHER, MS, PA-C
Assistant Professor, University of Detroit Mercy, Detroit, Michigan; Physician Assistant, Nephrology Division, University of Michigan, Ann Arbor, Michigan

FARAAZ SIDDIQUI, PA-S
University of Detroit Mercy, Detroit, Michigan

MELANIE T. STAPLETON, MS-PAS, PA-C
Nephrology Physician Assistant, HealthPartners Nephrology, Saint Paul, Minnesota

KELLY A. SWEENEY, PA-S
University of Detroit Mercy, Detroit, Michigan

KENDRA A. THOMSEN, MPAS, PA-C
Physician Assistant, Pulmonary Critical Care Medicine, Baylor Scott & White Health, Round Rock, Texas

JULIE C. UTLEY, MPAS, PA-C
Medical College of Wisconsin, Wisconsin

KARA-ANN VALENTINE, MMS, PA-C
Barry University Physician Assistant Program, Miami Shores, Florida

TROY ZIMMERMAN, BA
Special Projects Director, Government Relations, National Kidney Foundation, New York, New York

KIM ZUBER, PAC, MS
Executive Director, American Academy of Nephrology PAs, St Petersburg, Florida

Contents

There is an increased prevalence of chronic kidney disease (CKD) in the United States (US) and mortality is highly dependent on comorbidities. It is important to observe medical ethics in caring for patients with end-stage kidney disease (ESKD) especially regarding end-of-life care. The RPA has developed guidelines for shared decision making and appropriate initiation/withdrawal of dialysis. Incorporating palliative/hospice care, when appropriate, helps to maintain patients' goals of care and provide comfort to patients as they near EOL. Cultural and personal preferences should be incorporated into EOL discussions. Barriers to communication and establishing goals of care are important areas to identify and work to overcome any obstacles to provide the best possible quality patient care.

PHYSICIAN ASSISTANT CLINICS

FORTHCOMING ISSUES

July 2022
Obstetrics and Gynecology
Elyse Watkins, *Editor*

October 2022
Nutrition in Patient Care
Corri Wolf, *Editor*

January 2023
Emergency Medicine
Dan Tzizik, *Editor*

RECENT ISSUES

January 2022
Preventive Medicine
Stephanie Neary, *Editor*

October 2021
Gastroenterology
Jennifer R. Eames, *Editor*

July 2021
Behavioral Health
Kim Zuber and Jane S. Davis, *Editors*

SERIES OF RELATED INTEREST

Endocrinology and Metabolism Clinics
https://www.endo.theclinics.com/
Medical Clinics
https://www.medical.theclinics.com/
Primary Care: Clinics in Office Practice
https://www.primarycare.theclinics.com/

THE CLINICS ARE AVAILABLE ONLINE!
Access your subscription at:
www.theclinics.com

Foreword

Farewell

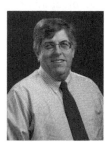

James A. Van Rhee, MS, PA-C
Consulting Editor

This is my final issue as consulting editor for *Physician Assistant Clinics*. In the summer of 2015, I first met with editors at Elsevier to discuss their plan for a *Clinics* journal series dedicated to the physician assistant (PA). We talked for over an hour outlining the topics we wanted to focus on, articles related to those topics, and possible editors. They called a week later asking if I wanted to be the first consulting editor, and I was honored to accept the position.

In the first issue, I described the *Physician Assistant Clinics* as being about providing the practicing PA a comprehensive review and the latest information they need for clinical practice. Issues would focus on a specific topic and provide the reader with detailed information on several subjects related to the issue topic. Plus, special topics related to latest trends in PA practice will be presented in each issue. I think we accomplished that. We covered all the major organ systems and covered special topics, such as hospice and palliative medicine, intrinsic skills for PAs, and primary care of the medically underserved.

Over these past 7 years, I have had the pleasure of working with and developing friendships with PAs around the country who have provided articles for this journal. The very first issue covered kidney disease, and the guest editors were Kim Zuber and Jane Davis. It is perfect then that my last issue also covers kidney disease once again with Kim Zuber and Jane Davis as guest editors.

It is also my pleasure to announce that Kim Zuber and Jane Davis will be taking over as consulting editors for *Physician Assistant Clinics*. The journal is in great hands, and I am sure they will continue to provide the readers with the latest information they need for clinical practice and maybe help to get the reader ready for any upcoming board exam. I will continue to enjoy each future issue, now as a reader and educator. I will continue to assign articles in *Physician Assistant Clinics* to my students as they progress through the curriculum in the Yale Physician Assistant Online Program.

Physician Assist Clin 7 (2022) xv–xvi
https://doi.org/10.1016/j.cpha.2022.01.002
2405-7991/22/© 2022 Published by Elsevier Inc.

physicianassistant.theclinics.com

Thank you to the staff at Elsevier for their assistance with getting the journal out every quarter. Thank you to all the guest editors and authors. Without your dedication to putting together the latest information for the practicing PA, this journal would not have been possible. Even during a pandemic, you each dedicated valuable time to putting together issues with comprehensive articles. A final thanks to you, the reader. It was for you we put these issues together so that you have the latest information available as you take care of patients every day. Thank you for allowing me to be a part of your clinical life in this small way.

James A. Van Rhee, MS, PA-C
Yale School of Medicine
Yale Physician Assistant Online Program
100 Church Street South, Suite A230
New Haven, CT 06519, USA

E-mail address:
james.vanrhee@yale.edu

www.paonline.yale.edu/

Preface

Nephrology 2022

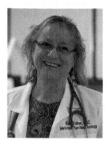 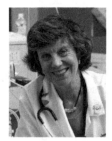

Kim Zuber, PAC, MS   Jane S. Davis, DNP
Editors

The kidneys get no respect.

A heart can be broken or can swell with delight.

A thing of beauty can take your breath away.

Our muscles can be so overcome with emotion that we are weak at the knees.

Even the adrenals get more respect; they can fire us up for fight or flight.

Yet all the while, the kidneys are silently working: cleaning the blood, eliminating waste, regulating blood pressure, encouraging red blood cells, balancing the see-saw of homeostasis.

Until they don't...

Welcome to *Physician Assistant Clinics*, Nephrology 2022.

In 2016, the inaugural issue of *Physician Assistant Clinics* focused on kidney disease.[1] In the ensuing 6 years, much as changed. Much is still the same.

The study of kidney disease is not new. Hippocrates (460–370 BC) recognized bubbles in the urine as a kidney disorder.[2]

But what to do about it? That took centuries of study, experiments, failures, and successes.

Today, 37 million Americans, or 15% of entire population, are living with kidney disease.[3] And yet, the study of nephrology is not as appealing to some as cardiology. After all, what is more dramatic on TV or film than a heart attack, asystole, and revival? Observing a patient during the dialysis session lacks drama and excitement. Of the myriad of programs with medical themes, how many have featured kidneys? Very few.

Yet how we got to here is a rich and colorful history. Kidney disease, earlier known as Bright disease, was known to be fatal and to affect all ages. Early attempts to treat were unsuccessful and even harmful. In the early 1900s, the medical community recognized if a diseased kidney could be replaced by a healthy one, the patient could live. In 1902, there began a series of attempts at transplant. First attempts were animal

Physician Assist Clin 7 (2022) xvii–xix

https://doi.org/10.1016/j.cpha.2022.01.001

2405-7991/22/© 2022 Published by Elsevier Inc.

physicianassistant.theclinics.com

to animal (1902) and then animal to human (1909). Unfortunately, the lifespan following a transplant was about an hour.

In 1933, we had the first human-to-human transplant; this failed because of rejection. The history of transplantation is often said to begin with a transplant between identical twins in 1954, but the first "successful" one was actually 1950, although the kidney functioned for only 53 days. So, what to do for those who did not have an identical twin? There were many attempts at blood cleaning.

Peritoneal dialysis actually preceded hemodialysis in 1959. The first successful hemodialysis (which lasted 76 hours) was in 1960, and the first outpatient hemodialysis was 1962.[4] One of the first "investigative reports" that changed minds and laws was regarding hemodialysis. "They decide who lives, who dies," was published in *Life Magazine* in November 1962.[5] This article caused such an uproar that payment for dialysis was built into Medicare, the only disease-specific program that Medicare pays for.[6]

So that is where we came from. Now, an outstanding list of authors will tell you where we are and where we are going.

Rosembaum and Utley will cover the what, where, when and how of kidney disease. This is followed by Maxson and Jackson discussing common medications, both prescription and over the counter, used by kidney patients. Not only is it educational but it is also a fun and interesting read. Thomsen, Ness, and Bone discuss the kidney in crisis, both in the intensive care unit and in acute injury. Rekow walks us through the interrelated changes of the kidney and other organs: the heart, the liver, and the gut. Gomez highlights the diabetic kidney and shares the newest research and guidelines for managing diabetic kidney disease. Feldman updates us on hypertension, both caused by and causing kidney disease. In 2021, new guidelines were published, and he discusses how these are different from the Heart Association standards.

Band reminds us that kids have kidney disease too, but pediatric disease looks very, very different than what we are all used to seeing in adults. Shaw-Gallagher and Davis along with students, Rangel, Sweeney, Digambaranath, Siddiqui, McKay, and Gadulka, take us off the beaten path with everything else. Kidney disease caused by diabetes and/or hypertension is common, but did you know about HIVAN? Eclampsia? Scleroderma? IgA? Myeloma? Rhabdo? This time we learn from the students.

Once the kidney fails, there are four options: Valentine and Mosman explain them to us. Grillo and Mitchell remind us that diet is important in all stages of chronic kidney disease. The military has been a "*behind the scenes*" force, and Ho and Zuber bring a light to shine on all things military. Racism, social determinants of health, and nephrology are all intertwined. Lyas manages to unwind the concepts, explaining where we are and how we are going to move from here. Park unravels the genetic basis of kidney disease and the newest breaking news from the genome projects.

Zimmerman explains Congress to us (a heavy lift, as one can imagine) along with how Medicare came to cover all patients with failed kidneys. We are still using similar treatments as we have for the last 50 years. Stapleton tells us about those treatments on the cutting edge and the KidneyX program to jumpstart treatment for kidney failure. As we all know, eventually all patients will die, and those with kidney disease have a higher death rate than oncology patients.[7] In that vein, Penninger and Collins tell us how to say good-bye.

The study of kidney disease may lack the glamor of some specialties, but it is fascinating and multifaceted and employs all the skills and knowledge as a practitioner. It is rumored to be the most complicated of all the internal medicine specialties, but we just consider it fun! Enjoy reading.

Kim Zuber, PAC, MS
American Academy of Nephrology PAs
131 31st Avenue North
St Petersburg, FL 33704, USA

Jane S. Davis, DNP
Division of Nephrology
University of Alabama at Birmingham
Birmingham, AL, USA

E-mail addresses:
zuberkim@yahoo.com (K. Zuber)
jsdavis@uabmc.edu (J.S. Davis)

REFERENCES

1. Davis J, Zuber K. Kidney disease. PA Clinics 2016;1(1).
2. Dunea G. History of nephrology: the beginning. Hektoen International. Available at: hekint.org/2017/01/30/history-of-nephrology-beginnings. Accessed August 26, 2021.
3. Chronic kidney disease in the United States, 2021. US Department of Health and Human Services, Center for Disease Control and Prevention. Available at: https://www.cdc.gov/kidneydisease/publications-resources/CKD-national-facts.html. Accessed May 1, 2021.
4. Blagg CR. The early history of dialysis for chronic renal failure in the United States: a view from Seattle. Am J Kidney Dis 2007;49(3):482–96.
5. Alexander A. They decide who lives and who dies. 1962. Available at: http://www.nephjc.com/news/godpanel. Life Magazine. Accessed July 25, 2021.
6. Center for Medicare and Medicaid Services (CMS). Fact sheet Medicare ESRD Program Network Organization Programs. Available at: https://www.cms.gov/Medicare/End-Stage-Renal-Disease/ESRDNetworkOrganizations/Downloads/ESRDNWBackgrounder-Jun12.pdf. Accessed July 24, 2021.
7. Naylor KL, Kim SJ, McArthur E, et al. Mortality in incident maintenance dialysis patients versus incident solid organ cancer patients: a population-based cohort. Am J Kidney Dis 2019;73(6):765–76.

Kidneys 101
A Bird's Eye View of Kidney Function, Disease, Classification, and Management

Dawn E. Rosenbaum, MHS, PA-C[a], Julie C. Utley, MPAS, PA-C[b,*]

KEYWORDS

- Chronic kidney disease • Acute kidney injury • KDIGO guidelines
- Kidney disease staging • Glomerular filtration rate

KEY POINTS

- Chronic kidney disease (CKD) diagnosis and staging uses measurements of estimated glomerular filtration rate and albuminuria. There are many causes of CKD, with diabetes and hypertension being most common in the United States
- Acute kidney injury diagnosis and staging uses urine output measurements and changes in creatinine
- Kidney Disease Improving Global Outcomes (KDIGO), an international expert organization, develops clinical practice guidelines for management of kidney disease based on current research

WHAT DO THE KIDNEYS DO, AND HOW DO THEY DO IT?

The primary functions of the kidneys are the filtering of blood and excreting waste products through the urine, balancing electrolytes, maintaining euvolemia through water regulation, and secreting hormones.[1]

The kidney is made up of nephrons, the collecting ducts, and a unique microvasculature.[1] The multi-papillary kidney of a human contains approximately 1 million nephrons.[2] This number varies a great deal, but the number of nephrons is established in the womb and no additional nephrons develop after birth. Nephrons are the cells that contain the primary filtration mechanism of the kidney, the glomerulus. Approximately 180 L of water is filtered by the glomeruli per day, but only approximately 1 L is excreted.[1,2]

HOW DO WE MEASURE KIDNEY FUNCTION?

Measuring kidney function is primarily done by analyzing the components of the urine and blood. The glomerular filtration rate (GFR) is widely accepted as the best overall index of kidney function in health and disease. The GFR can be assessed directly by measuring

[a] Geisinger Medical Group, 100 North Academy Avenue, Danville, PA 17821, USA; [b] Medical College of Wisconsin, W129 N7055 Northfield Drive, Menomonee Falls, WI 53051, USA
* Corresponding author.
E-mail address: jutley@mcw.edu

Physician Assist Clin 7 (2022) 201–213
https://doi.org/10.1016/j.cpha.2021.11.001
2405-7991/22/© 2021 Elsevier Inc. All rights reserved.
physicianassistant.theclinics.com

urinary clearance of inulin (gold standard) or plasma clearance measurements, but these tests are cumbersome and are therefore not widely used.[3] Most commonly, an estimated version is used, the eGFR, by inputting serum levels of endogenous filtration markers (eg, creatinine) into a calculator that factors in other biostatistics. Creatinine is useful as an initial assessment tool when used alongside an estimated GFR.[4]

There has been an evolution of formulas used for eGFR, including the 1976 Cockcroft-Gault (CG) formula (factors creatinine, age, sex, and weight). The CG formula was developed by measuring inulin excretion in 249 hospitalized White male patients and then extrapolating the data to include all races and genders.[5] The Modification of Diet in Renal Disease formula (which added urea, race, and albumin levels to the criteria used in CG) improved on the CG formula.[6] The Chronic Kidney Disease Epidemiology Collaboration Creatinine Equation (CKD-EPI$_{cr}$) is the current recommended eGFR equation used in the United States. This formula originally used creatinine, age, sex, and race to estimate GFR.[3–5]

After careful deliberation, in 2021, a task force formed by the National Kidney Foundation (NKF) and the American Society of Nephrology (ASN) recommended that the CKD-EPI should continue to be used, however the race coefficient (which designated African American vs non-African American) should be dropped.[7] This new calculator is referred to as the CKD-EPI (2021) to distinguish it from previous iterations. There are certain patients for whom the eGFR formulas using creatinine and demographic information have the potential to be skewed.[8] It is important to understand that creatinine is directly influenced by muscle mass, physical activity, dietary meat consumption, and overall state of good health.[8] Creatinine is best used in a steady state of generation and kidney elimination.[8] Some medications, such as trimethoprim, cimetidine, and fenofibrate, affect tubular secretion of creatinine and therefore have an effect on serum creatinine levels. Dialysis also lowers the creatinine by clearing it.[4]

Cystatin C is a kidney filtration marker that is independent of muscle mass. The eGFR using the CKD-EPI 2012 Cystatin C equation does not require a race coefficient and weighs the factors of age and sex less heavily than creatinine-based equations in formulas such as the 2009 CKD-EPI$_{cr}$. The role of using Cystatin C in the eGFR calculator, per Kidney Disease: Improving Global Outcomes (KDIGO, an organization dedicated to developing evidence-based practice guidelines) 2012 recommendations, is to confirm the presence of CKD in patients with a modest eGFR$_{cr}$ reduction. This may be a patient with an eGFR of 45 to 60 mL/min per 1.73 m^2 who does not have other manifestations of CKD (ie, albuminuria > 30 mg/g). In those patients, a Cystatin C–based GFR estimate (eGFR$_{cys}$) increases specificity. An eGFR$_{cys}$ less than 60 mL/min per 1.73 m^2, will confirm the diagnosis of CKD.[4]

Promising studies have shown superior accuracy of eGFR$_{cys}$ to eGFR$_{cr}$ in patients with malnutrition or human immunodeficiency virus (HIV), and in elderly individuals. It should be noted that eGFR$_{cys}$ is less accurate in situations in which there is rapid cell turnover, uncontrolled thyroid disease, or when patients are taking corticosteroids. Current limitations to widespread use of Cystatin C include cost and availability.[8] Though notably, the NKF-ASN taskforce suggests that using a combination of GFR estimates based on Creatinine (in CKD EPI) and Cystatin C would inrease accuracy compared to using any of these measures in isolation.[7]

Creatinine clearance (CrCl) is another way to estimate kidney function but requires a 24-hour urine collection along with a serum creatinine. CrCl is calculated as follows: urine creatinine × volume/serum creatinine. A 24-hour CrCl represents a slight overestimate of eGFR because of some tubular secretion of creatinine. The 24-hour collection and the requirement of the serum test make it impractical for most patients. Variance from day to day for the same patient can be as high as 25%.[6] Blood urea nitrogen (BUN) is reported on a metabolic panel, and although it does tend to rise with reduced GFR, other factors can cause changes. A high-protein diet, gastrointestinal bleeding, and/or corticosteroid therapy also can lead to a higher BUN. On the other hand, patients on a low-protein diet and those with liver disease tend to have a lower BUN. Although the role of the BUN in assessing a patient with kidney disease is often taught, the BUN is not an accurate marker of kidney function on its own. A mean of urea clearance and CrCl via a 24-hour collection is the recommended method for assessing residual kidney function in patients on dialysis.[6] The 24-hour urine collection can also be used to identify nephrotic syndrome, though a spot urine albumin or protein to creatinine ratio is a suitable alternative (and easier for your patients to provide).[4]

Accurate measurement of the patient's kidney function is crucial for proper dosing of many medications such as vancomycin and other antimicrobials, some antithrombotic and/or chemotherapies. The eGFR is also needed for prognostication, and in turn, education of patients about their condition.[9]

Assessing electrolyte abnormalities and albuminuria, and evaluating the volume status of a patient are also very helpful in determining functionality and treatment strategies in kidney disease states.[2]

HOW DO WE DEFINE KIDNEY DISEASE?

Kidney disease is a broad term encompassing acute and chronic diseases and disorders of the kidneys. There are a multitude of causes and categories. Acute kidney injury (AKI) is defined by the presence of any of the following (**Table 1**):

- Increase in serum creatinine by more than or equal to 0.3 mg/dL within 48 hours
- Increase in serum creatinine to more than or equal to 1.5 times baseline (within previous 7 days)
- Urine volume less than 0.5 mL/kg/h for 6 hours

Providers should include cause and stage of AKI when documenting if possible.[4]

CKD is defined as eGFR less than 60 mL/min per 1.73 m^2 or indicators of kidney damage lasting more than 3 months. Stage depends on eGFR, and risk category includes eGFR and amount of albuminuria. Both the eGFR and amount of albuminuria assist in prognostication. Although eGFR has an inverse relationship with risk of CKD progression (lower eGFR is worse disease state), the degree of albuminuria has a direct relationship with risk (**Table 2**).[10]

Further clarification of albuminuria stages is outlined in **Table 3**.

The time between AKI and progression to CKD is defined as acute kidney disease (AKD). AKD is functional kidney loss lasting more than 7 days but not more than 90 days. Research is under way to determine common causes, define factors, and develop prognostic calculators for this disease state.[12]

Although small fluctuations in eGFR are considered normal (a "sawtooth pattern"), in patients with CKD, their disease is considered to be progressing if their eGFR falls 25% or more from baseline. A sustained drop in eGFR of more than 5 mL/min per 1.73 m^2 per year is considered rapid progression.[4]

HOW IS KIDNEY DISEASE INVESTIGATED AND CAUSES IDENTIFIED?

A thorough review of the patient's past medical history, including medications and family history, are needed to identify the cause of kidney disease. Tests may include urinalysis, urine microscopy, and biochemistry; blood tests, including those that measure kidney function and electrolytes plus immunologic assays; imaging, including ultrasound, computed tomography, and magnetic resonance angiography; and in some

Table 1
Stages of AKI using KDIGO 2012 definitions[4]

Acute Kidney Injury Stages	Change in Serum Creatinine Criteria	Urine Output Criteria
1	1.5–1.9 × baseline or ≥0.3 mg/dL above prior level	<0.5 mL/kg/h for 6–12 h
2	2–2.9 × baseline	<0.5 mL/kg/h for 12 h or more
3	3 × baseline, creatinine rose to 4.0 mg/dL or higher, or renal replacement therapy started (*If patient is younger than 18, a decrease in eGFR to <35 mL/min per 1.73 m² meets criteria)	<0.3 mg/kg/h for 24 h or more or anuria for 12 h or more

cases, kidney biopsy.[11] We would add that although a family history is important to identify a cause of kidney disease, the patient description may need a bit of "translation" to identify disease states. An early cardiac death may be thought to be heart in origin, but may really be due to kidney disease; an early stroke or sudden death may be due to an aneurysm related to polycystic kidney disease.

WHAT ARE RISK FACTORS FOR ACUTE KIDNEY INJURY?

Exposure to certain medications, toxins, and conditions raises the likelihood of a patient developing AKI.[4] Conditions that lower blood pressure (BP), such as trauma,

Table 2
Stages of chronic kidney disease[10]

Prognosis of CKD by GFR and Albuminuria Categories: KDIGO 2012		Persistent albuminuria categories Description and range		
		A1	A2	A3
		Normal to mildly increased	Moderately increased	Severely increased
		<30 mg/g <3 mg/mmol	30-300 mg/g 3-30 mg/mmol	>300 mg/g >30 mg/mmol
GFR categories (ml/min/ 1.73 m²) Description and range	G1 Normal or high ≥90			
	G2 Mildly decreased 60-89			
	G3a Mildly to moderately decreased 45-59			
	G3b Moderately to severely decreased 30-44			
	G4 Severely decreased 15-29			
	G5 Kidney failure <15			

Table 3
Albuminuria/Proteinuria based on quantification using KDIGO 2012 criteria[4,11]

Albuminuria Categories	Abbreviation	Criteria
Normal		AER <10 mg/d; ACR <10 mg/d
Mildly increased (mild)		AER 10–29 mg/d; ACR 10–29 mg/g
Normal to mildly increased	A1	AER <30 mg/d; ACR <30 mg/g PER <150 mg/d; PCR <150 mg/g
Moderately increased	A2	AER 30–300 mg/d; ACR 30–300 mg/g PER 150–500 mg/d; PCR 150–500 mg/g
Severely increased	A3	AER>300 mg/d; ACR >300 mg/g PER >500 mg/d; PCR >500 mg/g
Nephrotic range proteinuria	A3	AER >2200 mg/d; ACR >2200 mg/g PER >3500 mg/d, PCR >3500 mg/g

Abbreviations: ACR, urinary albumin-creatinine ratio; AER, urinary albumin excretion rate; KDIGO, Kidney Disease: Improving Global Outcomes; PCR, urinary protein-creatinine ratio; PER, urinary protein excretion rate.

burns, dehydration, or surgery, can cause kidney injury or failure.[4] Medications may cause kidney impairment by inducing hypovolemia, decreasing kidney blood flow, inducing tubular necrosis, causing crystal nephropathies or interstitial nephritis. Urinary obstruction can lead to progressive rise in luminal pressure, compression of renal parenchyma, and rising creatinine if the obstruction is bilateral.[11] **Fig. 1** includes a nonexhaustive list of potential causes of AKI. AKI may or may not be reversible, and patients may be left with CKD or end-stage kidney disease (ESKD).[11]

WHO ARE THE TYPICAL PATIENTS WITH CHRONIC KIDNEY DISEASE? HOW COMMON IS CHRONIC KIDNEY DISEASE?

Patients with CKD stage 1 to 4 are approximately 14% of the US population.[13] As a group, patients with more advanced stages of CKD (CKD 3–5) tend to be older,

FACTORS ASSOCIATED WITH INCREASED RISK FOR ACUTE KIDNEY INJURY

Populations more susceptible:
 Advanced age
 Female
 Black
 Diabetics
 Patients with underlying kidney, heart, lung, or liver disease
 Patients with cancer

Urinary tract obstruction:
 Calculi
 Blood clots
 Tumor
 Stricture
 Prostatic enlargement
 Neurogenic bladder

Decreased renal perfusion:
 Dehydration
 Trauma
 Burns
 Sepsis
 Critical illness
 Major surgery (including cardiac, especially when using cardiopulmonary bypass)

Toxic exposures:
 Nephrotoxic drugs
 Radiocontrast agents
 Poisonous plants and animals

Fig. 1. Factors associated with nonspecific AKI.[4,11]

diabetic, and/or hypertensive. There is a higher prevalence of CKD 3 to 4 among Mexican American and non-Hispanic Black persons as compared with non-Hispanic White persons.[14]

In 2017, for every 1 million US residents, 2065 were receiving treatment for ESKD (approximately 670,000 people), with most ≥65 years old.[13] There is a lower mean age at onset of dialysis in Black and Hispanic individuals (58–59 years old) compared with White individuals (65 years old) and Asian individuals (62–63 years old).[15] In the United States, the causes of ESKD are, in order of significance, as follows[13]:

1) Diabetes
2) Hypertension
3) Glomerulonephritis
4) Cystic kidney disease

Cystic kidney disease is a condition characterized by cysts that grow in the kidneys over time, eventually destroying functional tissue.[16] Other causes of kidney disease and failure include lupus, immunoglobulin A nephropathy, anti-glomerular basement membrane disease (previously known as Goodpasture syndrome), lead and other heavy metal poisoning, genetic conditions, and renal artery stenosis.[16] Nephrotic syndrome may be seen in focal segmental glomerulonephritis (FSGS), membranous nephropathy, minimal change disease (MCD), amyloidosis, HIV/AIDS, or hepatitis B or C infections.[17]

Sometimes, AKI does not recover and the patient develops ESKD. Hemolytic uremic syndrome (HUS) is seen when toxins produced by *Escherichia coli* in the gut enter the bloodstream and cause hemolysis and damage to blood vessels, including those in the glomeruli. HUS is a rare but serious cause of ESKD in children and adults. Another uncommon (at least in the United States) cause of ESKD is poststreptococcal glomerulonephritis (PSGN), which can follow a streptococcal infection by 1 to 6 weeks. In PSGN, an overproduction of antibodies form damaging deposits in the kidneys.[18] Urine blockage or reflux can also cause kidney damage and/or failure.[11]

In 2013, approximately 10,000 children in the United States were receiving treatment for ESKD.[19] The leading cause of kidney failure in this population is cystic, hereditary, or congenital disorders, followed by glomerular diseases (such as MCD, FSGS, and membranoproliferative glomerulonephritis) and secondary causes of glomerulonephritis (eg, lupus). One genetic disorder of note is Alport syndrome, an X-linked collagen disease (affecting boys more severely), which leads to scarring and kidney failure, and vision and hearing loss.[18]

OK, NOW HOW DO I MANAGE PATIENTS WITH CHRONIC KIDNEY DISEASE?

Once you have identified patients with CKD and staged them according to the accepted stage 1 to 5 and albuminuria levels, efforts are aimed at slowing progression to ESKD. Minimizing progression and complications of CKD is best accomplished through identification, management, and surveillance of comorbidities.[4] Some of the most common management recommendations are listed in **Box 1** and are accompanied by their grading status, when provided by KDIGO.

There may be additional treatments indicated for certain underlying causes of kidney disease (eg, some glomerular diseases), and these will be covered in other articles in this issue.

ALBUMINURIA

An angiotensin converting enzyme inhibitor (ACEi) or angiotensin II receptor blocker (ARB) is recommended to treat adult diabetic patients with 30 to 300 mg of urine

---

Box 1
The grading system from Kidney Disease: Improving Global Outcomes[4]

A brief note on grading: each recommendation is accompanied by a level (number) and a grade (letter):

- Level 1: Most patients should receive the recommended course of action.
- Level 2: Different choices will be appropriate for different patents. Each patient needs help to arrive at a management decision consistent with their values and preferences.
- Grade A: Estimate of effect likely to represent true effect.
- Grade B: Estimate of effect likely to represent true effect, but may be substantially different.
- Grade C: Estimate of effect may be substantially different.
- Grade D: Estimate of effect is uncertain and often will be far from the truth.

---

albumin excretion (2D), and for all adult patients who have more than 300 mg of urinary albumin (1B).[4]

PATIENTS WITH DIABETES

In 2020, on the strength of multiple placebo-controlled, randomized trials, KDIGO stated that all patients with type 2 diabetes (T2DM) and an eGFR $\geq$ 30 mL/min per 1.73 m^2 be treated with metformin (1B) and a sodium-glucose cotransporter inhibitor (SGLT2i) (1A). For those patients unable to reach HbA1c goals or unable to take these agents, glucagonlike peptide 1 receptor agonists (GLP-1 RA) is recommended (1B). For patients with diabetic kidney disease, not on dialysis, a goal HbA1c between 6.5% and 8.0% should be individualized to the patient (1C).[20]

PROTEIN INTAKE

It is recommended that patients avoid greater than 1.3 g/kg per day in CKD stage G3 (2B, 2C) or more than 0.8 g/kg per day in CKD stage G4 (2C)[4] (see **Table 2** for definitions of CKD stages).

ANEMIA

For patients older than 15 years, hemoglobin (Hgb) is measured to identify anemia. Anemia in CKD is defined as less than 13.0 g/dL in male and less than 12.0 g/dL in female individuals. Patients with an eGFR greater than 60 mL/min per 1.73 m^2 should be screened for anemia only when clinically indicated. Patients with an eGFR 30 to 60 mL/min per 1.73 m^2 should be screened annually, whereas those with an eGFR less than 30 mL/min per 1.73 m^2 should be screened every 6 months. In addition, iron studies (t-sat, ferritin, total iron binding capacity) should be monitored, and supplementation added as needed.[4]

METABOLIC BONE DISEASE

In 2017, the Kidney Disease Outcomes Quality Initiative (the US version of KDIGO) proposed the following recommendations: check serum calcium and phosphate every 6 to 12 months in CKD 3, every 3 to 6 months in CKD 4, and every 1 to 3 months in CKD 5. Obtain a baseline intact parathyroid hormone (iPTH) in CKD 3, then repeat if there is CKD progression or if the baseline level is abnormal. Check PTH every 6 to 12 months in CKD 4 and every 3 to 6 months in CKD 5. Check alkaline phosphatase every 12 months or more often if the iPTH is elevated for patients with CKD stage 4 and 5. In patients with CKD and not on dialysis who have secondary hyperparathyroidism, it is not recommended to suppress elevated iPTH concentrations (2B) unless severely elevated and/or progressive (not graded). For dialysis patients with hyperparathyroidism, treatment with Vitamin D analogs, calcitriol, or calcimimetics may be used (2B).[21] Although standard teaching has been that bisphosphonates should be avoided in people with GFR less than 30 mL/min per 1.73 m^2 (2B) without a strong clinical rationale, a recent publication presents a different view.[4] For patients with CKD stage 4/5 and osteoporosis, an individualized plan is to be developed with the knowledge that falls and fractures are higher in this group, whereas antiresorptive agents are generally safe.[22]

METABOLIC ACIDOSIS

It is recommended that patients are treated with oral bicarbonate supplementation to maintain a goal serum bicarbonate $\geq$22 mmol/L, unless the medication is contraindicated (2B).[4] Fortunately, there has not been an association with alkali supplementation and an increase in BP, edema, or exacerbation of heart failure in studies of adding oral sodium bicarbonate.[23]

CARDIOVASCULAR DISEASE

Patients who have CKD are considered at increased risk for cardiovascular disease (CVD) (1A). It is recommended that patients be evaluated and treated for CVD and peripheral vascular disease as indicated (1B).[4] In adults with CKD who are aged 18 to 49 years and not on dialysis, treatment with a statin is recommended if the patient has known coronary artery disease, diabetes mellitus, prior ischemic stroke, or greater than 10% estimated 10-year incidence of coronary death or nonfatal myocardial infarction (2A). At age 50 and older, patients with CKD stages 3 through 5 (not on dialysis or transplant) should be treated with a statin or statin/ezetimibe combination (1A). The primary indication for statin use in these patients is their higher risk for future coronary events rather than only elevated low-density lipoprotein levels. For this reason, follow-up cholesterol levels are usually not indicated in these patients (not graded), in part because dose escalation is not recommended in CKD patients. To minimize harm and maximize benefit, it is recommended that statins NOT be initiated in adults with CKD on chronic dialysis (2A), although if the patient is already on the statin (+/− ezetimibe) at the onset of dialysis, then these drugs may be continued (2C). Adult patients who have received a kidney transplant should be treated with a statin (2A).[24]

MEDICATION MANAGEMENT

It is recommended that prescribers take eGFR into account when dosing medication. In people with an eGFR less than 60 mL/min per 1.73 m^2 (stages 3a–5) who have serious intercurrent illness that increases the risk of AKI, a temporary discontinuation of potentially nephrotoxic or renally excreted drugs is recommended (European "sick-day rules"). Agents that fall into this category, include, but are not limited to, ACEi, ARBs, aldosterone inhibitors, direct renin inhibitors, diuretics, nonsteroidal anti-inflammatory drugs, metformin, lithium, and/or digoxin (1C).[4]

SALT INTAKE

Target dietary intake for adults is <2 g sodium per day. These guidelines were reinforced in 2021, suggesting a sodium intake less than 2 g sodium per day (or <90 mmol sodium per day, or <5 g sodium chloride per day) in patients with high BP and CKD (2C).[25]

ADDITIONAL HEALTHY LIFESTYLE RECOMMENDATIONS

Patients with CKD need to maintain a healthy lifestyle to slow progression of the disease. Patients should be encouraged to follow healthy behaviors: achieving/maintaining a healthy body mass index, smoking cessation, routine exercise, and a low-salt diet along with cholesterol and glycemic control. Depending on the results of the laboratory tests, additional dietary advice might be needed to intervene on phosphate, potassium, and protein intake where indicated (1B). Patients need to be educated on avoidance of herbal supplements and encouraged to seek advice from their pharmacist or clinician before using over-the-counter medicines or nutritional protein supplements (1B).[4]

BLOOD PRESSURE

BP guidelines were updated in 2021. These recommendations included the use of both home BP monitoring and a standardized office BP measurement to diagnose high BP. For all patients with CKD and hypertension (HTN), it is suggested that they be treated with a target systolic BP of ≤120 mm Hg, when tolerated, using standardized office BP measurement (2B). In patients with ≥30 mg albuminuria, it is recommended that an ACEi or ARB be used in patients with and without diabetes. A dihydropyridine calcium channel blocker is recommended as first-line therapy in adult transplant recipients (1C). Pediatric guidelines are dependent on age, sex, and height.[25]

PHYSICAL ACTIVITY

Patients with HTN and CKD should be advised to undertake moderate-intensity physical activity for a cumulative duration of at least 150 minutes per week. This is to a level compatible with their cardiovascular and physical tolerance (2C).[25]

WHEN SHOULD PATIENTS BE REFERRED TO NEPHROLOGY?

The US Department of Health and Human Services (HHS) strongly recommends referring patients to nephrology before ESKD occurs.[15] Studies have shown the benefits of pre-dialysis nephrology care include improved preparation for dialysis, higher rates of transplantation, better patient survival, and reduced complications and hospitalizations.[15] Although continued management by a primary care provider is essential, referral to a nephrologist is currently recommended at an eGFR ≤30 mL/min per 1.73 m^2 if a patient has severely increased albuminuria or an abrupt decline in GFR. If the patient presents with hematuria or is experiencing complications of CKD, referral is recommended (**Fig. 2**). Common complications of advancing kidney disease include anemia due to kidney disease, electrolyte abnormalities, and/or resistant hypertension (requiring 4 or more antihypertensive agents to control).[15] Symptoms may not occur until late in the disease process and may include swelling in the lower extremities, itching, weakness, fatigue, loss of appetite, confusion, or memory loss.[26]

Although early referral to nephrology care has increased (defined as >12 mo before dialysis), it still falls woefully short of the HHS goal. As of 2015, only 31% of patients with ESKD were referred during the year before starting dialysis.[14]

WHAT SPECIAL CARE DOES THE NEPHROLOGY TEAM COORDINATE AS THE PATIENT PROGRESSES TO END-STAGE KIDNEY DISEASE?

Patients with progressive CKD should be managed from a multidisciplinary team approach, with access to dietary counseling, education, and counseling about

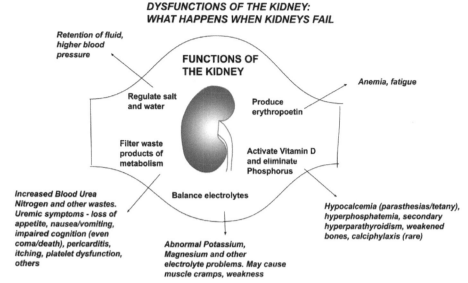

Fig. 2. Complications of renal disease are indications for referral to a nephrologist.[11,15,26]

different types of kidney replacement therapy (KRT) modalities; transplant options; vascular access surgery; and ethical, psychological, and social care. When patients develop an eGFR ≤20 mL/min per 1.73 m², and there is evidence of progressive and irreversible CKD over the preceding 6 to 12 months, discussions should begin to determine whether KRT or comprehensive conservative management should be pursued. If transplantation is intended, referral for preemptive kidney transplantation evaluation is considered, along with the opportunity to accrue "time" on the transplant list.[4,27]

Referral for planning for KRT is recommended in people with progressive CKD in whom the risk of kidney failure within 1 year is 10% to 20% or higher, as determined by validated risk prediction tools (1B).[4]

KRT modalities include hemodialysis, which is done either in a dialysis center or at home, or peritoneal dialysis (PD). PD can be performed at home through manual exchanges during the day, by a machine at night, or a combination of the two. Determination of the best modality for patients who wish to pursue KRT is influenced by multiple factors, including but not limited to the following:

- Comorbid conditions
- Home life/living situation
- Availability of support structure at home
- Patient ability to tolerate volume shifts
- Proximity to a dialysis facility
- Patient education and comprehension and preference

As preparing for a successful transition to KRT takes time, the aim is to avoid late referral and allow the patients time to decide on their plans.[27]

Starting KRT is not defined by a specific eGFR number, but instead by patient symptoms and complications. KRT is recommended for those who develop serositis, acid-base or electrolyte abnormalities, pruritus, inability to control volume status or BP, a progressive deterioration in nutritional status refractory to dietary intervention, and/

or cognitive impairment. Patients who are pursuing conservative management should have coordinated end-of-life care programs available to them. These programs should include protocols for symptom and pain management, psychological care, spiritual care, and culturally sensitive care for the dying patients and their family (whether at home, in a hospice, or a hospital setting), followed by the provision of culturally appropriate bereavement support.[4] Death from kidney failure can be managed in a holistic, peaceful manner with patient-centered medical care.

SUMMARY

A 2014 to 2015 study of more than 2 million Canadian patients found that those who were seen by nephrology providers (as compared with patients seen by other specialists/providers) had the highest rates of comorbidities, highest number of prescribed medications, highest placement in a long-term care facility, and highest incidence of death.[28] In this study, which looked at 13 different types of specialists, only one other group of providers saw patients with more consultants and who spent more days in the hospital than the group of patients seen by the nephrologists. This suggests that patients with kidney disease tend to be more complex than most.[28] Although they may require greater time and attention to be adequately cared for, the authors have found that treating patients with kidney disease is challenging yet rewarding, and certainly, never boring.

CLINICS CARE POINTS

- Consider expected muscle mass and other factors when assessing creatinine. Calculate GFR for identifying stages of CKD.
- BUN may be higher in kidney disease as well as high-protein diet, gastrointestinal bleeding, and with corticosteroid use.
- Proteinuria portends a higher risk of CKD progression.
- The first medication to treat hypertension in adults with any type of CKD and proteinuria greater than 300 mg per day should be an ACEi or ARB.
- Diabetic adults with proteinuria 30 to 300 mg per day should also be treated with an ACEi or ARB.
- Diabetic individuals with eGFR 30 mL/min per 1.73 m^2 or greater should be treated with a sodium-glucose cotransporter-2 (SGLT2) inhibitor unless contraindicated.
- Patients with CKD and HTN should be treated to a goal of less than 120 mm Hg systolic.

DISCLOSURE

The authors have nothing to disclose.

REFERENCES

1. Kriz W, Kaissling B. Structural organization of the mammalian kidney. In: The kidney. 3rd edition. Philadelphia, (PA): Lippincott Williams and Wilkens; 2000. p. 587–654.
2. Frehally J, Floege J, Tonelli M, et al. Comprehensive clinical nephrology. 6th edition. Philadelphia, (PA): Elsevier; 2019.
3. Levey AS, Stevens LA, Schmid CH, et al. Correction: a new equation to estimate glomerular filtration rate. Ann Intern Med 2011;155(6):408.

4. KDIGO 2012 Clinical Practice Guideline for the Evaluation and Management of Chronic Kidney Disease. Kidney Int 2017;19(1):22–206.

5. Levey AS, Stevens LA. Estimating GFR using the CKD Epidemiology Collaboration (CKD-EPI) creatinine equation: more accurate GFR estimates, lower CKD prevalence estimates, and better risk predictions. Am J Kidney Dis 2010;55(4): 622–7.

6. Traynor J, Fox JG, Geddes CC, et al. How to measure renal function in clinical practice. BMJ 2006;333(7577):733–7.

7. Delgado Cynthia, et al. A Unifying Approach for GFR Estimation : Recommendations of the NKF-ASN Task Force on Reassessing the Inclusion of Race in Diagnosing Kidney Disease. JASN 2021;32:2994–3015. https://doi.org/10.1681/ASN. 2021070988.

8. Shlipak MG, Mattes MD, Peralta CA. Update on cystatin c: incorporation into clinical practice. Am J Kidney Dis 2013;62(3):595–603.

9. Ebert N, Shlipak MG. Cystatin C is ready for clinical use. Curr Opin Nephrol Hypertens 2020;591–8.

10. Levey AS, Eckardt KU, Dorman NM, et al. Nomenclature for kidney function and disease: report of a Kidney Disease: Improving Global Outcomes (KDIGO) Consensus Conference. Kidney Int 2020;97(6):1117–29.

11. Kumar PJ, Yagoob MM, Ashman N. Kidney and urinary tract disease. In: Kumar & Clark's clinical medicine. Edinburgh: Elsevier; 2017. p. 721–93.

12. Chawla LS, Bellomo R, Bihorac A, et al. For the acute disease quality initiative workgroup. Acute kidney disease and renal recovery: consensus report of the Acute Disease Quality Initiative (ADQI) 16 Workgroup. Nat Rev Nephrol 2017; 13(4):241–57.

13. Chronic Kidney Disease (CKD) Surveillance System. Centers for Disease Control and Prevention. Available at: https://nccd.cdc.gov/ckd/default.aspx. Accessed June 28, 2020.

14. Vart P, Powe NR, McCulloch CE, et al. National trends in the prevalence of chronic kidney disease among racial/ethnic and socioeconomic status groups, 1988-2016. JAMA Netw Open 2020;3(7). https://doi.org/10.1001/jamanetworkopen. 2020.7932.

15. Purnell TS, Bae S, Luo X, et al. National trends in the association of race and ethnicity with predialysis nephrology care in the United States from 2005 to 2015. JAMA Netw Open 2020;3(8). https://doi.org/10.1001/jamanetworkopen. 2020.15003.

16. Causes of chronic kidney disease. National Institute of Diabetes and Digestive and Kidney Diseases. 2016. Available at: https://www.niddk.nih.gov/health-information/kidney-disease/chronic-kidney-disease-ckd/causes. Accessed June 13, 2021.

17. Nephrotic syndrome in adults. National Institute of Diabetes and Digestive and Kidney Diseases. 2020. Available at: https://www.niddk.nih.gov/health-information/kidney-disease/nephrotic-syndrome-adults#common. Accessed June 13, 2021.

18. Kidney disease in children. National Institute of Diabetes and Digestive and Kidney Diseases. 2014. Available at: https://www.niddk.nih.gov/health-information/kidney-disease/children. Accessed June 13, 2021.

19. Kidney disease statistics for the United States. National Institute of Diabetes and Digestive and Kidney Diseases. 2016. Available at: https://www.niddk.nih.gov/health-information/health-statistics/kidney-disease. Accessed Aug 17, 2021.

20. Ronco P. KDIGO 2020 clinical practice guideline for diabetes management in chronic kidney disease. Kidney Int 2020;9(4):221–33.
21. Ketteler MDM, Block MDGA, Evenepoel MD, et al. Diagnosis, evaluation, prevention, and treatment of chronic kidney disease-mineral and bone disorder. KDIGO. 2018. Available at: https://kdigo.org/guidelines/ckd-mbd/. Accessed August 4, 2021.
22. Evenepoel P, Cunningham J, Ferrari S, et al. Diagnosis and management of osteoporosis in chronic kidney disease stages 4 to 5D: a call for a shift from nihilism to pragmatism. Osteoporos Int 2021;32(12):2397–405. https://doi.org/10.1007/s00198-021-05975-7.
23. Dobre M, Rahman M, Hostetter TH. Current status of bicarbonate in CKD. American Society of Nephrology. 2015. Available at: https://jasn.asnjournals.org/content/26/3/515#sec-4. Accessed August 4, 2021.
24. Wanner C, Tonelli M. KDIGO clinical practice guideline for lipid management in CKD: summary of recommendation statements and clinical approach to the patient. Kidney Int 2014;85(6):1303–9.
25. Kidney Disease: Improving Global Outcomes (KDIGO) Blood Pressure Work Group. KDIGO 2021 clinical practice guideline for the management of blood pressure in chronic kidney disease. Kidney Int 2021;99(3S):S1–87.
26. What is kidney failure. National Institute of Diabetes and Digestive and Kidney Diseases. 2018. Available at: https://www.niddk.nih.gov/health-information/kidney-disease/kidney-failure/what-is-kidney-failure. Accessed June 13, 2021.
27. Lee MB, Bargman JM. Survival by dialysis modality-who cares? Clin J Am Soc Nephrol 2016;11(6):1083–7.
28. Tonelli M, Wiebe N, Manns BJ, et al. Comparison of the complexity of patients seen by different medical subspecialists in a universal health care system. JAMA Netw Open 2018;1(7). https://doi.org/10.1001/jamanetworkopen.2018.4852.

Medications and the Kidney

Rebecca Maxson, PharmD, BCPS*, Caroline Jackson, PharmD candidate

KEYWORDS

- Chronic kidney disease • Antibiotics • Gabapentin • SGLT-2 inhibitors
- Potassium binders • Herbal supplements • Medication dosing

KEY POINTS

- Optimal use of renin–angiotensin–aldosterone system (RAAS) inhibitors and SGLT-2 inhibitors are key to slowing CKD progression.
- Careful dosing of antibiotics, gabapentin, and pregabalin help avoid adverse drug reactions in patients with CKD.
- There is limited clinical evidence for herbal supplements/or marijuana use in patients with CKD.
- Herbal supplements can be harmful to patients with CKD.

INTRODUCTION

Patients with kidney disease often have a complicated relationship with their medications. Multiple medications are necessary to slow the progression of chronic kidney disease (CKD), treat secondary complications of CKD, and treat other comorbidities such as infections, pain syndromes, and other comorbidities.[1] Simultaneously, patients with kidney disease are at increased risk of harm from medications; these can range from acute kidney injury (AKI), adverse drug reactions (ADRs), inappropriate drug dosing, to omission of key therapies.[1–3] This article will provide a brief review of common medications used for patients with CKD including dosing considerations.

DOSING CONSIDERATIONS FOR CERTAIN MEDICATIONS THAT BENEFIT PATIENTS WITH CHRONIC KIDNEY DISEASE

The main therapeutic goal for patients with CKD is to prolong life and slow progression of CKD.[4] Several therapies have proven to slow CKD progression, by controlling diabetes and hypertension, inhibiting the renin–angiotensin–aldosterone system (RAAS), and correcting metabolic acidosis. In addition, losing weight and avoiding nephrotoxins can be beneficial.[2] In this section, clinical pearls related to dosing in CKD will be provided for certain key medications used to slow the progression or treat secondary complications of CKD. The evidence and efficacy supporting the therapeutic usefulness of these agents is discussed in other articles in this journal.

Auburn University Harrison School of Pharmacy, 2316 Walker Building, Auburn, AL 36849, USA
* Corresponding author.
E-mail address: maxsora@auburn.edu

Physician Assist Clin 7 (2022) 215–228
https://doi.org/10.1016/j.cpha.2021.11.002
2405-7991/22/© 2021 Elsevier Inc. All rights reserved.

Sodium–Glucose Cotransporter-2 Inhibitors

Sodium–glucose cotransporter-2 inhibitors (SGLT2i) were first FDA approved for treating diabetes through increasing glucosuria.[5] At that time, SGLT2i were contraindicated in patients with estimated glomerular filtration rate (eGFR) less than 60 mL/min/1.73 m^2, eliminating most of the patients with CKD. The more recent cardiovascular and kidney endpoint trials included patients with an eGFR lower than 60 mL/min/1.73 m^2 which have resulted in updated dosing recommendations. In the Credence trial, canagliflozin was initiated in patients with eGFR $\geq$ 30 mL/min/1.73 m^2 and continued until a patient started dialysis.[6] In the DAPA CKD trial, patients were included down to an eGFR of 25 mL/min/1.73 m^2.[7] Based on these 2 studies, clinicians now initiate these SGLT2i down to an eGFR of 25 mL/min/1.73 m^2 and continue it until the patient starts renal replacement therapy (RRT). The currently enrolling EMPA kidney trial includes patients with an eGFR of 20 mL/min/1.73 m^2.[8]

One of the concerns clinicians have with SGLT2i is the decrease in eGFR after initiation. Researchers have concluded that this "dip" is similar to that seen on the initiation of angiotensin-converting enzyme inhibitors (ACEi) and angiotensin receptor blockers (ARBs) and is an acute yet reversible 30% drop in eGFR. Current recommendations are to recheck eGFR at the patient's next scheduled visit after initiation of a SGLT2i.[9]

Insulin at Low Glomerular Filtration Rate

Insulin is a proven therapy for controlling hyperglycemia in patients with Type 1 and Type 2 diabetes. Hypoglycemia is a significant ADR from insulin and is defined as a blood glucose less than 80 mg/dL.[10] Even without insulin treatment, patients with CKD have an increased risk of hypoglycemia evidenced by a reported 1% to 3% rate of spontaneous hypoglycemia in patients with CKD and without diabetes.[11] Additionally, the incidence of hypoglycemia in patients with type 2 diabetes is much higher in patients with concomitant CKD versus those without, 10.7 versus 5.3 per 100 patient months.[11,12] This trend of increased hypoglycemia with CKD is also seen in patients with type 1 diabetes. The increased hypoglycemia risk for patients with CKD is the result of several possible factors including altered drug metabolism (decrease in insulin clearance when eGFR < 15–20 mL/min/1.73 m^2), interactions with ACEi, albuminuria, autonomic neuropathy, anorexia, infections, and/or impaired glucose release.[11] In patients with diabetes and CKD, clinicians must closely monitor for hypoglycemia as kidney function declines. Some experts suggest decreased insulin requirements by 20% or more when eGFR is < 45 mL/min/1.73 m^2.

Effectiveness of Thiazides at Lower Glomerular Filtration Rate

The choice of diuretics for patients with CKD is based on several factors: need for diuresis, need for blood pressure lowering, and current eGFR. Loop diuretics inhibit the Na+/K+/2Cl-pump in the loop of Henle and can increase the fractional excretion of sodium by 20%.[13] Conversely, thiazide diuretics inhibit the Na+/Cl-cotransporter of the distal convoluted tubule. Due to the decreased delivery of sodium to the distal convoluted tubule, thiazides increase the fractional excretion of sodium (FeNa) by only 5%.[14] The current consensus on thiazides is that they lose effectiveness at a GFR less than 30 mL/min/1.73 m^2.[14] The 2021 KIDGO blood pressure guidelines agree with this concept as they state that thiazides have reduced efficacy as diuretics and antihypertensives as GFR declines.[15] This conclusion is from a small study performed in 1961 whereby urine flow and sodium excretion were monitored closely after patients were administered a 500 mg intravenous dose of chlorothiazide. The 2 patients with the lowest clearance (6 and 11 mL/min) experienced minimal impact on urine flow or sodium excretion.[14]

Two small clinical trials question the belief that loop diuretics are more effective than thiazides at a lower eGFR. Both studies had a crossover design whereby each patient received either hydrochlorothiazide (HCTZ) 25 mg daily or furosemide 60 mg daily and then swapped to the other drug after an appropriate washout period. Primary outcomes included a change in blood pressure (BP) and FeNa. In the first study, 7 patients with a range of eGFR of 27 to 40 mL/min/1.73 m^2 had similar reductions in BP with furosemide and HCTZ.[16] When compared with baseline FeNa, furosemide had a nonstatistically significant increase, while HCTZ had a significantly increased FeNa. In the second study of 23 patients with a mean eGFR of 25 mL/min/1.73 m^2, mean BP reduction, and change in FeNa were similar after furosemide and HCTZ.[13] Both of these small studies question the conventional thought that thiazides are ineffective at lower GFR. To further investigate the effectiveness of thiazides at lower eGFR, a large randomized clinical trial is currently recruiting patients to study the effectiveness of chlorthalidone at reducing BP in patients with stage 4 CKD.[17]

Role of Potassium Binders

RAAS inhibitors are cornerstones in treating albuminuria and slowing the progression of CKD.[4] Hyperkalemia is a common and sometimes severe ADR from RAAS inhibitors and occurs in 5% to 10% of patients with CKD who take these medications.[18] A recent study investigated changes in RAAS inhibitor doses in patients with CKD stages 3 and 4 who experienced hyperkalemia events.[19] In patients on maximum RAAS inhibitor dose at baseline, mild hyperkalemia events (K$^+$ of 5.1–5.4 mEq/L) resulted in 22% discontinuation of RAAS inhibitor and 16% dose decreased. After a moderate to severe hyperkalemia event (K$^+$ $\geq$ 5.5 mEq/L), 26% had their drug discontinued and 21% had a dose decrease. The incidence of adverse cardiorenal outcome or death was higher in patients whose RAAS inhibitor was discontinued (54.4%) and those on submaximal dose (42.6%) when compared with those on maximum dose (42.6%) with all comparisons being statistically significant. This data shows that maximum doses of RAAS inhibitors are key for maximum benefit and that hyperkalemia interferes with maintaining patients on the maximum dose.

Currently, there are 3 FDA-approved potassium (K$^+$) binders, sodium polystyrene sulfate (SPS), patiromer, and sodium zirconium cyclosilicate (SZC); all bind potassium in the gastrointestinal (GI) tract to reduce the absorption of K$^+$ from the GI tract For the 2 new agents, patiromer and SZC, clinical trials showed benefit over placebo in maintaining normokalemia in patients with CKD and patients on dialysis.[20] While adding a K$^+$ binder can treat the ADR of hyperkalemia from RAAS inhibitors, they increase the pill burden for patients with CKD and are often costly. Further support for using K$^+$ binders to maintain RAAS inhibitor doses is currently under investigation in a randomized controlled trial which includes patients with CKD and heart failure.[21]

BENEFICIAL MEDICATIONS REQUIRING ATTENTION FOR DOSING WITH CHRONIC KIDNEY DISEASE

Antibiotics are lifesaving for patients with kidney disease as up to 33% of patients with diabetic kidney disease will die of infection before reaching end-stage kidney disease (ESKD).[22] Additionally, many patients with kidney disease, especially those with diabetes or ESKD, experience peripheral neuropathy which reduces the quality of life.[23] In this section, commonly used oral antibiotics that require special dosing considerations in patients with reduced kidney function will be described. Additionally, gabapentin and pregabalin will be discussed as they are widely used for the treatment of neuropathy and also require special dosing considerations in patients with reduced kidney function.

Trimethoprim–Sulfamethoxazole

Trimethoprim–sulfamethoxazole (TMP–SMX) is a broad-spectrum antimicrobial agent which synergistically inhibits the folate synthesis of many microorganisms, including many gram-positive and gram-negative pathogens. TMP–SMX is often used in the outpatient setting to treat urinary tract infections (UTI), cellulitis (due to the coverage of methicillin-resistant *staphylococcus aureus*), and as prophylaxis or treatment of *pneumocystis jiroveci* infections.[24–27]

Nephrotoxicity associated with TMP–SMX has been controversial. However, the most recently published study in 573 hospitalized patients found 5.8% experienced AKI likely caused by TMP–SMX.[26] The increase in serum creatinine resulting in AKI could be from interstitial nephritis caused by the sulfonamide moiety or from blocking creatine secretion by TMP with the later not being true AKI as eGFR is unchanged.[25,27] Additionally, TMP can result in an increase in serum potassium through an action similar to K-sparing diuretics.[28] As patients with CKD are at increased risk for hyperkalemia, additional monitoring and careful consideration of dosing for kidney function is critical (**Table 1**)

Selected Oral Beta-Lactam Antibiotics

Amoxicillin and amoxicillin-clavulanate are used in the outpatient setting primarily to treat upper and lower respiratory infections.[25,29] Oral cephalosporins have a slightly broader spectrum of activity and so are additionally used for treating UTIs and peritonitis. As beta-lactams have time-dependent pharmacokinetics and most are excreted renally, the dose of these medications should be decreased while maintaining the same dosing interval. This will achieve optimal safety and efficacy.[25,30] The concerning ADRs when dose adjustments are not made for kidney function are encephalopathy, confusion, and seizures (**Table 2**).[25,31]

Fluoroquinolones

Ciprofloxacin, levofloxacin, moxifloxacin, and ofloxacin are bactericidal agents which are commonly used for the treatment of upper and lower respiratory tract infections, UTIs, and bone, skin, and joint infections.[25] In a nested cohort study of men, ages 40 to 85, the fluoroquinolones (FQ) use resulted in a statistically significant 2.18-fold increase in incidence of AKI.[36] Additionally, a cohort study showed that within the 14 days after ciprofloxacin was initiated, there was a statistically significant 48% increase in the chance of AKI than amoxicillin.[37] An additional consideration for FQs is chelation with phosphate binders and oral iron products which reduces the absorption of FQ and can result in antibiotic failure.[25] All FQ's with the exception of moxifloxacin require dose adjustment for reduced kidney function (**Table 3**).

Gabapentin and Pregabalin

Gabapentin and pregabalin are analogs of gamma-aminobutyruc acid (GABA) an inhibitory neurotransmitter.[40,41] While gabapentin has FDA approval for postherpetic neuralgia and partial seizures, approximately 90% of gabapentin sales are off-label for a variety of pain syndromes including anxiety, neuropathic pain, restless leg syndrome, migraine headache, and trigeminal neuralgia.[40–42] Similarly, pregabalin is FDA approved for the treatment of neuropathic pain, spinal cord injury, postherpetic

Table 1
TMP–SMX dose adjustments for kidney function[24]

CrCl (mL/min)	Typical Dose Recommendation:			
	1 DS Tablet Every 24 h or 3 times per wk	1 DS Tablet Every 12 h	2 DS Tablet Every 12 h	2 DS Tablet Every 8 h
> 30	No dosage adjustment necessary			
15–30	1 SS every day or 3 times per wk (reduce dose to approximately 50%)	1 DS once then 1 SS every 12 h (reduce dose to approximately 50%)	1 DS every 12 h (reduce dose to approximately 50%)	2 DS every 12 h (reduce dose to approximately 50%)
< 15 Use appropriate caution and monitoring	1 SS every day or 3 times per wk (reduce dose to approximately 25% to 50%)	1 DS once then 1 SS every 12 or 24 h (reduce dose to approximately 25% to 50%)	1 DS every 12 h or 1 DS once then 1 SS every 12 h (reduce dose to approximately 25% to 50%)	1–2 DS every 12 h or 2 DS every 24 h (reduce dose to approximately 25% to 50%)

Abbreviations: CrCl, creatinine clearance; DS, double strength; SS, single strength; TMP–SMX, Trimethoprim/sulfamethoxazole.

Table 2 Dose adjustments in kidney impairment for selected oral beta-lactams[32–35]			
	Typical Dose Recommendation:		
Amoxicillin			
eGFR (mL/min)	250–500 mg every 8 h	875 mg to 1 g every 12 h	1 g every 8 h
≥ 30	No dosage adjustment necessary	No dosage adjustment necessary	No dosage adjustment necessary
10–30	250–500 mg every 12 h	500 mg every 12 h	1 g every 12 h
< 10	250–500 mg every 12–24 h	500 mg every 12–24 h	500 mg every 12 h
Hemodialysis, intermittent (thrice weekly)	250–500 mg every 12–24 h	500 mg every 12–24 h	500 mg every 12 h
Peritoneal dialysis	250–500 mg every 12 h	500 mg every 12 h	500 mg every 12 h
Amoxicillin-Clavulanate			
CrCl (mL/min)	*Avoid 875 mg IR and all ER tablets with CrCl < 30 mL/min*		
≥30	No dosage adjustment necessary		
10 to <30	250–500 mg every 12 h		
<10	250–500 mg every 12–24 h		
Hemodialysis, intermittent (thrice weekly)	250–500 mg every 12–24 h Administer dose after dialysis		
Peritoneal dialysis	250–500 mg every 12 h		
Cephalexin			
CrCl (mL/min)			
≥30	No dosage adjustment necessary		
15 to <30	250–500 mg every 8–12 h		
<15	250–500 mg every 12–24 h		
Hemodialysis, intermittent (thrice weekly)	250–500 mg every 12–24 h		
Peritoneal dialysis	250–500 mg every 12–24 h		
Cefdinir			
CrCl (mL/min)			
≥30	No dosage adjustment needed		
<30	300 mg once daily		
Hemodialysis, intermittent (thrice weekly)	300 mg once then 300 mg 3 times a week postdialysis on dialysis days with an additional 300 mg dose 48 h into each 72-h interdialytic period		
Peritoneal dialysis	300 mg every 48 h		

Abbreviations: CrCl, creatinine clearance; eGFR, estimated glomerular filtration rate.

neuralgia, fibromyalgia, and as an additional therapy for adults with partial-onset seizures.[43]

Gabapentin is not extensively metabolized and is primarily excreted by the kidneys.[41] Individuals with decreased kidney function are more susceptible to toxicity including dizziness, sedation, somnolence, ataxia, confusion, and asterixis **(Table 4)**.[40,41]

Table 3
Fluoroquinolone dose adjustments in altered kidney function[38,39]

Ciprofloxacin

CrCl (mL/min)	Oral, Immediate Release	Oral, Extended Release
>50 to <130	500–750 mg every 12 h	1 g every 24 h
30–50	250–500 mg every 12 h	1 g every 24 h
<30	500 mg every 24 h	500 mg every 24 h
Hemodialysis, intermittent (thrice weekly)	250–500 mg every 24 h	500 mg every 24 h
Peritoneal dialysis	250–500 mg every 24 h	500 mg every 24 h

Levofloxacin

CrCl (mL/min)	If usual recommended dose is 250 mg every 24 h	If usual recommended dose is 500 mg every 24 h	If usual recommended dose is 750 mg every 24 h
≥ 50	No dosage adjustment necessary		
20 to <50	No dosage adjustment necessary	500 mg initial dose, then 250 mg every 24 h	750 mg every 48 h
< 20	250 mg every 48 h[a]	500 mg initial dose, then 250 mg every 48 h	750 mg initial dose, then 500 mg every 48 h
Hemodialysis, intermittent (thrice weekly)	250 mg every 48 h	500 mg once then either 250 mg every 48 h or 125 mg every 24 h [b]	750 mg once then either 500 mg every 48 h or 250 mg every 24 h[b]
Peritoneal dialysis	250 mg every 48 h	500 mg once then either 250 mg every 48 h or 125 mg every 24 h[b]	750 mg once then either 500 mg every 48 h or 250 mg every 24 h[b]

Abbreviation: CrCl, creatinine clearance.
[a] Except for uncomplicated UTI, whereby no dosage adjustment is required).
[b] Daily dosing recommendations based on expert opinion to improve adherence.

Table 4
Gabapentin dose adjustments for kidney impairment[44]

CrCl (mL/min)	Maintenance Dose Adjustment	Maximum Maintenance Dose
> 79	No dose adjustment necessary	3600 mg/d in 3 divided doses
50–79	No dose adjustment necessary	1800 mg/d in 3 divided doses
30–49	~50% reduction	900 mg/d in 2–3 divided doses
15–29	~75% reduction	600 mg/d in 1–2 divided doses
< 15	~90% reduction	300 mg/d in 1 dose

Abbreviation: CrCl, creatinine clearance.

Pregabalin is well absorbed, readily crosses the blood–brain barrier, has limited metabolism and is primarily excreted unchanged from the kidneys.[43,45] As individuals with impaired kidney function may accumulate pregabalin, doses should be decreased by approximately 50% to ensure that patients will not experience toxicities such as somnolence, dizziness, blurred vision, dry mouth, weight gain, and difficulty concentrating (Table 5).[45]

HERBALS AND NUTRITIONAL SUPPLEMENTS IN CHRONIC KIDNEY DISEASE

The popularity of herbals and nutritional supplements increases every year. From 2010 to 2013, sales for herbal products increased by 8%.[47] Multiple herbals claim antiinflammatory properties that can be helpful in patients with CKD. As these agents are regulated as a food by the FDA, well-designed randomized controlled trials in humans are scarce.[48] Additionally in the generally small and short-term trials, patients with CKD are often not included leading to a lack of information on potential positive and negative effects.[49] There are herbal supplements that should be avoided in CKD (Table 6).

Turmeric

Turmeric is known to have autoimmune and antiinflammatory properties and is often recommended for arthritis pain.[50] However, turmeric reduces inflammation and pain through inhibition in the production of prostaglandins (PG). This is a similar mechanism of action as nonsteroidal antiinflammatory (NSAIDS) drugs. NSAIDS are known to increase the risk of AKI due to the imbalance of PG resulting in impaired auto-control of eGFR at the level of the glomerulus.[51] Thus, turmeric has a similar risk profile to NSAIDs in patients with CKD.

Cannabis

Cannabis, also known as marijuana, pot, or weed, is used to self-treat psychiatric conditions including depression, anxiety, and insomnia as well as treating symptoms of chronic pain, nausea, or loss of appetite.[52] The 2 main active ingredients of cannabis are cannabidiol (CBD) and delta-9 tetrahydro-cannabidiol (THC). The CBD component has analgesic, antianxiety, and antiinflammatory properties, but does not have psychoactive properties, while the THC component has psychoactive properties.[53] Compared with recreational cannabis which typically has a higher content of THC and is usually smoked, medical cannabis typically has a higher CBD content and can be administered orally or can be vaporized.[52]

Table 5 Pregabalin dose adjustments in altered kidney function[46]									
	Immediate Release					Extended Release			
CrCl (mL/min)	Usual Recommended Dose (mg/d)				Dosing Frequency	Usual Recommended Dose (mg/d)			Dosing Frequency
≥ 60	150	300	450	600	2–3 divided doses	165	330	495 660	Once daily
30 to < 60	75	150	225	300	2–3 divided doses	82.5	165	247.5 330	Once daily
15 to < 30	25–50	75	100–150	150	1–2 divided doses	Use not recommended.			
< 15	25	25–50	50–75	75	Single daily dose				

Abbreviation: CrCl, creatinine clearance.

Table 6 Herbal supplements to avoid in CKD[48]			
Dangerous for Patients with CKD	**Contain Potassium**	**Contain Phosphorus**	**Act as Water Pill**
Astragalus	*Avoid in patients with*	*Avoid in patients with*	*Can cause kidney*
Barberry	*hyperkalemia or on*	*hyperphosphatemia*	*irritation or*
Cat's claw	*RAAS inhibitors*		*damage*
Apium graveolens	Alfalfa	American ginseng	Bucha leaves
Creatine	American ginseng	Bitter melon	Juniper berries
Goldenrod	Bai Zhi (root)	Borage (leaf)	Uva ursi
Horsetail	Bitter melon (fruit, leaf)	Buchu (leaf)	Parsley
Huperzinea	Black mustard (leaf)	Coriander (leaf)	
Java tea leaf	Blessed thistle	Evening primrose	
Licorice root	Chervit (leaf)	Feverfew	
Nettle, stinging nettle	Chicory (leaf)	Flaxseed (seed)	
Oregon grape root	Chinese boxthorn (leaf)	Horseradish (root)	
Parsley root	Coriander (leaf)	Indian sorrel (seed)	
Pennyroyal	Dandelion (root, leaf)	Milk thistle	
Ruta Graveolens	Dulse	Onion (leaf)	
Uva ursi	Evening primrose	Pokeweed (shoot)	
Yohimbe	Feverfew	Purslane	
	Garlic (leaf)	Shepherd's purse	
	Genipap (fruit)	Silk cotton tree (seed)	
	Goto kola	Stinging nettle (leaf)	
	Japanese honeysuckle (flower)	Sunflower (seed)	
	Kelp	Turmeric (rhizome)	
	Kudzu (shoot)	Water lotus	
	Lemongrass	Yellow dock	
	Mugword		
	Noni		
	Papaya (leaf, fruit)		
	Purslane sage (leaf)		
	Safflower (flower)		
	Sassafras		
	Scullcap		
	Shepherd's purse		
	Stinging nettle (leaf)		
	Turmeric (rhizome)		
	Water lotus		

Abbreviation: CKD, chronic kidney disease; RAAS, renin-angiotensin-aldosterone system.

Three studies have compared the effect of medical cannabis on kidney function. The Coronary Artery Risk Development in Young Adults (CARDIA) study followed healthy individuals who used cannabis and did not find an association between cannabis use and change in eGFR, rapid decline in eGFR ($\geq$3% per year), or albuminuria over a 15-year period.[54] Similarly, the National Health and Nutrition Examination Survey (NHANES) analyzed 13,995 adults between 2007 and 2014 and did not find any clinically significant difference between the effect of past or present cannabis use on eGFR, microalbuminuria, serum creatinine in stage 2 or higher CKD.[55] Finally, the Chronic Renal Insufficiency Cohort (CRIC) Study analyzed 3939 adults with an eGFR between 20 and 70 mL/min/1.73 m^2 between 2003 and 2008 and did not find a link between the use of cannabis and the progression of CKD.[56] While cannabis

Table 7
Evidence for beneficial effects of cannabis[23]

Condition Treated	Evidence	Conclusion
Neuropathic pain	No studies in patients with CKD Moderate pain relief from inhaled cannabis in patients with normal kidney function (30% reduction, NNT = 6, brief treatment duration) Conflicting evidence in other pain syndromes for patients with normal kidney function	Less risk than opioids for patients with CKD. Unknown if effective at treating nonneuropathic pain or long-term use.
Nausea and Vomiting	No studies in patients with CKD Strong data for treating CINV for synthetic cannabinoids Conflicting data for nonsynthetic cannabis use in CINV, small study size, low dose of THC	Benefit for CINV, mostly for synthetic cannabinoids. No data for uremic nausea and vomiting
Anorexia	No studies in uremic anorexia Insufficient data in AIDS and HIV wasting syndrome, cancer, and anorexia nervosa	No data to support use
Uremic pruritus	Small study in patients on HD with topical endocannabinoids with support for reducing uremic pruritus	Topic product (Physiogel AI cream®) helpful for patients on HD No evidence for patients with CKD not on HD
Insomnia	No evidence of benefit for patients with normal kidney function in treating primary insomnia or insomnia from chronic pain	No evidence for use

Abbreviation: CINV, Chemotherapy-induced nausea and vomiting; CKD, chronic kidney disease; HD, hemodialysis; NNT, number to treat.

has not been shown to be nephrotoxic, it can still cause adverse effects such as impaired cognition, dizziness, or drowsiness, orthostatic hypotension, and cannabinoid hyperemesis syndrome.[23] Additionally, smoked cannabis increases the risk of developing chronic bronchitis, lung cancer, and mortality after a myocardial infarction. **Table 7** provides the current evidence supporting benefits from cannabis use in patients with CKD.

SUMMARY

Medications are key for slowing the progression of CKD and improving mortality. At the same time, patients with kidney disease are at increased risk from medications due to several factors: kidney elimination of medications necessitates careful dosing, taking multiple medications, and nephrotoxicity of some medications. Thus, beneficial medications such as SGLT2 inhibitors, RAAS inhibitors, diuretics, antibiotics, and GABA analogs require careful dosing and close monitoring of changes to kidney function. Additionally, due to the need to avoid nephrotoxic medications, sensitivity to K^+ and phosphorus ingestion, and lack of studies containing patients with kidney disease, most herbal medications have unproven efficacy and safety profiles for patients with CKD.

CLINICS CARE POINTS

- RAAS inhibitors and SGLT2 inhibitors help slow progression for patients with chronic kidney disease with albuminuria.
- Potassium binders are useful for patients to continue their RAAS inhibitor in the setting of hyperkalemia.
- Data supports continuing thiazides for patients with lower eGFR.
- Insulin doses may need to be reduced as eGFR declines.
- Careful monitoring of kidney function is needed when dosing antibiotics.
- Herbal supplements are not studied in patients with kidney disease.
- Many herbal supplements are eliminated by the kidneys and can be harmful to CKD patients.

DISCLOSURE

The authors have no conflicts to disclose.

REFERENCES

1. Whittaker CF, Miklich MA, Patel RS, et al. Medication safety principles and practice in CKD. Clin J Am Soc Nephrol 2018;13:1738–46.
2. Chen TK, Sperati CJ, Thavarajah S, et al. Reducing kidney function decline in patients with CKD: core curriculum 2021. Am J Kidney Dis 2021;77:969–83.
3. Khalili H, Bairami S, Kargar M. Antibiotics induced acute kidney injury: incidence, risk factors, onset time and outcome. Acta Med Iran 2013;51:871–8.
4. Kidney Disease Improving Global Outcomes (KDIGO). KDIGO 2012 clinical practice guideline for the evaluation and management of chronic kidney disease. Kidney Int 2013;1:1–150.
5. Maxson RA, McCoy EK. Noninsulin therapy for diabetes. PA Clin 2020;5:153–65.
6. Perkovic V, Jardine MJ, Neal B, et al. Canaglifozin and renal outcomes in type 2 diabetes and nephropathy. N Engl J Med 2019;380:2295–306.
7. Heerspink HJL, Stefansoon BV, Caorrea-Rotter R, et al. Dapaglifozin in patients with chronic kidney disease. N Engl J Med 2020;383:1436–46.
8. Herrington WG, Preiss D, Haynes R, et al. The potential for improving cardio-renal outcomes by sodium-glucose co-transporter-2 inhibition in people with chronic kidney disease: a rationale for the EMPA-KIDNEY study. Clin Kidney J 2018;11:749–61.
9. Heerspink HJL, Cherney DZI. Clinical implications of an acute dip in eGFR after SGLT2 inhibitor initiation. Clin J Am Soc Nephrol 2021. https://doi.org/10.2215/CJN.02480221.
10. American Diabetes Association. Glycemic targets: standards of medical care in diabetes – 2021. Diabetes Care 2021;44(Supp 1):S73–84.
11. Alsahli M, Gerich JE. Hypoglycemia in patients with diabetes and renal disease. J Clin Med 2015;4:948–64.
12. Mauricio D, Gourdy P, Bonadonna RC, et al. Glycaemic control with insulin glargine 300 U/mL in inidividuals with type 2 diabetes and chronic kidney disease: a REALI European pooled data analysis. Diabetes Ther 2021;12:1159–74.

13. Dussol B, Moussi-Frances J, Morange S, et al. A pilot study comparing furosemide and hydrochlorothiazide in patients with hypertension and stage 4 or 5 chronic kidney disease. J Clin Hypertens 2012;14:32–7.
14. Sinha AD, Agarwal R. Thiazide diuretics in chronic kidney disease. Curr Hypertens Rep 2015;17:13.
15. Kidney Disease Improving Global Outcomes (KDIGO). KDIGO 2021 Clinical practice guideline for the management of blood pressure in chronic kidney disease. Kidney Int 2021;35:S1–87.
16. Dussol B, Moussi-Frances J, Morange S. A randomized trial of furosemide vs hydrochlorothiazide in patients with chronic renal failure and hypertension. Nephrol Dial Transpl 2005;20:349–53.
17. Agarwal R, Cramer AE, Balmes-Fenwick M, et al. Design and baseline characteristics of the chlorthalidone in chronic kidney disease (CLICK) trial. Am J Nephrol 2020;51:542–52.
18. Palmer BF. Potassium binders for hyperkalemia in chronic kidney disease – diet, renin-angiotensin-aldosterone system inhibitor therapy, and hemodialysis. Mayo Clin Proc 2020;95:339–54.
19. Epstein M, Reaven NL, Funk SE, et al. Evaluation of the treatment gap between clinical guidelines and the utilization of renin-angiotensin-aldosterone system inhibitors. Am J Manag Care 2015;21:S212–20.
20. Cogle SV, Maxson R. Common medication issues in dialysis patients. Support Line 2021;43:10–6.
21. Murphy D, Ster IC, Kaski JC. The LIFT trial: study protocol for a double-blind, randomized, placebo-controlled trial of K$^+$-binder Lokelma for maximization of RAAS inhibition in CKD patients with heart failure. BMC Nephrol 2021;22:254.
22. Alicic RZ, Rooney MT, Tuttle KR. Diabetic kidney disease: challenges, progress, and possibilities. Clin J Am Soc Nephrol 2017;12:2032–45.
23. Ho C, Martinusen D, Lo C. A review of cannabis in chronic kidney disease symptom management. Can J Kidney Health Dis 2019;6:1–14.
24. Sulfamethoxazole and Trimethoprim. Lexi-drugs. Hudson. OH: Lexicomp; 2021. Available at: http://online.lexi.com/. [Accessed 4 August 2021].
25. Eyler RF, Shvets K. Clinical pharmacology of antibiotics. Clin J Am Soc Nephrol 2019;14:1080–90.
26. Fraser TN, Avellaneda AA, Graviss EA, et al. Acute kidney injury associated with trimethoprim/sulfamethoxazole. J Antimicrob Chemother 2012;67:1271–7.
27. MacDougall C. Sulfonamides, Trimethoprim-Sulfamethoxazole, Quinolones, and Agents for Urinary Tract Infections. In: Brunton LL, Hilal-Dandan R, Knollmann BC, editors. Goodman & Gilman's: the Pharmacological Basis of therapeutics. 13th ed. McGraw Hill; 2021. Available at: Accesspharmacy.mhmedical.com/content.aspx?bookid=2189&sectionid=172484698.
28. Nickels LC, Jones C, Stead LG. Trimethoprim-sulfamethoxazole-induced hyperkalemia in a patient with normal renal function. Case Rep Emerg Med 2012;815907.
29. Jordan E, Voide C, Petignat PA, et al. Cephalosporins in clinical practice. Med Suisse 2020;16:1906–11.
30. MacDougall C. Penicillins, cephalosporins, and other β-lactam antibiotics. In: Brunton LL, Hilal-Dandan R, Knollmann BC, editors. Goodman & Gilman's: the Pharmacological Basis of therapeutics. 13th ed. McGraw Hill; 2021. Available at: Accesspharmacy.mhmedical.com/content.aspx?bookid=2189&sectionid=172484867.

31. Anthony C, Sharma M, Spina R, et al. Dose-adjusted beta-lactam antibiotic-induced encephalopathy in a patient with end-stage renal impairment: a case report. Euro J Case Rep Int Med 2015;2:172.
32. Amoxicillin. Lexi-drugs. Hudson, OH: Lexicomp; 2021. Available at: http://online.lexi.com/. [Accessed 4 August 2021].
33. Amoxicillin and clavulanate. Lexi-drugs. Hudson, OH: Lexicomp; 2021. Available at: http://online.lexi.com/. [Accessed 4 August 2021].
34. Cephalexin. Lexi-drugs. Hudson, OH: Lexicomp; 2021. Available at: http://online.lexi.com/. [Accessed 4 August 2021].
35. Cefdinir. Lexi-drugs. Hudson, OH: Lexicomp; 2021. http://online.lexi.com/. [Accessed 4 August 2021].
36. Bird ST, Etminan M, Brophy JM, et al. Risk of acute kidney injury associated with the use of fluoroquinolones. CMAJ 2013;185:E475–82.
37. Crellin E, Mansfield KE, Leyrat C, et al. Trimethoprim use for urinary tract infection and risk of adverse outcomes in older patients: cohort study. BMJ 2018;360:k341.
38. Ciprofloxacin (systemic). Lexi-drugs. Hudson, OH: Lexicomp; 2021. http://online.lexi.com/. [Accessed 4 August 2021].
39. Levofloxacin (systemic). Lexi-drugs. Hudson, OH: Lexicomp; 2021. http://online.lexi.com/. [Accessed 4 August 2021].
40. Bassilios N, Launay-Vacher V, Khoury N, et al. Gabapentin neurotoxicity in a chronic haemodialysis patient. Nephrol Dial Transpl 2001;16:2112–3.
41. Miller A, Price G. Gabapentin toxicity in renal failure: the importance of dose adjustment. Pa Med 2009;10:190–2.
42. Fukada C, Kohler JC, Boon H, et al. Prescribing gabapentin off label: perspectives from psychiatry, pain and neurology specialists. Can Pharm J 2012;145:280–4.
43. Lyrica [package insert]. Vega Baja(PR): Pfizer Pharmaceuticals LLC; 2011. Available at: https://www.accessdata.fda.gov/drugsatfda_docs/label/2011/021446s026,022488s005lbl.pdf. [Accessed 6 August 2021].
44. Gabapentin. Lexi-drugs. Hudson, OH: Lexicomp; 2021. Available at: http://online.lexi.com/. [Accessed 4 August 2021].
45. Lee D, Lee HJ, Kim HJ, et al. Two cases of pregabalin neurotoxicity in chronic kidney disease patients. NDT Plus 2011;4:138.
46. Pregabalin. Lexi-drugs. Hudson, OH: Lexicomp; 2021. Available at: http://online.lexi.com/. [Accessed 4 August 2021].
47. Rashrash M, Schommer JC, Brown LM. Prevalence and predictors of herbal medicine use among adults in the United States. J Patient Exp 2017;4:108–13.
48. National Kidney Foundation. Herbal supplements and kidney disease. Available at: https://www.kidney.org/atoz/content/herbalsupp. [Accessed 23 July 2021].
49. Asgharpour M, Alirezaei A. Herbal antioxidants in dialysis patients: a review of potential mechanisms and medical implications. Ren Fail 2021;43:351–61.
50. Marton LT, Barbalho SM, Sloan KP, et al. Curcumin, autoimmune and inflammatory diseases: going beyond conventional therapy – a systematic review. Crit Rev Food Sci Nutr 2020. https://doi.org/10.1080/10408398.2020.1850417.
51. Fournier JP, Sommet A, Durrieu G, et al. More on the "Triple Whammy": antihypertensive drugs, non-steroidal anti-inflammatory agents and acute kidney injury – a case/non-case study in the French pharmacovigilance database. Ren Fail 2014;36:1166–8.
52. Rein JL. The nephrologist's guide to cannabis and cannabinoids. Curr Opin Nephrol Hypertens 2020;29:248–57.

53. Canadian Public Health Association. Cannabasics. 2018. Available at: https://www.cpha.ca/sites/default/files/uploads/resources/cannabis/cannabasics-2018-fact-sheets-e.pdf. [Accessed 1 July 2021].

54. Ishida JH, Auer R, Vittinghoff E, et al. Marijuana use and estimated glomerular filtration rate in young adults. Clin J Am Soc Nephrol 2017;12:1578–87.

55. Lu C, Papatheodorou SI, Danziger J, et al. Marijuana use and renal function among US adults. Am J Med 2018;131:408–14.

56. Bundy JD, Bazzano LY, Xie D, et al. Self-reported tobacco, alcohol, and illicit drug use and progression of chronic kidney disease. Clin J Am Soc Nephrol 2018;13:993–1001.

Kidneys in the Danger Zone

Kendra A. Thomsen, MPAS, PA-C

KEYWORDS

• Acute kidney injury • ICU • Critically ill patient • Kidney replacement therapy

KEY POINTS

• The incidence of acute kidney injury (AKI) is increasing due to the increasing prevalence and incidence of chronic kidney disease (CKD)
• Critically ill patients are at higher risk for AKI
• AKI has many causes, some of which are preventable
• AKI in a critically ill patient worsens prognosis, particularly in COVID-19 acute respiratory distress syndrome
• Determining when to initiate kidney replacement therapy can be difficult, but there are guidelines

INTRODUCTION

Acute kidney injury (AKI) is the rapid decrease in kidney function. There are multiple causes and varied outcomes within a patient population. AKI can occur in anyone with injury to the kidneys but has an increased prevalence and incidence in those with existing chronic kidney disease (CKD) and increases with worsened CKD.[1] Worldwide, the prevalence and incidence of CKD are on the rise because of higher rates of hypertension (HTN), diabetes mellitus type 2 (T2DM), obesity, and aging.[2] People with CKD have a higher burden of chronic illness: heart disease, HTN, T2DM, and/or cerebrovascular disease, making this a bidirectional disease. AKI patients are 3 to 5 times more likely to require hospitalization.[3] The requirement for intensive care unit (ICU) support for AKI is on the rise.[4] Once within the ICU, AKI increases the morbidity and mortality in the critically ill patient population.[5]

A hospitalized patient's decline in kidney function can range from mild impairment to kidney failure. Various staging systems have been developed in the last 20 years (**Fig. 1**). The most recent well-accepted classification comes from the *Kidney Disease: Improving Global Outcomes (KDIGO) Group* (2012), which defines AKI as follows:

• Increase in serum creatinine (SCr) by $\geq$0.3 mg/dL within 48 hours; OR
• Increase in SCr to $\geq$1.5 times the baseline within the prior 7 days; OR

Pulmonary Critical Care Medicine, Baylor Scott & White Health, 302 University Blvd., Round Rock, TX 78665, USA
E-mail address: kendrapa07@yahoo.com

Physician Assist Clin 7 (2022) 229–237
https://doi.org/10.1016/j.cpha.2021.11.010
2405-7991/22/© 2021 Elsevier Inc. All rights reserved.

physicianassistant.theclinics.com

Abbreviations	
AKI	acute kidney injury
ATN	acute tubular necrosis
CKD	chronic kidney disease
HF	heart failure
HTN	hypertension
ICU	intensive care unit
IHD	Intermittent hemodialysis
KRT	kidney replacement therapy
T2DM	type 2 diabetes mellitus
UA	urinalysis

- Urine volume less than 0.5 mL/kg/h for 6 hours[6]

As the stage of AKI progresses, the risk of hospital mortality increases.

CLASSIFICATION OF AKI

In a critically ill patient, the etiology of the AKI is paramount. There are 3 main etiologies:

1. Prerenal AKI: impaired kidney perfusion without cellular injury. The kidney is functionally normal.
   - Causes include: decreased blood volume (hemorrhage, dehydration, and diuresis), decrease in effective arterial volume (heart failure [HF] and hepatorenal syndrome), medications (nonsteroidal anti-inflammatories or renin-angiotensin-aldosterone system inhibitors).

Stage	Urine output	RIFLE[b]	AKIN	KDIGO
1	<0.5 mL/kg/h for 6 h	Risk: increase in SCr of 1.5x or decrease in GFR >25%	Increase in SCr 1.5 x baseline or ≥3.0 mg/dL	Increase in SCr of 1.5-1.9 x baseline or >0.3 mg/dL increase in SCr
2	<0.5 mL/kg/hr for 12 h	Injury: Increase in SCr 2x or decrease in GFR >50%	Increase in SCr 2x baseline	Increase in SCr of 2-2.9x baseline
3	<0.3 mL/kg/h for 24 h or anuria for 12 h	Failure: Increase in SCr 3x or decrease in GFR >75%	Increase in SCr 3x baseline or ≥4 mg/dL (with acute rise of >0.5 mg/dL)	Increase in SCr of >3x baseline or increase in SCr ≥4.0 mg/dL or initiation of KRT

Fig. 1. Classifications of AKI.[a] [a]Information adapted from the RIFLE (Risk, Injury, Failure, Loss of kidney function, and End-stage kidney disease) 2004, AKIN (Acute Kidney Injury Network) 2007, and KDIGO (Kidney Disease, Improving Global Outcomes) 2012 classifications. [b]Loss and ESRD of the RIFLE criteria are not included in this classification chart as they are considered outcome variables. KRT, kidney replacement therapy; SCr, serum creatinine.

2. Intrinsic AKI: disorders of the kidney itself, including vasculature, glomerulus, interstitium, and tubules.
   • Causes include: glomerulonephritis, interstitial nephritis, acute tubular necrosis
   (ATN), atheroembolic disease, vasculitis, or multisystem disorders (thrombotic
   thrombocytopenic purpura or hemolytic uremic syndrome).
3. Postrenal AKI: disorders of the "plumbing system," such as obstructive uropathies.
   • Causes include: bladder outlet obstruction, benign prostatic hypertrophy, bilateral ureteral obstruction or unilateral in the case of only one kidney from nephrolithiasis, or obstruction of urinary catheter.

In the ICU, prerenal AKI is usually secondary to decreased blood flow to the kidneys,
hypotension, dehydration, bleeding, and/or shock. The most common cause of
intrinsic (ATN) is from prolonged prerenal AKI, hypotension, sepsis, and/or nephrotoxic medications including contrast media.[7] Prerenal AKI and ATN account for nearly
75% of all cases of AKI in hospitalized patients and 85% to 90% of AKI in the ICU patient.[8] As for postrenal AKI in the ICU, it is commonly caused by obstruction of the urinary catheter or a history of urinary retention before admission. There is no recent
research in postrenal AKI in the ICU patient.

EPIDEMIOLOGY

AKI is seen in 8% to 16% of hospital admissions and, as previously mentioned, increases mortality.[9] In critically ill patients, the complication of AKI has a prevalence
of 25% to 50%.[10] AKI is an equal opportunity complication occurring in both surgical
and nonsurgical patients. Cardiac surgery patients on cardiopulmonary bypass have a
higher incidence of AKI due to surgical episodes of hypotension and the monophasic
flow of the pump. In the septic patient, the incidence of AKI increases with the delay of
administration of appropriate antibiotics.[11] In patients postcardiac arrest, the requirement of vasopressors for more than 24 hours after resuscitation correlates with a
higher incidence of AKI. This is likely due to overall systemic injury.[12] Less than
50% of AKI patients are discharged from a hospital with a follow-up with nephrology.
In 2013, the International Society of Nephrology launched the Oby25 Initiative with the
goal of eliminating worldwide preventable deaths from AKI by 2025.[13] The most common cause of AKI in high-income and upper-middle-income countries is hypotension
and shock, whereas the most common cause in lower-middle-income and lower-
income countries is dehydration.[14] In high-income and upper-middle-income countries, HF, postoperative AKI, and nephrotoxic agents often intersect with a population
of older, comorbid patients. In lower-middle-income and lower-income countries, the
AKI patient is younger and dehydration, infection, toxin exposure, and/or pregnancy
complications were the more common causes of AKI.
For treatment, continuous renal replacement therapy (CRRT) machines are not
commonly used in lower-income countries, likely due to cost and resources. Peritoneal
dialysis, a more affordable and convenient form of kidney replacement therapy (KRT), is
used more frequently but still remains underutilized. Half of the patients in the ICU will
develop AKI and the mortality rate for these critically ill patients is 6 times higher than
the hospitalized mortality rate. Patients in the ICU on vasopressors and/or mechanical
ventilators who develop AKI requiring KRT have a higher rate of mortality.[15]

DIAGNOSIS OF AKI

In hospitalized patients, prerenal AKI and ATN account for two-thirds of the patients
with AKI. The 3 most common causes in an ICU patient are as follows:

- Infection (sepsis)
- Hypotension
- Medication exposure.

On presentation, the clinician should assess, to the extent possible, the patient's history such as drug exposure, regular medications including over-the-counter and supplements/vitamins, as well as prior kidney disease. Physical examination should evaluate for volume overload with edema, jugular venous distension, pulmonary rhonchi, and/or ascites. Hypovolemia from fluid losses, HF, or cirrhosis can contribute to diminished kidney function. Monitor for signs of infection. When ordering a urinalysis (UA), specify microscopic to look for proteinuria, hematuria, pH, and casts. Proteinuria or albuminuria can indicate intrinsic kidney disease. Hematuria can indicate glomerulonephritis or vasculitis.

Obstructive uropathies causing postrenal AKI are evaluated by a bladder ultrasound, kidney ultrasound, and/or a detailed physical examination. The prerenal and intrinsic disease can be harder to differentiate in some patients. As the most common causes of AKI in a critically ill patient are prerenal and intrinsic, the fractional excretion of sodium (FE_{NA}) can be used to help determine the etiology. In a healthy kidney faced with prerenal causes such as hypotension, the kidney will conserve sodium (Na), so the FE_{NA} will be low (<1%). A value of greater than 2% is indicative of intrinsic kidney disease. To calculate the FE_{NA}, the serum sodium, SCr, urine sodium, and urine creatinine must be collected at the same time.

There are some caveats to this general rule. As previously mentioned, patients with prolonged prerenal AKI can progress to intrinsic AKI. The FE_{NA} may still be less than 1%; however, the patient has developed ATN. This can also be true of patients who develop contrast-induced AKI. On the flip side, patients on diuretic therapy may have an elevated FE_{NA} because of the drug-induced sodium excretion. For patients on diuretics, a fractional excretion of urea (FE_{UREA}) may be more useful in differentiating the etiology. Urine output should be monitored in critically ill patients. A minimum of 0.5 mL/kg/h is considered adequate urine output suggesting stable kidney function.

FINDINGS FOR PRERENAL AKI

- BUN:SCr ratio greater than 20:1
- Fe_{NA} less than 1
- Fe_{UREA} less than 35%
- Urine osmolality (Ur osmo) 500 mOsm/kg
- UA micro can show hyaline casts.

FINDINGS FOR INTRINSIC AKI

- BUN:SCr ratio less than 20:1
- Fe_{NA} greater than 2
- Fe_{UREA} greater than 50%
- Ur Osmo less than 300 mOsm/kg
- UA micro can show cellular debris, muddy brown casts, red cell casts, eosinophils, proteinuria, and albuminuria

FINDINGS FOR POSTRENAL AKI

- BUN:SCr ratio less than 20:1
- Fe_{NA} greater than 2
- Ur Osmo less than 300 mOsm/kg

- Urine micro can show white blood cell casts
- *Imaging findings*: pyelonephritis, nephrolithiasis, and bladder mass.

In recent years, expanding research into newly identified biomarkers have helped diagnose AKI and aid in determining the timing of the initiation of KRT.[16]
These markers include:

- Functional biomarkers (*cystatin C and proenkelphalin*)
- Urinary low-molecular-weight protein that undergoes glomerular filtration and re-absorbed without secretion (*α_1-microglobulin, β_2-microglobulin, retinol-binding protein, adenosine deaminase-binding protein, and cystatin C*)
- Cellular injury/stress-associated protein (*neutrophil gelatinase-associated lipo-calin, kidney injury molecule-1, liver-type fatty-acid-binding protein, tissue inhib-itor of metalloproteinase 2, and insulin-like-growth-factor-binding protein 7*)
- Urinary tubular enzyme (*proximal renal tubular epithelial antigen, α-glutathione S-transferase, pi-glutathione S-transferase, γ-glutamyltranspeptidase, alanine aminopeptidase, lactate dehydrogenase, N-acetyl-beta-glucosaminidase, and alkaline phosphatase*)
- Inflammatory markers released by renal cells (*interleukin-18*).

Using biomarkers in the critically ill patient may prevent delay of maneuvers to lessen the assault on the kidneys, improve kidney function, and identify AKI hours to days before clinical AKI has manifested (**Fig. 2**)[17]. The challenge is that many of the biomarkers are not specific enough in the critically ill population and the ideal cut-off for the range to determine significance is not known. Biomarker testing is also expensive and not available in every laboratory.

Functional testing includes the furosemide stress test.[18] Patients are administered a large dose of intravenous (IV) furosemide (1 mg/kg for diuretic-naïve patients and 1.5 mg/kg for diuretic-exposed patients). Urine output is monitored. If urine output is less than 200 mL 2 hours after administration of the IV furosemide, then the patient is more likely to require KRT.

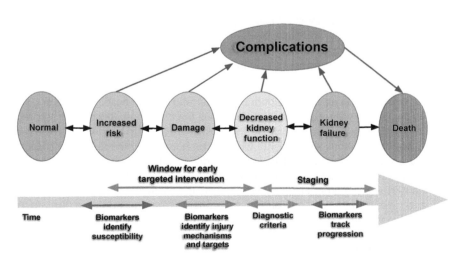

Fig. 2. Conceptual model for the progression of chronic kidney disease and the role of bio-markers in diagnosis. (*Adapted and modified from* image in[17] Levey AS, Coresh J. Chronic kidney disease. Lancet. 2012;379(9811):165-180. Reprinted with permission of Elsevier.)

TREATMENT OF AKI

The current treatment of AKI in the ICU involves recognition of patients at risk for AKI and prophylactically treating any conditions that can contribute to kidney injury. Prevention is more effective than treatment. Preventing hypoperfusion to the kidneys with IV fluids and vasopressors, treating infection, avoiding nephrotoxic medications, diuresing the cardiorenal patient to improve perfusion to the kidneys, and the judiciously using KRT are effective in the ICU. To prevent intrinsic AKI, avoid nephrotoxic medications and avoid contrast media. Monitor postrenal AKI to differentiate between decreasing urine output and urinary obstruction (may need a bladder scan).[19]

Drug-induced AKI accounts for up to 20% of AKI in the ICU.[20] In one study, 3-year follow-up on the results of a quality improvement program showed a decrease of AKI by 64% in hospitalized children by drawing a SCr daily in children deemed high risk for AKI.[21] Some have recommended criteria to determine causality of AKI including:

- Drug exposure duration of at least 24 hours preceding evidence of AKI
- Biological plausibility that the suspected drug can cause AKI
- An assessment of the suspected drug causing AKI versus the risk of other causes of AKI[22]

Early preventative measures can decrease the severity and duration of drug-induced AKI.

KIDNEY REPLACEMENT THERAPY

Among critically ill patients with AKI, more than 20% of them will require KRT within the first week of being in the ICU.[15] With the significant increased risk for mortality in this population, the timing of initiation of KRT is vital but the exact indicators are often been debated. Indications for KRT include hyperkalemia, volume overload, metabolic acidosis, or signs of uremia.[23] A common pneumonic used is *AEIOU*.

A: acidosis: metabolic, pH less than 7.1
E: electrolyte imbalances: hyperkalemia greater than 6.5 meq/L or rapidly rising and refractory to treatment
I: intoxications/ingestions: toxic alcohols, salicylates, lithium, dialyzable magnesium-containing laxatives
O: overload, volume: oliguria or anuric, HF, pulmonary edema
U: uremia: pericarditis, encephalopathy, gastrointestinal bleeding, seizures, intractable nausea/vomiting.

Note that neither an elevated SCr nor BUN:SCr ratio is an indication for starting KRT. Many patients' AKI will resolve without KRT, thus the challenge. It is difficult to predict which AKI patients would be harmed by unnecessary KRT when their AKI is on the verge of recovery versus those AKI patients who will be harmed by the delay of initiation of KRT.[24] Delay could increase the risk of mortality due to volume overload or toxin buildup.

Multiple studies have looked at KRT initiation. Results of some recent trials favor delaying KRT without urgent indications because the mortality rate between early initiation and delayed initiation were similar and patients randomized to the delayed initiation arm did not need KRT.[24] The hemodynamic stability of the patient may affect the initiation of KRT as well. The patient requiring vasopressors to maintain blood pressure may not tolerate hemodialysis.

The choice of hemodialysis modality for KRT in the ICU depends on the patient, the staff, and the level of ICU care. For hemodynamically stable critically ill patients, intermittent hemodialysis (IHD) is usually initiated. IHD requires less equipment, less staff training, and less cost. The most common complication from IHD is hypotension caused by fluid removal outpacing the refilling of the vascular space from intracellular and inter-stitial compartments but this can be decreased with slow, daily IHD. For those hemody-namically unstable requiring vasoactive drips, CRRT is more often a better option because of the slower, continuous rate of fluid removal. However, because CRRT is continuous, it can filter out treatment medications (most commonly antibiotics) and interfere with other diagnostic procedures, imaging and/or procedures. Hybrid modal-ities are now being used where patients will undergo prolonged IHD or a shortened run of CRRT depending on the patients' needs, hospital/ICU staffing, and resources.[25]

Special Considerations

Since 2020, the SARS-CoV-2 virus and its effect on kidneys have increased the inci-dence of AKI in the ICU. One study shows that about 50% of patients with COVID-19 acute respiratory distress syndrome (ARDS) develop AKI.[26] COVID-19 ARDS patients with AKI were generally older, had underlying CKD, sicker at admission, more likely to require mechanical ventilation, and more likely to continue onto end-organ dysfunc-tion. When they developed AKI, they also presented at a more advanced stage, stage 3 versus stage 1 or 2. AKI often developed after initiation of mechanical ventilation with 75% of patients developing AKI after intubation.[26] COVID-19 ARDS patients with AKI had a significantly higher rate of mortality: in stage 3 AKI, the mortality rate was an astounding 93%. Even within stage 1 (69% mortality) or stage 2 (70% mortality), the combination of COVID-19 and AKI had poor outcomes.[26] There are 2 areas of thought regarding why so many COVID-19 ARDS patients develop AKI and the mortality rate is so high. One belief is that increased intrathoracic pressure with mechanical ventilation leads to impaired gas exchange, poor lung compliance in turn causes an increase in kidney vascular resistance decreasing kidney perfusion. The second belief is that SARS-CoV-2 attacks the kidneys directly through the angiotensin-converting enzyme 2 receptors in the lungs and kidneys. Ultimately, it may be a combination of these two that is the cause of AKI and the increased mortality in COVID-19. This is a bidirectional issue as poorer kidney function decreases cytokine clearance, contributing to volume overload in critically ill patients with many IV drips, which in turn make ARDS worse.

SUMMARY

To eliminate preventable AKI worldwide one needs to consider differences in etiology based on location and resources. National and international prevalence and incidence are increasing because of comorbidities, including CKD, HTN, and T2DM. Within the ICU, identification of AKI and its cause is tantamount. Although serum and urine labora-tory testing can help determine the cause of AKI, there is promising research with the use of biomarkers. Biomarkers are promising in identifying AKI earlier, which may mitigate some kidney damage. Some of the causes of AKI can be eliminated; others can be mini-mized. Treatment should be tailored to each patient. Determining when to initiate KRT is difficult to determine in the critically ill patient, but there are clear indications for KRT. A spike in the incidence of AKI in 2020 and 2021 can be attributed to COVID-19 ARDS. Crit-ically ill patients with COVID-19 ARDS have a higher risk of developing AKI, particularly AKI stage 3 and an extraordinarily high risk of mortality associated with AKI.

CLINICS CARE POINTS

- The combination of vancomycin and piperacillin/tazobactam is associated with increased AKI risk and should be avoided if possible, especially in patients who have other risk factors for AKI.

- When using estimated glomerular filtration rate (eGFR) in very large or very small patients, it should be adjusted to the body surface area.
- In prerenal AKI, IV resuscitation should not be delayed.
- IV iodinated contrast can be given safely to most patients with end stage kidney disease (ESKD) who are maintained on hemodialysis. Immediate post–contrast dialysis is unnecessary as a routine practice.

DISCLOSURE

The author has nothing to disclose.

REFERENCES

1. Hsu RK, Hsu CY. The role of acute kidney injury in chronic kidney disease. Semin Nephrol 2016;36(4):283–92.
2. Lv JC, Zhang LX. Prevalence and disease burden of chronic kidney disease. Adv Exp Med Biol 2019;1165:3–15.
3. United States Renal Data System. CKD in the general population. 2020 Annual Data Report. Available at: https://adr.usrds.org/2020/chronic-kidney-disease/1-ckd-in-the-general-population. Accessed June 5, 2021.
4. Fortrie G, de Geus HRH, Betjes MGH. The aftermath of acute kidney injury: a narrative review of long-term mortality and renal function. Crit Care 2019;23(1):24.
5. Makris K, Spanou L. Acute kidney injury: definition, pathophysiology and clinical phenotypes. Clin Biochem Rev 2016;37(2):85–98.
6. Levey AS, Eckardt KU, Dorman NM, et al. Nomenclature for kidney function and disease: report of a Kidney Disease: Improving Global Outcomes (KDIGO) Consensus Conference. Kidney Int 2020;97(6):1117–29.
7. Hanif MO, Bali A, Ramphul K. Acute renal tubular necrosis. Treasure Island (FL): StatPearls; 2021.
8. Uchino S, Kellum JA, Bellomo R, et al. Acute renal failure in critically ill patients: a multinational, multicenter study. JAMA 2005;294(7):813–8.
9. Sawhney S, Fraser SD. Epidemiology of AKI: utilizing large databases to determine the burden of AKI. Adv Chronic Kidney Dis 2017;24(4):194–204.
10. Case J, Khan S, Khalid R, et al. Epidemiology of Acute Kidney Injury in the Intensive Care Unit. Crit Care Res Pract 2013;2013:479730.
11. Bagshaw SM, Lapinsky S, Dial S, et al. Acute kidney injury in septic shock: clinical outcomes and impact of duration of hypotension prior to initiation of antimicrobial therapy. Intensive Care Med 2009;35(5):871–81.
12. Chua HR, Glassford N, Bellomo R. Acute kidney injury after cardiac arrest. Resuscitation 2012;83:721–7.
13. International Society of Nephrology. Oby25 Initiative. Available at: https://www.theisn.org/initiatives/the-0by25-initiative/. Accessed June 21, 2021.
14. Mehta RL, Burdmann EA, Cerda J, et al. Recognition and management of acute kidney injury in the International Society of Nephrology 0by25 Global Snapshot: a multinational cross-sectional study. Lancet 2016;387(10032):2017–25.
15. Hoste EAJ, Bagshaw SM, Bellomo R, et al. Epidemiology of acute kidney injury in critically ill patient: the multinational AKI-EPI study. Intensive Care Med 2015;41(8):1411–23.
16. Rizvi MS, Kashani KB. Biomarkers for early detection of acute kidney injury. J Appl Lab Med 2019;2(3):386–99.

17. Levey AS, Coresh J. Chronic kidney disease. Lancet 2012;379(9811):165–80.
18. Koyner JL, Davison DL, Brasha-Mitchell E, et al. Furosemide stress test and bio-markers for prediction of AKI severity. J Am Soc Nephrol 2015;26:2023–31.
19. Vijayan A. Tackling AKI: prevention, timing of dialysis and follow-up. Nat Rev Nephrol 2021;17(2):87–8.
20. Kane-Gill SL, Goldstein SL. Drug-induced acute kidney injury: a focus on risk assessment for prevention. Crit Care Clin 2015;31(4):675–84.
21. Goldstein SL, Mottes T, Simpson K, et al. A sustained quality improvement pro-gram reduces nephrotoxic medication-associated acute kidney injury. Kidney Int 2016;90(1):212–21.
22. Awdishu L. Drug-induced kidney disease in the ICU: mechanisms, susceptibility, diagnosis and management strategies. Curr Opin Crit Care 2017;23(6):484–90.
23. Rachoin JS, Weisberg LS. Renal replacement therapy in the ICU. Crit Care Med 2019;47(5):715–21.
24. Gaudry S, Hajage D, Benichou N, et al. Delayed versus early initiation of renal replacement therapy for severe acute kidney injury: a systematic review and in-dividual patient data meta-analysis of randomised clinical trials. Lancet 2020; 395(10235):1506–15.
25. Fathima N, Kashif T, Janapala RN, et al. Single-best choice between intermittent versus continuous renal replacement therapy: a review. Cureus 2019;11(9): e5558.
26. Wang F, Ran L, Qian C, et al. Epidemiology and outcomes of acute kidney injury in COVID-19 patients with acute respiratory distress syndrome: a multicenter retrospective study. Blood Purif 2021;50(4–5):499–505.

Acute Kidney Injury
When the Kidneys Go South

Becky Ness, PA-C, MPAS, DFAAPA, FNKF[a],*, Brittany Heady, PA-C[b]

KEYWORDS

- Acute kidney injury (AKI) • Chronic kidney disease (CKD) • Biomarkers
- Community-acquired AKI • Hospital-acquired AKI

KEY POINTS

- Acute kidney injury (AKI) is more prevalent than initially thought.
- Early recognition of AKI improves patient outcomes.
- The diagnosis of AKI, community or hospital acquired, places patients at increased risk of earlier diagnosis/progression of underlying CKD.
- Biomarkers are being investigated as a means of earlier diagnosis and as improved prognostic indicators of needs for kidney replacement therapy as well as potential for kidney recovery.

INTRODUCTION

Acute kidney injury (AKI) is commonly encountered in the hospital setting with an incidence approaching 20%.[1] It is associated with both considerable morbidity and mortality and is characterized by rapid loss of kidney function resulting in retention of waste products. Patients who develop AKI are at increased risk of development, or worsening of, chronic kidney disease (CKD). Early recognition of AKI and identification of the underlying cause are essential in guiding management.

Definition

AKI, previously referred to as acute renal failure (ARF), has been defined and revised several times over the last decades. The original attempt to define AKI was the RIFLE (risk, injury, failure, loss of kidney function, end stage) criteria but this mixed laboratory evaluation and outcomes. Currently the AKIN (Acute Kidney Injury Network) or KDIGO (Kidney Disease Improving Global Outcomes) definitions of acute kidney injury are the standard definitions used in identifying AKI[1,2] (**Table 1**).

[a] Mayo College of Medicine, Mayo Clinic Health System - SW Region, 1025 Marsh Street, Mankato, MN 56001, USA; [b] St. Louis Kidney Consultants, 456 North New Ballas Road, Suite 348, St Louis, MO 63141, USA
* Corresponding author.
E-mail address: ness.becky@mayo.edu

Physician Assist Clin 7 (2022) 239–250
https://doi.org/10.1016/j.cpha.2021.11.014
2405-7991/22/© 2021 Elsevier Inc. All rights reserved.

Table 1				
Definition of acute kidney injury				
Stage	**Urine Output**	**RIFLE**	**AKIN**	**KDIGO**
1	<0.5 mL/kg/h for 6 h	*RISK*: increase in SCr of 1.5x baseline or decrease in eGFR > 25%	Increase in SCr 1.5 x baseline or ≥ 3.0 mg/dL	Increase in SCr of 1.5–1.9 x baseline or ≥ 0.3 mg/dL increase in SCr
2	<0.5 mL/kg/h for 12 h	*Injury*: increase in SCr 2x or decrease in GFR > 50%	Increase in SCr 2x baseline	Increase in SCr of 2–2.9 x baseline
3	<0.3 mL/kg/h for 24 h or anuria for 12 h	*Failure*: increase in SCr 3x or decrease in GFR > 75%	Increase in SCr 3x baseline or ≥ 4 mg/dL (with an acute increase of > 0.5 mg/dL)	Increase in SCr of > 3x baseline or increase in SCr ≥ 4.0 mg/dL or initiation of RRT

Abbreviations: SCr, serum creatinine.
Table recreated and used with permission from Erica Davis, PA-C, Acute Kidney Injury; The Ugly Truth, Elsevier

There are important nuances to consider regarding the differences in a community-acquired (CA-AKI) versus a hospital-acquired (HA-AKI) AKI. In CA-AKI, a reduction in kidney function is present initially, whereas in HA-AKI, the condition develops during a hospital stay. Unfortunately, HA-AKI is often iatrogenic secondary to treatments and/or procedures implemented while treating a separate condition. As the incidence of CA-AKI increases, more attention is being directed to this phenomenon. Recent meta-analysis supports existing theory that CA-AKI patients tend to have a better prognosis, less severe clinical manifestations, a lower incidence of oliguria, and less demand for hospital stays or intensive care unit (ICU) care as compared with patients with HA-AKI.[3] Interestingly, there does not seem to be a significant difference in regard to the degree of recovery of kidney function.

COVID-19 has had an impact on the incidence of AKI with worse outcomes for patients of color, those with multiple comorbid conditions (ie, heart failure, diabetes, hypertension, and/or obesity), as well as those with a lower socioeconomic status. As in non-COVID–related AKI, those with an HA-AKI fared worse regarding clinical outcomes than those with CA-AKI.[4]

EPIDEMIOLOGY

AKI is estimated to occur in 10% to 18% of all hospitalized patients and approaches 40% of patients who are critically ill in the ICU. In addition, 10% of patients in the ICU will require kidney replacement therapy (KRT).[5]

The incidence of AKI has increased by more than 4-fold in the United States since 2000. The total number of hospitalizations with AKI increased from 953,926 in 2000 to 3,959,560 in 2014, a 76% increase over 14 years.[6]

CLASSIFICATION

The causes of AKI have traditionally been classified into 3 categories: prekidney, intrinsic, and postkidney. The cause of AKI in ICU patients is often multifactorial.

> **Box 1**
> **Causes of prekidney acute kidney injury**
>
> Decrease in effective circulating volume
>   *Gastrointestinal losses*: vomiting, diarrhea, loss of fluids via nasogastric suction or intestinal
>   stoma losses: diabetes insipidus, osmotic diuresis (mannitol or glycosuria), diuretic-induced,
>   adrenal insufficiency
>   *Skin losses*: burns
>   *Hemorrhage*: surgical, gastrointestinal, trauma
>   *Third-space losses*: hypoalbuminemia
>
> Afferent arteriolar vasoconstriction
>   *Drugs*: NSAIDs, calcineurin inhibitors
>   Hypercalcemia
>
> Efferent arteriolar vasodilatation
>   ACEI and ARB
>
> Decreased effective circulatory volume
>   Congestive heart failure
>   Liver failure
>   Sepsis
>
> *Abbreviations:* ACEI, angiotensin-converting enzyme inhibitor; ARB, angiotensin receptor
> blocker; NSAIDs, nonsteroidal antiinflammatory drugs.

PREKIDNEY AZOTEMIA

Prekidney azotemia is the most common cause of AKI and occurs with inadequate kidney blood flow. There is no parenchymal damage to the kidney, and normalization of kidney function occurs once kidney perfusion is restored.

Prekidney azotemia may be seen in both hypovolemic and hypervolemic patients (**Box 1**). Optimization of volume status is the treatment of prekidney azotemia. In patients who are hypovolemic, isotonic fluids typically result in a rapid improvement in kidney function. In patients who are hypervolemic (heart failure, cirrhosis), the treatment is directed at the underlying disease state.[7]

It is important to differentiate between prekidney azotemia and intrinsic causes of AKI, as repletion of intravascular volume will not result in improved kidney function and may exacerbate volume overload in the later.

INTRINSIC ACUTE KIDNEY INJURY

The most common causes of intrinsic AKI are sepsis, ischemia, and nephrotoxins. Intrinsic kidney causes can be grouped by the site of the kidney that is primarily affected: tubular, glomerular, vascular or interstitium (**Box 2**).

Acute Tubular Necrosis

Acute tubular necrosis (ATN) is the most common type of intrinsic AKI in hospitalized patients, and ischemia and nephrotoxins are the most common causes of ATN. Risk factors for development of ATN include advanced age, preexisting kidney disease, hypertension, diabetes, and/or heart disease.

Numerous medications as well as endogenous and exogenous toxins can cause ATN. Some examples include the following:

- Vancomycin
- Contrast media

> **Box 2**
> **Causes of intrinsic acute kidney injury**
>
> Vascular
>   Renal artery/vein thrombosis
>   Malignant hypertension
>   Scleroderma renal crisis
>   Vasculitis
>   HUS/TTP
>
> Glomerulus
>   Glomerulonephritis
>
> Tubule
>   *Ischemia*: hypotension, sepsis
>   *Endogenous toxins*: hemolysis, myeloma, rhabdomyolysis, intratubular crystals
>   *Exogenous toxins*: contrast, nephrotoxic drugs
>
> Interstitium
>   Acute interstitial nephritis
>   Infiltrative malignancies
>   Acute pyelonephritis
>
> *Abbreviations*: HUS, hemolytic uremic syndrome; TTP, thrombotic thrombocytopenic purpura.

- Aminoglycosides
- Foscarnet
- Cidofovir
- Cisplatin
- Heavy metals
- Heme pigments
- Paraproteins

Urinary fractional excretion of sodium (FENa), urinalysis, and urine sodium can all be helpful in differentiating ATN and prekidney AKI. Most patients with ATN will have FENa greater than 2%. Urine sodium tends to be less than 40 mEq/L in ATN, as tubules are unable to conserve sodium due to tubular injury. Urinalysis is often normal in ATN although muddy brown granular casts may be present. To decrease the risk of ATN, it is important to maintain adequate hydration and, if possible, avoid nephrotoxic agents and hypotension.

ACUTE INTERSTITIAL NEPHRITIS

Acute interstitial nephritis (AIN) is a common cause of AKI in hospitalized patients, estimated to occur in 10% to 27% of patients. It is characterized by inflammation of the kidney interstitium. Medications are the most common cause of AIN (70% of cases) but it can also be seen in the setting of infections and systemic diseases. The most commonly implicated drugs are antibiotics and nonsteroid antiinflammatory drugs (NSAIDs). In addition, new chemotherapies, such as checkpoint, have a 2% to 4% incidence of AIN.[8] Causes of drug-induced AIN are listed in **Box 3**.

Drug-induced AIN can develop over weeks or months after exposure to the inciting agent. Flank pain, gross hematuria, and arthralgia may also occur.[9] The classic triad of fever, rash, and eosinophilia is not always present.

Urinalysis may reveal nonspecific findings including sterile pyuria and/or hematuria. Mild proteinuria is common with nephrotic range proteinuria being unusual outside of

---

Box 3
Causes of acute interstitial nephritis[8]

Medications
  Penicillins
  Cephalosporins
  Ciprofloxacin
  Sulfonamides
  NSAIDs
  Proton Pump inhibitors
  Diuretics
  Allopurinol

Systemic diseases
  Sarcoidosis
  Sjogren syndrome
  Systemic lupus erythematosus
  Tubulointerstitial nephritis and uveitis syndrome

Infectious
  Bacterial
  Viral
  Parasitic

Abbreviations: NSAIDs, nonsteroidal antiinflammatory drugs.

NSAID-induced AIN. Eosinophiluria may be observed in patients with AIN; however, the test is neither sensitive nor specific for the diagnosis. Some hospitals use the Wright stain instead of the Hansel stain for their urinalysis. The Wright stain is less specific. Eosinophiluria can also be seen in other conditions including urinary tract infections and atheroembolic disease.[8]

Kidney biopsy is the gold standard for definitive diagnosis of AIN. The mainstay of therapy is the discontinuation of potential offending agents. Underlying infections and systemic diseases associated with AIN should be treated. The benefit of glucocorticoids remains unproved although they have been beneficial in some studies, especially when initiated early in the disease. In a retrospective, multicenter study of 61 patients with biopsy-proven AIN, 52 were treated with steroids. Those who were treated with steroids had lower frequency of dialysis (4% vs 44%) and lower serum creatinine (2.1% vs 3.7%).[10]

Atheroembolic Disease

Atheroembolic kidney disease occurs when an aortic plaque ruptures releasing cholesterol crystals into the small kidney arteries. Although it can occur spontaneously, it usually develops in those on anticoagulation or after vascular surgery or cardiac cath. Patients may develop blue discoloration of their toes. Low complements, eosinophilia, and increasing creatinine are possible signs. Treatment is supportive therapy.[11]

Contrast-Induced Nephropathy

Iodinated contrast can lead to a (usually) reversible cause of AKI referred to as contrast-induced nephropathy (CIN). CIN is commonly seen 48 to 72 hours after administration of intravenous (IV) or intraarterial contrast. Patient tend to be asymptomatic and nonoliguric. In patients with normal kidney function, the risk of CIN is negligible at less than 1%. In patients with CKD, the risk of CIN increases in proportion to the severity of underlying kidney dysfunction.[12] Risk factors for CIN include diabetes, contrast volume, heart failure, volume depletion, and advanced age.

Multiple studies have evaluated type, amount, and duration of volume replacement to prevent CIN. IV fluid replacement before contrast is standard of care.[1] IV hydration is recommended over oral hydration due to increased volume expansion. Initially, isotonic bicarbonate was thought to be more efficacious by reducing reactive oxygen species. However, the PRESERVE trial, which included 4993 patients, compared isotonic bicarbonate with normal saline and showed no benefit with isotonic bicarbonate.[13] Because of lack of benefit of the bicarbonate solution and higher cost, normal saline is preferred.

Postkidney Acute Kidney Injury

Postkidney AKI occurs from blockage of urine flow in both ureters, the bladder and/or urethra (**Box 4**). For obstruction to cause AKI, the obstruction must involve both normal kidneys or be unilateral in a solitary or nonfunctional contralateral kidney.

In addition to anatomic causes of obstruction, functional disturbances of bladder emptying must be considered as well. Anticholinergic agents or neurogenic bladder secondary to diabetes or spinal cord trauma can cause urinary retention and lead to postkidney AKI.

Postkidney AKI is most commonly seen in older men due to prostatic disease (hypertrophy or cancer). Gynecologic malignancies arising from pelvic organs may result in azotemia secondary to bilateral ureteral obstruction.

Because benign prostate hypertrophy is the most common cause of obstruction, it is important to inquire about urinary symptoms.[1] Patients may experience hesitancy, weak stream, frequency, nocturia, or urgency. Flank or suprapubic pain may suggest obstruction.

Box 4
Causes of postrenal acute kidney injury

Ureteral obstruction
  Stone
  Tumor
  Retroperitoneal fibrosis
  Papillary necrosis
  Accidental ureteral ligation

Bladder neck obstruction
  Prostatic hypertrophy
  Prostate cancer
  Neurogenic bladder
  Bladder carcinoma
  Clot

Functional
• Anticholinergic agents
• Neurogenic bladder

Urethral obstruction
  Stricture
  Tumor
  Obstructed foley catheter

Developed by Bone B, Ness B.

DIAGNOSIS

A decrease in urine output or increase in serum creatinine should prompt further evaluation. A careful history and thorough chart review along with a comprehensive physical examination are essential to recognize and correct the cause or causes leading to AKI.

Chart review and careful history can identify the use of nephrotoxic medications or preexisting conditions such as diabetes or congestive heart failure that increases the risk of kidney injury. Review of the urine output and elicitation of any history of urgency, frequency, or weak stream can point toward prostatic hypertrophy as a cause of postkidney AKI.

The history, chart review, and physical examination along with laboratory results will often identify the cause and direct the treatment.

URINALYSIS

In prekidney and postkidney AKI, the urine sediment is usually bland without protein, hematuria, or casts. The urine sediment in ATN can contain renal tubular epithelial cells with granular casts. Findings on review of urine sediment can help build the differential diagnoses (**Box 5**). If examined properly, the presence of dysmorphic red cells or red cell casts is diagnostic of glomerulonephritis.[14]

URINE ELECTROLYTES

In patients with oliguria, FENa is helpful in distinguishing prekidney from intrinsic causes of AKI. The FENa is the percentage of sodium filtered at the glomerulus and excreted in the urine. In prekidney azotemia (especially hypotension), the tubules will increase sodium reabsorption to help restore perfusion. In this state, the FENa will decrease to less than 1%, suggesting tubular sodium reabsorption or normal kidney function. In contrast, in ATN, as tubular function is impaired, this will result in elevated FENa greater than 2%.

$$FENa = \frac{urine\ sodium \times serum\ creatinine}{serum\ sodium \times urine\ creatinine} \times 100$$

An FENa less than 1% is not always diagnostic of prekidney disease. For example, the FENa may be greater than 1% in patients with prekidney azotemia who are on diuretics. In these patients the FEUrea may be helpful in differentiating prekidney azotemia from ATN.

$$FEUrea = \frac{urine\ urea \times serum\ creatinine}{serum\ urea \times urine\ creatinine} \times 100$$

In prekidney azotemia FEUrea is usually less than 35% and greater than 50% in ATN.

Box 5
Urinary casts
Hyaline—can be a normal finding or seen in patients with dehydration
Granular—acute tubular injury or necrosis (ATN)
White blood cell—Acute interstitial nephritis (AIN), pyelonephritis
Red blood cell—glomerulonephritis (GN)
Fatty—nephrotic syndrome

BIOMARKERS

In light of the known limitations surrounding serum creatinine as a marker of kidney function, there has been ongoing research into novel biomarkers for kidney disease, including predictive biomarkers in the setting of AKI. These markers need to predict those at risk as well as the likelihood of recovery. There are several factors that need to be considered for an "ideal" biomarker for AKI:[15]

- Easily measured, a rapid test from readily available sample (blood/urine)
- Cost-effective biological/physiologic assay with a high degree of sensitivity and specificity
- Rapid and dynamic changes in levels available that would correlate with progression and or improvement of kidney function
- Have prognostic value

Over the last number of years, there have been several biomarkers identified that are predictive to some extent. Some of these biomarkers predict development of AKI, whereas others are better at predicting the need for some form of KRT (**Table 2**). There continues to be ongoing research in identifying the ideal biomarker, with promise being shown with the following:[16]

- MicroRNAs
  - ○ Potential early detection and/or prognosis in AKI
- Development-related molecules—Wnt/β-catenin: DKK (Dickkopf)
- Hemojuvelin (HJV)
  - ○ Early AKI biomarker in response to iron homeostasis in the setting of AKI
- Osteopontin
  - ○ Potential role in sepsis-related AKI

IMAGING

Kidney ultrasound is performed in patients with AKI to rule out obstruction. It is noninvasive, less costly than computed tomography or MRI, and avoids contrast exposure.

Table 2 Classification of available biomarkers[15,16]			
Functional Biomarkers	**Tubular Enzymes**	**Biomarkers of Damage**	**Pre-AKI Biomarkers**
Creatinine	Alkaline phosphatase (urine)	KIM-1 (urine)	TIMP-2 + IGFBP7 (urine)
Cystatin C	α-GST (urine)	NGAL (serum/urine)	MicroRNAs (urine)
—	NAG	IL-18 (urine)	Wnt (serum/urine)
—	—	L-FABP (urine)	DKK (urine)
—	—	HJV (urine)	—
—	—	Cystatin C (urine)	—
—	—	Osteopontin (serum/urine)	—
—	—	Albumin (urine)	—

Abbreviations: DKK, Dickkopf; HJV, hemojuvelin; IGFBP7, insulin-like growth factor-binding protein 7; IL-18, interleukin-18; KIM-1, kidney injury molecule 1; L-AFBP, liver-type fatty acid binding protein; NAG, N-acetyl-β-glucosaminidase; NGAL, neutrophil gelatinase-associated lipocalcin; TIMP-2, tissue inhibitor of metalloproteinase-2; Wnt, wingless-related integration site; α-GST, alpha-glutathione S-transferase.

It is useful in evaluating the size of the kidneys and their echotexture. Increased renal parenchymal echogenicity and decreased kidney size are consistent with CKD.

KIDNEY BIOPSY

Kidney biopsy may be indicated after the cause of AKI is narrowed down to intrinsic causes. It is rarely done in critically ill patients due to risk of bleeding complications. An active urine sediment with proteinuria or hematuria should prompt serologic evaluation and may require kidney biopsy.

MANAGEMENT

There is a general paradigm regarding the management of an AKI regardless of whether it is CA-AKI or HA-AKI:

- Discontinue all nephrotoxic agents
- Ensure volume status and perfusion pressure (HA-AKI)
- Consider functional hemodynamic monitoring
- Monitor serum creatinine and urine output
- Avoid hyperglycemia
- Consider alternatives to radiocontrast procedures
- Check for changes in medication dosing
- Consider KRT

There are some variations in treatment based on patient's location (outpatient vs inpatient) and stable versus unstable (**Tables 3** and **4**).

The optimal time to initiate KRT in the setting of AKI is not well defined. Multiple studies have been completed without clear recommendations regarding earlier versus later initiation.[17] There are number of concerns:

- Escalation of hypotension potentially requiring greater vasopressor support
- Initiation of cardiac arrhythmias
- Complications acquiring and accessing vascular access
- Need to administer anticoagulation to maintain dialysis access
- Potential for membrane incompatibility
- Could potentially delay recovery of kidney function
- Could potentiate progression of CKD in patients with baseline CKD

There are clear indications for the prompt initiation of kidney replacement therapy:

- Severe/refractory hyperkalemia (potassium >7 mEq/L is the usual criteria)
- Severe/refractory metabolic acidosis
- Volume overload resistant/nonresponsive to aggressive diuresis
- Significant uremic complications

Table 3 Outpatient treatment	
Stable	**Unstable**
STOP offending medications	ED evaluation or direct admission
Hydration—increase oral fluids	—
Close laboratory follow-up	—

Abbreviation: ED, emergency department

Table 4 Inpatient treatment	
Med Surg	**ICU/PCU**
STOP offending medications	STOP offending medications
Assess for obstruction—if present treat with urinary catheter	Assess for obstruction—if present treat with urinary catheter
CLOSELY monitor I/Os	CLOSELY monitor I/Os
Routine schedule laboratory tests	Routine schedule laboratory tests
Monitor vitals	Monitor vitals
Consider diuretic therapy to help with UOP, managing fluid overload, and/or abnormal electrolytes	Consider diuretic therapy to help with UOP, managing fluid overload, and/or abnormal electrolytes
Kidney replacement therapy	Vasopressors
—	Kidney replacement therapy

Abbreviations: I/O, intake/output; ICU, intensive care unit; PICU, pediatric intensive care unit; UOP, urine output.

Other consideration regarding the timing of initiation of KRT include

- Severity of underlying illnesses
- Degree of multiorgan dysfunction
- Solute burden
- Need for additional intake (ie, IV medications and/or parental nutrition

Once the decision has been made to proceed with KRT, there are a few modalities to be considered, with severity of patient's illness, available modalities, and experience of treating nephrology provider being the primary deciding factors (**Table 5**).

PROGNOSIS

There is a linear relationship between the stage of AKI and mortality, that is, the greater the stage of AKI, the higher the risk of mortality/morbidity. Currently reported rates regarding mortality in the setting of an AKI range from 40% to 70% with age, the presence of sepsis, respiratory failure, liver failure, or thrombocytopenia as features associated with higher mortality.[12]

Table 5 Kidney replacement therapy options	
Inpatient	**Outpatient**
IHD (intermittent hemodialysis)	IHD
PD (peritoneal dialysis)	PD
CRRT • CVVH (continuous venous venous hemofiltration) • CVVHD (continuous venous venous hemodialysis) • CVVHDF (continuous venous venous hemodiafiltration) • SCUF (slow continuous ultrafiltration)	
SLED (sustained low-efficiency daily diafiltration) EDD (extended daily dialysis)	

Recovery from AKI varies based on the stage of AKI, presence or absence of moderate to severe CKD at the onset of AKI, and whether KRT was initiated. Approximately 25% of patients with AKI experience a recurrent hospitalization within 1 year of discharge following their initial AKI diagnosis.[12] In the subgroup of patients with diabetes and CKD, more than 33% of patients experienced a recurrent AKI hospitalization within 1 year. In review of the competing events of death versus end-stage kidney disease (ESKD), the incidence of death was far greater than the incidence of ESKD. The relative incidence of death versus ESKD steadily increases with increasing age.[12]

SUMMARY

Given the linear relationship between AKI staging and mortality, the prompt recognition of an AKI followed by implementation of appropriate interventions improves patient outcomes, reduces related medical costs, and can decrease length of stay in the hospitalized patient.

CLINICS CARE POINTS

- AKI is a common, yet underrecognized syndrome affecting 20% of hospitalized patients.
- AKI is often under reported/coded, especially when kidney function improves prior to discharge. Reviewing patient labs from admission to discharge will help avoid missing this crucial diagnosis.
- It can take up to 90 days for kidney function to recover following an AKI. Make sure to follow SCr for a minimum of 3 months following AKI diagnosis.
- Multiple risk factors for the development of acute kidney injury exist which includes advanced age and diabetes. The most important risk factor for acute kidney injury is preexisting chronic kidney disease.
- Early education regarding hydration, low sodium diet, and avoidance of NSAIDs are key to preserving/maintaining kidney function moving forward.

DISCLOSURE

The authors have nothing to disclose.

REFERENCES

1. KDIGO AKI Work Group. KDIGO clinical practice guideline for acute kidney injury. Kidney Int Suppl 2012;17:1–138.
2. Mehta RL, Kellum JA, Shah SV, et al, Acute Kidney Injury Network. Acute kidney injury network: report of an initiative to improve outcomes in acute kidney injury. Crit Care 2007;11(2):R31.
3. Huang L, Xue C, Kuai J, et al. Clinical characteristics and outcomes of community-acquired versus hospital-acquired acute kidney injury: a meta-analysis. Kidney Blood Press Res 2019;44(5):879–96.
4. Pelayo J, Lo KB, Bhargav R, et al. Clinical Characteristics and Outcomes of Community- and Hospital-Acquired Acute Kidney Injury with COVID-19 in a US Inner City Hospital System. Cardiorenal Med 2020;10(4):223–31.
5. Sawhney S, Fraser SD. Epidemiology of AKI: utilizing large databases to determine the burden of AKI. Adv Chronic Kidney Dis 2017;24(4):194–204.

6. Pavkov ME, Harding JL, Burrows NR. Trends in Hospitalizations for Acute Kidney Injury - United States, 2000-2014. MMWR Morb Mortal Wkly Rep 2018;67(10): 289–93.
7. Belcher JM, Parikh CR. Is it time to evolve past the prerenal azotemia versus acute tubular necrosis classification? Clin J Am Soc Nephrol 2011;6(10):2332–4.
8. Nussbaum EZ, Perazella MA. Diagnosing acute interstitial nephritis: considerations for clinicians. Clin Kidney J 2019;12(Issue 6):808–13.
9. Raghavan R, Eknoyan G. Acute interstitial nephritis - a reappraisal and update. Clin Nephrol 2014;82(3):149–62.
10. González E, Gutiérrez E, Galeano C, et al. Early steroid treatment improves the recovery of renal function in patients with drug-induced acute interstitial nephritis. Kidney Int 2008;73(8):940–6.
11. Scolari F, Ravani P. Atheroembolic renal disease. Lancet 2010;375(9726): 1650–60.
12. United States Renal Data System. 2020 USRDS annual data report: epidemiology of kidney disease in the United States. Bethesda (MD): National Institutes of Health, National Institute of Diabetes and Digestive and Kidney Diseases; 2020. Acute Kidney Injury.
13. Weisbord SD, Gallagher M, Jneid H, et al, PRESERVE Trial Group. Outcomes after Angiography with Sodium Bicarbonate and Acetylcysteine. N Engl J Med 2018;378(7):603–14.
14. Bagshaw SM, Gibney RT. Acute kidney injury: clinical value of urine microscopy in acute kidney injury. Nat Rev Nephrol 2009;5(4):185–6.
15. Shah N, Lerma E. Novel biomarkers of renal function introduction and overview, characteristics of an ideal marker for kidney disease, biomarkers of acute kidney injury. Available at: https://emedicine.medscape.com/article/1925619-overview#a4. Accessed Apr 26, 2021.
16. Oh DJ. A long journey for acute kidney injury biomarkers. Ren Fail 2020;42(1): 154–65.
17. Feng YM, Yang Y, Han XL, et al. The effect of early versus late initiation of renal replacement therapy in patients with acute kidney injury: a meta-analysis with trial sequential analysis of randomized controlled trials. PLoS One 2017;12(3): e0174158.

The Kidney and Friends
The Heart, Liver, and Gut

Michaela Rekow, PA-C

KEYWORDS

- Cardiorenal syndrome • Hepatorenal syndrome • Gut microbiome • Gut kidney axis
- Acute kidney injury

KEY POINTS

- The kidney system is involved in cardiac, hepatic, and gut disease processes.
- Cardiorenal syndrome encompasses a spectrum of disorders between the heart and kidneys and requires a multidisciplinary team for optimal management.
- Hepatorenal syndrome is a complication of severe liver disease and confers a poor prognosis, and timely diagnosis and treatment are crucial to improve outcomes.
- Experimental research has shown that the gut microbiome affects outcomes in acute and chronic renal dysfunction and may offer novel therapeutic strategies.

INTRODUCTION

The kidney is an organ of paramount physiologic importance. Practicing nephrology requires an in-depth knowledge of the relationships among the kidney and multiple organ systems and, most importantly, how they work together to maintain homeostasis. Dysfunction in any one organ can lead to physiologic derangements in others, and managing the multiple systemic consequences is complex. Highlighting how the kidney system is involved in cardiac, hepatic, and gut disease processes along with current management strategies will help guide practitioners, of all specialties, to optimize care for their patients.

HEART

Cardiorenal syndrome (CRS) is a bidirectional disorder involving the heart and kidneys whereby acute or chronic dysfunction in one organ may induce acute or chronic dysfunction in the other.[1] The relationship between the heart and kidneys was described as early as 1836, although a formal definition was not developed until 2004 by the Working Group of the National Heart, Lung, and Blood Institute.[2] In

Nephrology Department, Medical College of Wisconsin, 8701 W Watertown Plank Rd, Wauwatosa, WI 53226, USA
E-mail address: Krekow10@gmail.com

Physician Assist Clin 7 (2022) 251–260
https://doi.org/10.1016/j.cpha.2021.11.011
2405-7991/22/© 2021 Elsevier Inc. All rights reserved.
physicianassistant.theclinics.com

2008 the Acute Dialysis Quality Initiative defined CRS as 2 phenotypes based on the primary organ of dysfunction: the heart or the kidney. These definitions have been further divided into 5 subtypes, which constitute the consensus definition of CRS.[1,3]

DEFINITION

CRS exists on a spectrum and is characterized by 5 subtypes that reflect the bidirectional and temporal nature of the kidney and heart interactions (**Table 1**). The purpose of defining CRS in this way is to assist clinicians to categorize patients based on phenotype, guide diagnostic and therapeutic management, and support the design of future clinical trials.[1] This definition uses the standardized criteria for diagnosis of acute kidney injury (AKI) as put forth by the Kidney Disease: Improving Global Outcomes (KDIGO) in 2012.[4] Differentiating between phenotypes can be challenging, and evolution from one phenotype to another is common as disease progresses. CRS-1 and 2 are the focus of this section because they are the most commonly encountered and studied phenotypes.

PATHOPHYSIOLOGY

The traditional explanation for the development of CRS-1 and 2 focuses on poor forward flow (due to heart failure) leading to hypoperfusion of the kidneys. Decreased kidney perfusion activates the renin-angiotensin-aldosterone system (RAAS) and sympathetic nervous system (SNS), leading to extracellular volume expansion and worsening heart failure.[1] However, the Acute Decompensated Heart Failure National Registry (ADHERE) showed no significant difference in increasing serum creatinine (SCr) levels between patients with acute heart failure with reduced versus preserved ejection fraction suggesting there is more to the story.[5]

Table 1
Classification of cardiorenal system based on the Consensus Conference of the Acute Dialysis Quality Initiative[4]

Phenotype	Definition	Pathophysiology
CRS type 1 (acute CRS)	Acute cardiac impairment resulting in AKI	Cardiogenic shock, acute decompensated heart failure, ACS, cardiac surgery
CRS type 2 (chronic CRS)	Chronic cardiac impairment resulting in progressive renal impairment	Diastolic heart failure, systolic heart failure
CRS type 3 (acute renocardiac syndrome)	AKI resulting in acute cardiac impairment	AKI due to hypervolemia or hypovolemia, glomerulonephritis, metabolic disturbances
CRS type 4 (chronic renocardiac syndrome)	CKD resulting in cardiac impairment	CKD contributing to increased risk of adverse cardiovascular events, cardiac hypertrophy
CRS type 5 (secondary CRS)	Systemic conditions that lead to both cardiac and renal impairment	Diabetes mellitus, amyloidosis, sepsis, drug toxicity

Abbreviations: ACS, acute coronary syndrome; CKD, chronic kidney disease.

Increased Central Venous Pressure

The focus on low ejection fraction as the driving factor of CRS has shifted to elevated central venous pressure (CVP), which is a key finding in CRS. Kidney perfusion depends on a large difference between arterial driving pressures and venous outflow pressures. Thus, an elevated CVP can lead to kidney hypertension and impaired intrarenal blood flow. In one study in patients undergoing right heart catheterization, an elevated CVP was associated with reduced estimated glomerular filtration rate and all-cause mortality.[6]

Neurohormonal Activation

In patients with severe HF, there is upregulation of the neurohormonal systems, RAAS and SNS, which are responsible for maintaining homeostasis during low-flow or hypotensive states. RAAS is activated in response to perceived decreased perfusion in the kidneys and leads to volume expansion via sodium retention and systemic vasoconstriction. In addition, neurohormonal pathways can worsen clinical outcomes and organ injury by activating inflammatory and oxidative pathways.[7]

DIAGNOSIS

To diagnose CRS there must be clinical signs and symptoms present as well as evidence of structural or functional abnormalities of the heart and kidneys. Diagnostic tools that demonstrate such findings include biomarkers, imaging, and invasive hemodynamic measurement techniques.

Biomarkers

Many patients with heart failure or chronic kidney disease (CKD) are on diuretics, and in the setting of CRS small fluctuations in SCr levels may not represent true renal tubular injury. The clinician must then distinguish between AKI and increasing SCr levels with or without tubular injury. Kidney biomarkers of glomerular integrity include cystatin C (CysC) and albuminuria, whereas markers of tubular injury can be seen on urine microscopy in the form of casts. Neutrophil gelatinase-associated lipocalin (NGAL) is a novel biomarker that has been shown to be a significant predictor of true worsening kidney function; tests for this biomarker are not available for clinical use in the United States.[8]

Commonly tested cardiac biomarkers include N-terminal (NT)-pro hormone BNP (B-type natriuretic peptide) (indicates myocardial stretching) and high-sensitivity troponin I and T (indicates myocardial injury).[1] Of note, patients with CKD have higher baseline BNP and troponin levels due to impaired kidney clearance and chronic volume overload.[9]

Imaging and Volume Assessment

Various modalities can be used to determine congestive state and guide therapeutic management. Noninvasive imaging such as echocardiography (ECHO) and kidney ultrasonography can demonstrate the severity of venous congestion. An ECHO will also provide hemodynamic measurements such as CVP, pulmonary capillary wedge pressure, and left ventricular ejection fraction. Kidney ultrasonography can provide information on chronicity of kidney disease using echogenicity, kidney mass, and cortical thickness. Intrarenal Doppler ultrasonography is an emerging modality used to identify kidney venous congestion.[1]

In patients in whom intravascular volume status is difficult to ascertain, invasive techniques such as right heart catheterization can be helpful for accurate hemodynamic measurements. However, The Evaluation Study of Congestive Heart Failure and Pulmonary Artery Catheterization Effectiveness trial (ESCAPE) showed no benefit of pulmonary artery catheter-guided therapy in terms of incidence of worsening kidney function during hospitalization and after discharge; therefore, it is not routinely performed.[10]

TREATMENT
Diuresis

The cornerstone of therapy is management of congestion and volume status with diuretics. Loop diuretics are most often prescribed and lead to natriuresis and volume loss.[1] Diuretic resistance is commonly encountered and can often be overcome by increasing the diuretic dose, frequency, or adding a thiazide diuretic. Sodium glucose cotransporter 2 (SGLT2) inhibitors are novel medications that improve mortality in patients with heart failure and advanced CKD and have recently been shown to significantly increase kidney free water excretion when used in combination with a loop diuretic.[11] There are general guidelines for goals of volume management in CRS (**Box 1**).

If a patient fails maximal diuretic therapy, the final option is mechanical ultrafiltration (UF), which removes isotonic plasma through a dialysis machine. The Ultrafiltration versus Intravenous Diuretics for Patients Hospitalized for Acute Decompensated Heart Failure (UNLOAD) trial showed that ultrafiltration performed better than loop diuretics at producing fluid loss and that patients had a lower 90-day readmission rate.[13] However, the Cardiorenal Rescue Study in Acute Decompensated Heart Failure (CARESS-HF) study found no difference in outcomes in ultrafiltration versus pharmacologic diuresis.[14] Further studies are needed on risk versus benefit of UF.

Inotropes

Inotropes such as dobutamine and milrinone can be used to improve cardiac index and kidney blood flow. Although effective at maintaining hemodynamic stability, they have not been shown to improve clinical outcomes or reduce mortality.[15]

Angiotensin-Converting Enzyme Inhibitors and Angiotensin Receptor Blockers

RAAS inhibition, including angiotensin-converting enzyme inhibitor (ACEi) and angiotensin receptor blockers (ARBs), has been shown to decrease mortality in patients with heart failure and CKD in multiple studies, and RAAS inhibitors are recommended

---

Box 1
Goals with diuresis in cardiorenal syndrome[12]

Avoid hypotension and underfilling, goal MAP greater than 65 mm Hg

Determine high-dose versus low-dose diuretics and if they should be a continuous infusion versus IV bolus

Monitor weight and urine output

Removal of third space fluid: paracentesis if needed, lower extremity compression

Decrease afterload: vasodilators (if MAP >65). Increase contractility: inotropes

Increase effective circulatory volume: inotropes to increase contractility, vasodilators to decrease afterload

Abbreviations: IV, intravenous; MAP, mean arterial pressure.

by both US and European guidelines.[8] However, there is a lack of data using patients with significant kidney impairment or acutely decompensated heart failure. Adverse effects of ACEis or ARBs include hyperkalemia and worsening kidney function, and caution should be used when initiating these medications in patients with advanced CKD.[7]

Mineralocorticoid Receptor Antagonists

Mineralocorticoid receptor antagonists (MRAs) can provide additional suppression of RAAS activity and have been shown to have long-term cardiorenal benefits.[1] As with RAAS inhibition, patients treated with MRAs had higher rates of hyperkalemia. Of note, the addition of newer potassium-binding agents such as patiromer or sodium zirconium cyclosilicate allow for continued guideline-directed therapy. A more recent nonsteroidal MRA, finerenone, has been shown to shown to delay the progression of kidney disease and have cardiac benefits.[16]

Tolvaptan

Vasopressin is a hormone released by the posterior pituitary and acts on vasopressin receptor 2 (V2) in the kidneys leading to reabsorption of free water in response to perceived hypovolemia. Tolvaptan is a V2 receptor antagonist and leads to increased free water excretion and an increased serum sodium level. Although tolvaptan can help with volume status and hyponatremia, studies have failed to show any long-term benefits in CRS.[15]

LIVER

Kidney dysfunction is common in patients with liver disease, and hepatorenal syndrome (HRS) is a serious complication of advanced cirrhosis or acute liver failure and associated with high short-term mortality.[17] In 2007 the International Club of Ascites defined HRS as 2 phenotypes:[18]

- HRS-1: A rapid decline in kidney function often due to a precipitating event
- HRS-2: A more gradual increase in SCr level, does not meet criteria for HRS-1

Of note, it has been proposed (but not uniformly accepted) that HRS-1 be renamed HRS-AKI and HRS-2 be renamed HRS-NAKI (non-AKI). Regardless of the name, timely diagnosis and treatment of HRS is critical to improving clinical outcomes.

APPROACH TO KIDNEY DYSFUNCTION IN DECOMPENSATED CIRRHOSIS

HRS is a diagnosis of exclusion; thus, other causes of AKI must first be ruled out. The most common causes of AKI in patients with liver disease are prerenal azotemia, acute tubular necrosis (ATN), and HRS-1.[19] To correct prerenal AKI, diuretics should be stopped and intravascular volume expanded with albumin (1 g/kg) for at least 48 hours. If kidney function does not improve and other causes of AKI have been excluded, the differential can be narrowed to ATN versus HRS-1.[20]

Differentiating ATN from HRS-1 is challenging because SCr is not a marker of tubular injury; thus it cannot be used to distinguish among causes of AKI. A search for novel biomarkers of tubular injury is ongoing. As previously mentioned, NGAL is a tubular protein that is upregulated by kidney injury and urinary NGAL has been shown to have high accuracy in differentiating ATN from HRS-1. Unfortunately, NGAL and other novel biomarker tests are not clinically available.[21] The diagnostic criteria for HRS-1, the most studied type of HRS, is summarized in **Box 2**.

> **Box 2**
> **European Association for the Study of the Liver 2018 hepatorenal syndrome-1 diagnostic criteria[20]**
>
> Presence of cirrhosis and ascites
>
> Diagnosis of AKI according to ICA-AKI criteria; increase in SCr levels greater than 0.3 mg/dL within 48 hours
>
> Absence of shock
>
> No response after 2 consecutive days of diuretic withdrawal and plasma volume expansion with albumin
>
> No current or recent use of nephrotoxic drugs (NSAIDs, aminoglycosides, iodinated contrast)
>
> No macroscopic signs of structural kidney injury, defined as
> • Absence of proteinuria (>500 mg/d)
> • Absence of microhematuria (>50 RBCs per high-power field)
> • Normal findings on renal ultrasonography
>
> *Abbreviations:* ICA, International Club of Ascites; NSAIDs, nonsteroidal anti-inflammatory drugs; RBCs, red blood cells.

HRS-2 is vaguely characterized by a gradual increase in SCr level that does not meet criteria for HRS-1. The newly proposed HRS-NAKI attempts to clarify the definition by further classifying as HRS-CKD or HRS-AKD (acute kidney disease) based on duration of elevated SCr levels.[21] HRS exists on a spectrum, thus it is possible to have HRS-1 superimposed on HRS-2, and the definition is evolving as we learn more about the syndrome.

PATHOPHYSIOLOGY

The hallmark of HRS is circulatory dysfunction characterized by renal vasoconstriction and peripheral vasodilation. In patients with advanced cirrhosis and portal hypertension, the effective arterial blood volume decreases secondary to systemic and splanchnic vasodilation. This in turn activates the RAAS axis and SNS leading to sodium retention, renal vasoconstriction, and decreased kidney perfusion.[18]

Newer research has shown that systemic inflammation is also a component of HRS pathophysiology. Two groups of molecules are known to play a role in driving inflammation: pathogen-associated molecular patterns (PAMPs) and damage-associated molecular patterns (DAMPs). Bacterial translocation or infection (such as spontaneous bacterial peritonitis) leads to production of PAMPs. DAMPs are molecules released from damaged hepatocytes. In addition, these molecules may directly damage the kidney via immune activation.[21]

TREATMENT

Once the criteria for HRS-1 are met, the first line of treatment involves administration of vasoconstrictors and albumin in an attempt to reverse HRS-1. Vasoconstrictors target splanchnic vasodilation and can significantly increase mean arterial pressure (MAP) and kidney perfusion. In the United States, midodrine plus octreotide or norepinephrine are the 2 vasopressor options available.[22] Studies have shown that a small increase in MAP (5–15 mmHg) from baseline is associated with improved kidney function. Volume expansion with albumin is part of the criteria for diagnosis of HRS-AKI and is essential for treatment of HRS-1. In addition, albumin has antioxidant and immunomodulatory effects that may impact systemic inflammation and improve outcomes in patients with HRS.[18] Ultimately the only definitive treatment of HRS is liver transplant.

The use of kidney replacement therapy (KRT) for AKI in patients with HRS is becoming more common. The same standard indications for KRT apply as with any patient: uremia, volume overload, and/or electrolyte derangements. Continuous renal replacement therapy is used in patients in the intensive care unit with hypotension rather than the standard intermittent hemodialysis. Most clinicians agree that KRT is appropriate in patients who are candidates for liver transplant with KRT used as a bridge to transplant. In patients who do not meet criteria for liver transplant, the risks and benefits of dialysis must be carefully evaluated.[23]

HRS-2 can generally be managed in the outpatient setting if otherwise stable. These patients often present with refractory ascites and should be treated with diuretics if they achieve natriuresis in addition to implementing a sodium restriction of 40 to 80 mmoles per day. Scheduled paracentesis with concomitant intravenous albumin can be used to treat tense or refractory ascites. In patients with hypervolemic hyponatremia, a fluid restriction of roughly 1 L/d is recommended. In addition, timely diagnosis and treatment of spontaneous bacterial peritonitis is key to prevent development of HRS-1.[17]

GUT

There are an estimated 10^{13} microbes that inhabit the human digestive tract, collectively referred to as the "gut microbiome," and our knowledge about the link between the microbiome and disease is progressing rapidly.[24] The intestines are home to the largest reservoir of immune cells in the body and play an important role in immune and metabolic homeostasis. Research has shown that gut dysbiosis, or alterations in the microbiome, can exacerbate and increase susceptibility to metabolic and immune dysfunction.[25] These alterations can be caused by Western diets, retention of uremic toxins, and/or frequent antibiotic use. In addition, we know that CKD and AKI are associated with systemic inflammation, including activation of innate and adaptive immune cells.[24,26] Thus, it is possible that intestinal dysbiosis, and resulting changes in immune response, can have a significant impact on kidney disease, and vice versa.[27]

MICROBIOME AND ACUTE KIDNEY DISEASE

Experimental data have shown that the gut microbiota can significantly affect outcomes in AKI.[28] Yang and colleagues[29] investigated the relationship between AKI, the gut microbiome, and immune response in mouse models. The investigators found that the intestinal microbiota in those with AKI differed from that of the control group and that this different microbiome was associated with dysbiosis. The intestinal dysbiosis was causally linked to the severity of kidney injury, highlighting a bidirectional relationship between the kidneys and intestines. Dysbiosis was measured as relative increases in *Escherichia* and *Enterobacter* and decreases of *Lactobacillus* bacteria, as well as reduced levels of short-chain fatty acids (SCFAs).[30] SCFAs are fermentation products of dietary fiber and have a role in regulating host and microbiome homeostasis. Experimental data have shown beneficial effects of treatment with SCFAs in kidney injury.[29] Although these studies are in mice, it is expected that the human biome would respond in a similar way.

MICROBIOME AND CHRONIC KIDNEY DISEASE

Urea nitrogen is a normal waste product found in the blood that comes from the breakdown of protein and is filtered across the glomerulus and secreted in the urine. Kidney disease progression leads to retention of blood urea nitrogen and eventually uremia. Vaziri and colleagues[31] studied the intestinal microbiota of uremic versus nonuremic humans and rats and found that uremia was associated with an increased number of pathologic intestinal organisms. The investigators hypothesize that the hydrolysis of urea by urease expressed in the gut flora results in increased quantities of ammonia, which alters the luminal pH and may disrupt the intestinal barrier. This disruption can lead to bacterial translocation and persistent systemic inflammation. Indoxyl sulfate is one proinflammatory uremic toxin derived from gut microbes that has been shown to accumulate in patients with CKD. We know that diet impacts the health of our gut flora, and patients with CKD often follow strict diets that limit the intake of fruits, vegetables, fiber, and dairy products, which contain nutrients for beneficial microbes. One small study in patients with end-stage kidney disease showed that increasing dietary fiber reduced plasma levels of indoxyl sulfate, suggesting a therapeutic role for fiber to ameliorate uremia.[32]

MICROBIOTA AS A THERAPEUTIC TARGET

These experimental findings suggest that strategies targeting dysbiosis and altered gut immunity can lead to the development of novel therapies, that is, probiotics, for the prevention or treatment of kidney disease. However, more research is needed to identify causal pathogens and underlying molecular mechanisms as well as translational studies in human models.

SUMMARY

The kidneys interact with all organ systems in the body, and dysfunction of any of these systems can contribute to kidney impairment, or vice versa. It is important that clinicians understand and recognize the mechanisms by which the kidneys and other organ systems interact. This allows one to intervene early and reduce complications while improving outcomes for our patients. As with many areas of medicine, there is much to be learned. Exciting research is taking place to elucidate therapy optimization, novel biomarkers, and improved patient outcomes related to kidney dysfunction.

CLINICS CARE POINTS

- An elevated serum creatinine compared to baseline in patients with known heart failure is often a sign of cardiorenal syndrome and management is with diuresis.
- Serum creatinine elevation during diuresis may not be due to true kidney injury, and if no other causes of elevated creatinine are found and the patient is clinically improving, diuresis can be continued.
- Hepatorenal syndrome is seen in patients with advanced liver disease due to circulatory dysfunction, and confers high morbidity and mortality.
- Treatment of HRS in admitted patients consists of holding nephrotoxic medications including diuretics and administering albumin and vasoconstrictors with a goal MAP >85 mmHg.
- Experimental data suggests a bidirectional relationship between gut dysbiosis and severity of kidney injury.
- Novel probiotics or increasing dietary fiber in patients with AKI or CKD might be a therapy for chronic inflammation and immune dysregulation, however it is unclear if this effects outcomes and more studies are needed.

DISCLOSURE

None.

REFERENCES

1. Rangaswami J, Bhalla V, Blair JEA, et al. Cardiorenal syndrome: classification, pathophysiology, diagnosis, and treatment strategies: a scientific statement from the American Heart Association. Circulation 2019;139(16):840–78.
2. National Institute of Health. National heart, Lung and Blood Institute, Bethesda, MD. https://www.nhlbi.nih.gov/events/2004/cardio-renal-connections-heart-failure-and-cardiovascular-disease. Accessed July 31, 2021.
3. Ronco C, McCullough P, Anker SD, et al. Cardio-renal syndromes: report from the Consensus Conference of the Acute Dialysis Quality Initiative. Eur Heart J 2010; 31:703–11.
4. Kidney Disease: Improving Global Outcomes (KDIGO) Acute Kidney Injury Work Group. KDIGO clinical practice guideline for acute kidney injury. Kidney Int 2012;(suppl 4):1–138.
5. Adams KF Jr, Fonarow GC, Emerman CL, et al, for the ADHERE Scientific Advisory Committee and Investigators. Characteristics and outcomes of patients hospitalized for heart failure in the United States: rationale, design, and preliminary observations from the first 100,000 cases in the Acute Decompensated Heart Failure National Registry (ADHERE). Am Heart J 2005;149:209–16.
6. Damman K, van Deursen VM, Navis G, et al. Increased central venous pressure is associated with impaired renal function and mortality in a broad spectrum of patients with cardiovascular disease. J Am Coll Cardiol 2009;53:582–8.
7. Raina R, Nair N, Chakraborty R, et al. An Update on the Pathophysiology and Treatment of Cardiorenal Syndrome. Cardiol Res 2020;11(2):76–88.
8. Zannad F, Rossignol P. Cardiorenal syndrome revisited. Circulation 2018;138(9): 929–44.
9. McCullough PA, Neyou A. Comprehensive review of the relative clinical utility of B-type natriuretic peptide and N-terminal Pro-B-type natriuretic peptide assays in cardiovascular disease. Arterioscler Thromb Vasc Biol 2020;40(9):2018–32.
10. The ESCAPE Investigators and ESCAPE Study Coordinators. Evaluation study of congestive heart failure and pulmonary artery catheterization effectiveness: the ESCAPE trial. JAMA 2005;294(13):1625–33.
11. Mordi NA, Mordi IR, Singh JS, et al. Renal and cardiovascular effects of SGLT2 inhibition in combination with loop diuretics in patients with type 2 diabetes and chronic heart failure: the RECEDE-CHF trial. Circulation 2020;142(18): 1713–24.
12. Verbrugge FH, Grieten L, Mullens W. Management of the cardiorenal syndrome in decompensated heart failure. Cardiorenal Med 2014;4(3–4):176–88.
13. Costanzo MR, Guglin ME, Saltzberg MT, et al, for the UNLOAD Trial Investigators. Ultrafiltration versus intravenous diuretics for patients hospitalized for acute decompensated heart failure. J Am Coll Cardiol 2007;49(6):675–83.
14. Bart BA, Goldsmith SR, Lee KL, et al, for the Heart Failure Clinical Research Network. Ultrafiltration in decompensated heart failure with cardiorenal syndrome. N Engl J Med 2012;367(24):2296–304.
15. Kim CS. Pharmacologic management of the Cardio-renal Syndrome. Electrolyte Blood Press 2013;11(1):17–23.

16. Rico-Mesa JS, White A, Ahmadian-Tehrani A, et al. Mineralocorticoid receptor antagonists: a comprehensive review of finerenone. Curr Cardiol Rep 2020; 22(11):140.

17. Ginès P, Guevara M, Arroyo V, et al. Hepatorenal syndrome. Lancet 2003; 362(9398):1819–27.

18. Simonetto DA, Gines P, Kamath PS. Hepatorenal syndrome: pathophysiology, diagnosis, and management. BMJ 2020;1–14.

19. Allegretti AS, Ortiz G, Wenger J, et al. Prognosis of acute kidney injury and hepatorenal syndrome in patients with cirrhosis: a prospective cohort study. Int J Nephrol 2015;2015:108139.

20. European Association for the Study of the Liver, European Association for the Study of the Liver. EASL clinical practice guidelines for the management of patients with decompensated cirrhosis. J Hepatol 2018;69(2):406–60.

21. Angeli P, Garcia-Tsao G, Nadim MK, et al. News in pathophysiology, definition and classification of hepatorenal syndrome: a step beyond the International Club of Ascites (ICA) consensus document. J Heptol 2019;71(4):811–22.

22. Velez J. Transplanting new guidelines into practice in hepatorenal syndrome and acute kidney injury *everything is fixed, right?* Oral presentation at national kidney foundation spring clinical meeting. New Orleans: Louisiana; 2020.

23. Regner KR. Patients with hepatorenal syndrome should be dialyzed? Commentary. Kidney360 2020;2(3):413–4.

24. Anders HJ, Andersen K, Stecher B. The intestinal microbiota, a leaky gut, and abnormal immunity in kidney disease. Kidney Int 2013;83(6):1010–6.

25. Bull MJ, Plummer NT. Part 1: the human gut microbiome in health and disease. Integr Med (Encinitas) 2014;13(6):17–22.

26. Noel S, Martina-Lingua MN, Bandapalle S, et al. Intestinal microbiota-kidney cross talk in acute kidney injury and chronic kidney disease. Nephron Clin Pract 2014;127:139–43.

27. Jo SK. Kidney-Gut crosstalk in acute kidney injury. Kidney360 2021;1(5):886–9.

28. Rabb H, Griffin M, McKay D, et al. Inflammation in AKI: current understanding, key questions, and knowledge gaps. J Am Soc Nephrol 2016;27:371–9.

29. Yang J, Kim CJ, Go YS, et al. Intestinal microbiota control acute kidney injury severity by immune modulation. Kidney Int 2020;98(4):932–46.

30. Gong J, Noel S, Pluznick JL, et al. Gut microbiota-kidney cross-talk in acute kidney injury. Semin Nephrol 2019;39(1):107–16.

31. Vaziri ND, Wong J, Pahl M, et al. Chronic kidney disease alters intestinal microbial flora. Kidney Int 2013;83(2):308–15.

32. Sirich TL, Plummer NS, Gardner CD, et al. Effect of increasing dietary fiber on plasma levels of colon-derived solutes in hemodialysis patients. Clin J Am Soc Nephrol 2014;9(9):1603–10.

Diabetic Kidney Disease

Dale Marie Gomez, PA-C

KEYWORDS

- CKD • Diabetes • Diabetic kidney disease • DKD • SGLT2 inhibitors
- GLP-1 inhibitors

KEY POINTS

- Diabetes is the leading cause of chronic kidney disease in the United States (CDC, 2019).
- Diabetes (Hajar, 2017) and chronic kidney disease (Sarnak, 2003) are both risk factors for coronary artery disease
- Research into biomarkers and the introduction of new medications have the potential to significantly shift the diagnosis and management of DKD in the coming years
- KDIGO has issued new guidelines for management of DKD

INTRODUCTION AND BACKGROUND

Research on new diabetes medications and their interaction with the kidney has resulted in a shifting diabetic kidney disease (DKD) treatment paradigm. The most recent Kidney Disease Improving Global Outcomes (KDIGO) published in 2020 highlighted these data.[1] The incidence of diabetes has continued to increase across the past 30 years, and DKD is the leading cause of end-stage kidney disease (ESKD) worldwide.[2,3] Implementation of these guidelines may prevent or significantly delay ESKD.

Adoption by clinicians of the new KDIGO guidelines is vital given the potential burden of disease in the future. In particular, the efficacy of sodium glucose cotransporter-2 inhibitors (SGLT2i) will be key to reducing the incidence of ESKD in the future (**Fig. 1**).

Despite new medications to fight this battle, there are vast nonrandom variations in geographic distribution of people with diabetes who reach ESKD, thus pointing to environmental and/or genetic factors that may impact disease presentation as well.[4]

Chronic kidney disease (CKD) is defined as the presence of kidney damage, physiologic changes, and/or persistently low estimated glomerular filtration rate (eGFR) of less than 60 mL/min per 1.73 m^2 body surface area for more than 3 months.[5] Once CKD is identified, it is staged according to eGFR and the presence and/or amount of albuminuria (**Fig. 2**).

Mid Atlantic Nephrology Associates, 7106 Ridge Road, Suite 155, Baltimore, MD 21237, USA
E-mail address: Dgomez@MANAPA.com
Twitter: @dalegomez (D.M.G.)

Physician Assist Clin 7 (2022) 261–272
https://doi.org/10.1016/j.cpha.2021.11.015
2405-7991/22/© 2021 Elsevier Inc. All rights reserved.
physicianassistant.theclinics.com

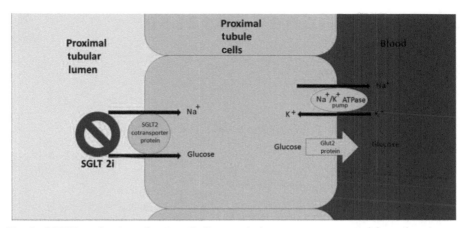

Fig. 1. SGLT2i mechanism of action. Sodium and glucose are transported from the glomerular filtrate by the SGLT2 transmemebrane protein into the interior of proximal convoluted tubule (PCT) cells as it passes through the PCT. The Glut2 protein then passes the glucose from inside the PCT cells back into the blood. The sodium is then exchanged for potassium via an enzyme that requires energy from ATP. These activities conserve sodium and glucose, while eliminating excess potassium. The SGLT2i prevents the initial step of this process, resulting In a loss of sodium and glucose via urine.

As eGFR decreases and/or albuminuria increases, risk of progression to ESKD increases. To determine a cause of the kidney disease, urinalysis/serologic testing/imaging and/or biopsy are used. Albuminuria in a patient with diabetes and kidney disease often indicates that the cause of the kidney disease is diabetes.[6] A kidney biopsy is the gold standard for determining if CKD is the result of a patient's comorbid diabetes, but the risk of this invasive procedure is often not warranted and likely will not change the management plan for the patient[7]; this presents a dilemma because studies have shown that many patients with diabetes mellitus type 2 (T2DM) have nondiabetic kidney disease (NDKD) or mixed DKD/NDKD, making clinical diagnosis of DKD in the absence of a biopsy suspect in regard to accuracy.[3] As a result the true incident rate of DKD is not known.

Research suggests that development of DKD is associated with genetic and epigenetic factors and that not all patients with T2DM will develop DKD, even with poor glycemic control.[3] The current state of research has not teased out the precise role of environmental versus genetic factors that contribute to the development of CKD.[8] However, familial clustering of CKD/ESKD, with an estimated incidence rate of 30% to 75%, is observed with all prevalent causes of the disease.[9] As such, it is reasonable to use family history as an alternative marker for risk of future nephropathy or even as indication for risk of progression of the disease.

It is estimated that about 25% of patients with diabetes have DKD.[10] In 2020, approximately 34.2 million Americans had diabetes (90%–95% T2DM) while another 88 million were prediabetic.[11] Overall, an estimated 70% of patients with prediabetes will develop diabetes in the long term.[12] Therefore, in 2020, an estimated 8.55 million Americans had DKD, with potentially another 15.4 million developing DKD in coming years. Note that this calculation does not include patients with type 1 diabetes.

In the United States, diabetes disproportionately affects African Americans, Hispanics, and persons with low socioeconomic status (SES). These groups are also disproportionately impacted by barriers to care, which can include[10]

				Persistent albuminuria categories Description and range		
				A1	**A2**	**A3**
Prognosis of CKD by GFR and Albuminuria Categories: KDIGO 2012				Normal to mildly increased	Moderately increased	Severely increased
				<30 mg/g <3 mg/mmol	30-300 mg/g 3-30 mg/mmol	>300 mg/g >30 mg/mmol
GFR categories (ml/min/ 1.73 m²) Description and range	G1	Normal or high	≥90			
	G2	Mildly decreased	60-89			
	G3a	Mildly to moderately decreased	45-59			
	G3b	Moderately to severely decreased	30-44			
	G4	Severely decreased	15-29			
	G5	Kidney failure	<15			

Fig. 2. Stages of kidney disease. (Inker LA, Astor B, Fox CH, et al. Evaluation and management of CKD. AJKD vol 63 (5), pg713–735. 2014)

- Low awareness of CKD
- Education/SES
- Health care literacy
- Health insurance/cost
- Access to health care
- Inadequate screening
- Delayed nephrology referral
- Fragmented care

SGLT2i medications are renoprotective and are the main intervention for the patient with DKD.[1] Despite the greater risk of DKD in racial minorities and those with lower SES, evidence is already mounting that there are gender and racial disparities in the use of SGLT2i in the United States. Women, Black, Asian, and lower-income patients with T2DM were less likely to receive the SGLT2i according to a recent published retrospective study.[13] However, due to study design, it is unclear if these disparities are a reflection of treatment bias or represent a barrier to care (ie, cost). The increasing incidence of diabetes, coupled with a high prevalence in populations that face disproportionate barriers to care, will result in a considerable increase in DKD in the future if changes are not implemented now.

Initially, the pathology of DKD was thought to primarily involve glomerular damage based on the early glomerular changes seen in kidney biopsies.[3] Based on more current research, the primary pathology responsible for decline in kidney function seems to be tubulointerstitial damage, with glomerular damage occurring secondary to changes brought on by tubulointerstitial damage.[3] Animal studies indicate that albuminuria is a sensitive marker for tubular toxicity even without glomerular damage present. Urinary biomarkers in humans support proximal tubular damage as a primary factor in early diabetic nephropathy.[14]

Ongoing research has improved our understanding of the pathophysiology of DKD and may provide alternatives for diagnosis with less invasive means than the kidney biopsy. Our improved understanding of the pathology also helps target therapies to improve outcomes. The SGLT2i medications are proving to be beneficial in protecting the kidney from damage and may prevent a tsunami of new cases of DKD-related ESKD in our future.[1] However, as of yet, we do not fully understand the kidney protective mechanisms of action of these medications. Reports have surfaced in the public literature citing hesitancy to prescribe SGLT2i by cardiology and nephrology despite mounting evidence that they provide cardio/renal protection.[15,16] Recent trials have noted the renoprotective qualities of SGLT2i, and on that data, the US Food and Drug Administration (FDA) approved dapagliflozin for use in the treatment of CKD *without* diabetes.[17]

KIDNEY DISEASE IMPROVING GLOBAL OUTCOMES GUIDELINES

The most current expert international guideline for management of diabetes in the patient with CKD was published in October 2020.[1] This version includes *Recommendations* and newly added *Practice Points* to guide medical personnel in the care of patients with DKD. *Recommendations* are evidenced based and the preferred action over alternatives, whereas *Practice Points* do not have the level of evidence of recommendations but are generally supported by consensus. If implemented in the patient with DKD, evidence suggests these new guidelines will help considerably in the battle against DKD, and even CKD in the absence of comorbid diabetes. However, as these medications were originally marketed for the control of hyperglycemia, and there are risks to using them, there has been reported hesitancy on the part of cardiology and nephrology providers to adopt their usage.[15,16] The recent FDA approval of dapagliflozin to slow CKD progression in nondiabetic patients with CKD may provide the catalyst to remove this hesitancy to prescribe, at least on the part of nephrology providers.

DKD is a complex medical condition requiring a comprehensive approach to care.[1] Under the KDIGO guidelines, all patients with CKD and diabetes should be encouraged to exercise, focus on good nutrition, control blood pressure and blood sugar, and manage lipids. It is recommended that all patients quit smoking. Most patients should be taking an angiotensin-converting enzyme inhibitor (ACEi) or angiotensin receptor blocker (ARB). KDIGO recommends that an SGLT2i be concurrently started with metformin,[1] although this may prove a little more difficult in the United States where often metformin therapy must fail or the patient be intolerant to it before most insurances will pay for the addition of an SGLT2i.

Because ACEi and ARBs have proven efficacy in protecting the kidney, it is recommended they be used, at their highest tolerated dose, for hypertensive patients with diabetes and albuminuria. ACEi and ARBs may be used in normotensive patients as well, especially those with albuminuria. Potassium levels and serum creatinine (SCr) should be monitored after initiation of either of these medications and during dose adjustments due to the risk of hyperkalemia and/or kidney function decline. The consensus is to continue use of the ACEi or ARBs unless SCr level increases by more than 30% after starting these medications. Dose decrease or stopping of ACEi/ARBs is advised in the setting of hypotension or hyperkalemia not controlled with the use of potassium-binding medications. Given their teratogenicity, women of childbearing age should be on birth control, and these medications must be stopped in the event of pregnancy.

KDIGO recommends that hemoglobin A_{1c} (HbA_{1C}) be used to monitor glycemic control twice a year in patients who are within glycemic goal, and quarterly in patients who are not at goal or who are undergoing medication adjustments.[1] Providers should be aware that use of HbA_{1C} is significantly less reliable in patients with later stages of CKD due to the impact of anemia, use of erythropoiesis-stimulating agents, and/or use of iron replacement therapy, all of which cause the HbA_{1C} to be falsely low. Inflammation, oxidative stress, and metabolic acidosis, all prevalent in patients with kidney disease, can cause HbA_{1C} to be falsely high. In general, HbA_{1C} tends to run artificially low in later stages of CKD (stage 4 and higher), especially in patients on dialysis. To mitigate the risk of suspected inaccurate HgA_{1C} measurements, continuous glucose monitoring (CGM) is recommended to derive a glucose management indicator (GMI). GMI is a blood glucose average calculated from CGM that is expressed in units of HbA_{1C} (%). CGM is then compared with the measured HbA_{1C} to enable more accurate interpretation of the laboratory-reported value.

Patients who are on medications that place them at higher risk of hypoglycemia (insulin, sulfonylureas and/or meglitinides) should use a CGM or daily self-monitoring of blood glucose (SMBG). Providers should be aware of the newer products available for CGM because they may be beneficial for certain members of their patient population. It is advisable, if possible, to avoid using medications with high hypoglycemia risks in patients unwilling or unable to use a CGM or SMBG. As always, diabetes medications should be dosed according to eGFR. There is no clear value to doing this sort of monitoring in patients on antiglycemic medications with a low risk of hypoglycemia (metformin, SGLT2i, glucagonlike peptide 1 receptor agonist [GLP1-RA], or dipeptidyl peptidase 4 [DPP-4] inhibitors).

In nondialysis patients, KDIGO recommends an HbA_{1C} between 6.5% and 7% individualized for each patient.[1] Studies have shown that in the general diabetes population, there is a U-shaped association between HbA_{1C} levels and adverse outcomes. Higher levels increase the risk of microvascular and macrovascular complications, whereas lower targets for HbA_{1C} may place patients at risk of dangerous hypoglycemic events. In managing patients with DKD, the HbA_{1C} goal selected should take into consideration patient preferences, risks to the patient, life expectancy, medical therapy burden, and disease burden. A lower target may be more appropriate for patients with concerns of onset and progression of albuminuria, or who have experienced nonfatal myocardial infarction, as well as those with a lower risk of hypoglycemia. A higher HbA_{1C} may be more appropriate for a patient with a lower eGFR and/or use of medications with a greater risk of hypoglycemia, because both these situations may place them at greater risk for more hypoglycemic events. Patients with a shorter life expectancy and significant comorbidities may warrant a higher goal as well. For those with a lower HbA_{1C} goal, mitigation of risk of hypoglycemic events is possible by using CGM, SMBG, and/or medications with a lower risk of hypoglycemia.[1]

Lifestyle factors such as diet, exercise, and weight loss are an important component of DKD care.[1] Patients should have an individualized diet high in vegetables, whole grains, fruits, fiber, legumes, unsaturated fats, and plant-based proteins. Patients should avoid sugared beverages, refined carbohydrates, and processed meats, and in later stages of CKD, foods with a high potassium content.

Patients with kidney disease are often provided lists of acceptable and unacceptable foods that usually do not take into account culture, income, food availability, cooking skills, family food needs, patient dentition, or patient diet needs for comorbid conditions.[1] The kidney diet is restrictive and complex, making implementation difficult when considering all the aforementioned factors which serve to further increase complexity. However, diet can greatly modify HbA_{1C} levels and prevent acidosis or hyperkalemia. Providing nutrition education and working to develop an individualize diet plan via a shared decision-making process with patients is an important step in care.[1]

KDIGO recommends protein intake of 0.8/g protein/kg body weight/d for nondialysis patients with DKD, despite the fact that lower protein intake may reduce glomerular hyperfiltration (in the general population) and therefore slow progression of kidney damage. The rationale is that given carbohydrate restriction for these patients, a lower protein intake could result in unintended weight loss and increase the risk of hypoglycemia.[1] Furthermore, there is only weak to very weak evidence in the literature that supports lower protein diets for slowing the progression of kidney disease. Even if intended for weight loss, a high protein diet is also not recommended for these patients, especially protein loads of greater than 1 g protein/kg of body weight/d. A high protein diet may harm the kidneys and increase acid load, which in turn increases the risk of metabolic acidosis; this is especially true in later stages of CKD. Patients with high body mass index (BMI) should have their protein needs calculated based on ideal body weight, not actual body weight, to avoid excessively high protein intake. On the contrary, patients on hemodialysis or peritoneal dialysis should have a protein intake of 1.0 to 1.2 g/kg/d to counteract the impact of uremia and increased risk of hypoglycemia.

The KDIGO guideline recommends a sodium-restricted diet for patients with DKD.[1] Patients should limit their daily sodium to no more than 2 g. High sodium increases blood pressure and by extension, cardiovascular risk. Salt load can impact volume status and increase proteinuria. Lower sodium also improves the benefits of ACEi and ARBs. Salt substitutes should be avoided because they are generally potassium based and place patients with later-stage CKD at increased risk for hyperkalemia. The dietary approaches to stop hypertension, also known as the DASH diet may increase risk of hyperkalemia and should be avoided in later stages of kidney disease. If a patient suffers from orthostatic hypotension, salt intake limits may need to be guided for these patients by a health care professional. If salt is the primary source of iodine for a patient, for example, people who do not have access to saltwater seafood, 2 g per day of iodinated salt will only meet two-fifth of their iodine needs.[1] An alternate plan may be needed for these patients to prevent goiters. Patient sodium taste thresholds can be changed, and it takes about 4 to 6 weeks to do so; however, a variety of factors may impede a patients' ability to adjust their diet including food insecurity or high-sodium foods of cultural significance.

Physical activity is the second component of lifestyle factors that patients with DKD should endeavor to incorporate into their habits. Patients should be advised to avoid a sedentary lifestyle. KDIGO recommends 150 minutes per week of moderate-intensity physical activity or at a level compatible with a patient's cardiovascular and physical tolerance.[1] Studies have recently shown that physical activity can slow the decline in eGFR.[1] Exercise also improves insulin sensitivity, mood, and cognition. Even in low-resource situations, exercise regimens are feasible. Because patients with CKD are often older, they may have an increased risk of falls or physical limitations that might hinder their participation in activity; this should be taken into consideration.

Patients with DKD who are overweight should be encouraged to lose weight, especially those with mild to moderate kidney disease. Weight loss can lower blood pressure, improve albuminuria, and may deliver some kidney benefits to those with mild to moderate disease. However, in later stages of CKD weight loss may be unintentional, and a higher BMI is associated with better outcomes in dialysis patients. Therefore, the benefit to the individual patient needs to be considered before advising weight loss for a patient in a later stage of CKD.[1]

Glycemic control for DKD should always start with lifestyle changes, but when this is not effective, KDIGO recommends the initial use of metformin and an SGLT2i in patients with an eGFR greater than or equal to 30 mL/min/1.73 m^2. Additional medications, preferably a GLP-1 RA, may be added as needed to meet HbA$_{1C}$ goals. These medications present less risk of hypoglycemia than insulin or sulfonylureas.

Metformin is inexpensive, may help with weight loss, may provide cardiovascular benefits, and is safe and effective at lowering HbA$_{1C}$ levels. Metformin has significantly less risk of hypoglycemia than sulfonylureas or insulin. Metformin is also acceptable for use in patients who have undergone transplant who meet eGFR limits. However, the gastrointestinal effects of metformin may cause issues for the patient and an extended-release version tends to be better tolerated. The eGFR of patients treated with metformin should be monitored at least annually and every 3 to 6 months once eGFR drops below 60 mL/min/1.73 m^2.[1] At an eGFR of 30 to 45 mL/min/1.73 m^2, metformin dosing should be reduced to half and be completely stopped below 30 mL/min/1.73 m^2. Metformin interferes with intestinal absorption of B$_{12}$, and B$_{12}$ levels should be monitored at 4 years of dosing.[1] Supplementation is not routinely necessary.

The SGLT2i drugs have less impact on HbA$_{1C}$, especially at an eGFR less than 60 mL/min/1.73 m^2, but maintain significant kidney and cardioprotective benefits independent of glycemic impact[1]; this suggests that an alternative mechanism, outside of glycemic control, is responsible for these benefits. In light of this, it is recommended to use SGLT2i with metformin in T2DMs with CKD even if HbA$_{1C}$ goals are met with metformin alone.[1] If needed, one can reduce the metformin dose or reduce or eliminate other antiglycemic medication to add on the SGLT2i. Risk of hypoglycemia is generally low with the SGLT2i class, particularly if used as monotherapy, because glycosuria produced by the blocking of the sodium-glucose transporters in the proximal tubule decreases as blood glucose normalizes. However, risk of hypoglycemia is higher when used with sulfonylureas or insulin.[1] Once eGFR drops below 30 mL/min/1.73 m^2, metformin is stopped to reduce the risk of lactic acidosis. At present, SGLT2i should continue until kidney replacement therapy begins.[1]

In patients with type 1 diabetes (T1DM) and kidney transplant recipients, safety and efficacy of SGLT2i drugs are less known and trials are underway.[1] At present, KDIGO does not recommend the SGLT2i class of drugs for transplant recipients due to the increased risk of mycotic infections.[1] Patients who are at high risk of side effects, such as those with infection or urinary tract infection, or who face cost barriers may opt for alternative medications.

At times, it is necessary to alter medication regimens to reduce risks and harm when using SGLT2i. When a patient faces a period of low oral intake, illness, surgery, or prolonged fasting states, one needs to hold the SGLT2i to reduce the risk of euglycemic diabetic ketoacidosis. Patients who are on thiazide or loop diuretics and start an SGLT2i may need medication adjustments to prevent hypovolemia. Patients with tenuous volume status may also be at risk of hypovolemia. These patients should have close follow-up to monitor volume status, and education on symptoms of volume depletion and low blood pressure. A modest, reversible drop in eGFR when initiating an SGLT2i is expected, which is not an indication for discontinuing the medication.[1]

If the HbA$_{1C}$ is still elevated while using metformin and an SGLT2i, KDIGO recommends adding a GLP-1 RA to the medication regimen.[1] However, comorbid conditions, patient preference, cost, and eGFR should be considered in the final decision for which medication to choose (**Table 1**).

KDIGO guidelines recommend the GLP-1 RA class due to their cardiovascular and possible kidney benefits.[1] Randomized controlled trials show that 4 of the GLP-1 RA-

Table 1
Considerations in selection of antiglycemic medications when metformin and sodium–glucose cotransporter-2 inhibitors do not meet glycemic goals alone

Factors in Selection of Antiglycemic Therapy	Preferable Medication	Least Preferred Medication
Weight loss	• Glucagonlike peptide 1-receptor agonist	• Sulfonylurea • Insulin • Thiazolidinedione
Low cost	• Sulfonylurea • Thiazolidinedione • Alpha-glucosidase inhibitor	• Glucagonlike peptide 1-receptor agonist • Insulin • Dipeptidyl peptidase-4 inhibitor
Heart failure	• Glucagonlike peptide 1-receptor agonist	• Thiazolidinedione
High atherosclerotic cardiovascular disease (ASCVD) risk	• Glucagonlike peptide 1-receptor agonist	
Potent glucose lowering	• Glucagonlike peptide 1-receptor agonist • Insulin	• Dipeptidyl peptidase-4 inhibitor • Thiazolidinedione • Alpha-glucosidase inhibitor
Avoiding hypoglycemia	• Dipeptidyl peptidase-4 inhibitor • Thiazolidinedione • Alpha-glucosidase inhibitor • Glucagon-like peptide 1-receptor agonist	• Sulfonylurea • Insulin
Avoid Injections	• Dipeptidyl peptidase-4 inhibitor • Oral glucagonlike peptide-1 receptor agonist • Sulfonylurea • Thiazolidinedione • Alpha-glucosidase inhibitor	• Glucagonlike peptide-1 receptor agonist • Insulin
eGFR < 15 mL/min/1.73 m^2 or on dialysis	• Dipeptidyl peptidase-4 inhibitor • Thiazolidinedione • Insulin	• Sulfonylurea • Alpha-glucosidase inhibitor

Adapted from KDIGO Guidelines.

injectable medications (liraglutide, semaglutide, albiglutide, dulaglutide) significantly reduce major cardiac adverse events in patients with T2DM and a HbA_{1C} persistently greater than 7.0%.[1] These medications also promote weight loss, reduce blood pressure, reduce albuminuria, and probably preserve eGFR. To prevent gastrointestinal side effects, these medications should be started at a low dose and titrate slowly. Because DDP-4i stimulates the body's natural release of GLP-1, these medications should not be used in conjunction with GLP-1 RAs.[1] Contraindications to both GLPs and DPP4i include a history of medullary thyroid cancer, multiple endocrine neoplasia syndrome 2, and acute pancreatitis. Care should be taken when using with medications with a high risk of hypoglycemia such as insulin or sulfonylureas because doses may need adjustment to reduce risks, especially as kidney function declines.[1]

The management of patients with DKD is clearly a complex undertaking for both the patient and the health care providers. Given the complexity, KDIGO recommends that patients have access to self-management educational programs that include educators trained in the delivery of diabetes and CKD lifestyle management.[1] These programs should take into account local context, culture, and resources. To mitigate the challenges health care providers face when caring for such complex patients, a team-based integrated care model is preferred with a structured care paradigm that incorporates accountability to prevent gaps in care.

The previous information summarizes the main points of the current KDIGO DKD guideline. **Box 1** lists the guideline recommendations.[1]

To access the complete KDIGO guideline, please refer to KDIGO 2020 Clinical Practice Guidelines for Diabetes Management in Chronic Kidney Disease.

What future changes in clinical management might be in store for patients with DKD? As noted earlier, because of the risks and limited clinical benefit of biopsy it is not routinely done and as a result, the true incidence of DKD is not well known. However, a wide variety of clinical factors including family history, albuminuria onset, anemia, among others present differently in patients with DKD. Using these clinical factors as a noninvasive means of predicting the presence of DKD versus NDKD would be possible if enough evidence is gathered to thoroughly define these changes in the DKD population.[3] In addition, as we more extensively identify the genetic and epigenetic milieu of DKD, we should be able to identify early serum biomarkers for the presence of DKD thereby creating a far less risky means of accurate diagnosis than kidney biopsies.[18]

This would allow earlier, more aggressive interventions that could impact the epigenetic changes responsible for "*metabolic memory*" that leads to worse disease across time. In the long run, genetic and epigenetic research will provide information on the role of heritability versus environmental factors that impact presentation of the disease. This knowledge may tease out subsets of pathophysiology, as of yet unidentified, that would impact our ability to develop more precise and, as a result, more efficacious and less risky treatment regimens, for individuals based on their specific epigenetic signature.

We can expect some more immediate changes in regard to treatment of DKD/CKD. With the recent FDA approval of dapagliflozin for use in CKD without comorbid diabetes, we should expect to see more patients with kidney disease prescribed SGLT2i.[17,19,20] Although dapagliflozin is the first of the SGLT2i for CKD without diabetes, it will not be the last. At present, trials for other SGLT2i are underway. This new indication for CKD in the patient without diabetes may wind up being the key to preventing a large increase in our dialysis population in the coming years.

Box 1
Recommendations from Kidney Disease Improving Global Outcomes 2020 Clinical Practice Guideline for diabetes management in chronic kidney disease

KDIGO recommends treatment with an angiotensin-converting enzyme inhibitor (ACEi) or angiotensin II receptor blocker be initiated in patient with diabetes, hypertension, and albuminuria, and that these medications be titrated to the highest approved dose that is tolerated. (1B)[a]

KDIGO recommends advising patient with diabetes and CKD who use tobacco to quit using tobacco products. (1D)

KDIGO recommends using hemoglobin A_{1c} to monitor glycemic control in patients with diabetes and CKD (1c)

KDIGO suggests maintaining a protein intake of 0.8 g protein/kg body weight/d for those with diabetes and CKD not treated with dialysis. (2C)

KDIGO suggests that sodium intake be <2 g sodium per day (of < 90 mmol of sodium per day, or <5 g of sodium chloride per day) in patients with diabetes and CKD. (2C)

KDIGO recommends that patients with diabetes and CKD be advised to undertake moderate-intensity physical activity for a cumulative duration of at least 150 minutes per week, or to a level compatible with their cardiovascular and physical tolerance. (1D)

KDIGO recommends treating patients with T2D, CKD, and an eGFR $\geq$ 30 mL/min per 1.73 m_2 with metformin. (1B)

KDIGO recommends treating patients with T2D, CKD, and an eGFR $\geq$ 30 mL/min per 1.73 m_2 with an SGLT2i. (1A)

In patients with T2D and CKD who have not achieved individualized glycemic targets despite use of metformin and SGLT2i, or who are unable to use those medications, KDIGO recommends using a long-acting GLP-1 RA. (1B)

KDIGO recommends that a structured self-management educational program be implemented for care of people with diabetes and CKD. (1C)

KDIGO suggests that policy makers and institutional decision makers implement team-based integrated care focused on risk evaluation and patient empowerment to provide comprehensive care in patients with diabetes and CKD. (2B)

[a]Ratings: Level 1: most patients should follow the recommendation; 2, many should but other options may be better on a case-by-case basis. A–D is the quality of evidence supporting the recommendation with A being the highest and D the lowest.

CLINICS CARE POINTS

1. Prescribe an ACEi or ARB to all patients with CKD, except those who experience a greater than 30% increase in SCr levels after starting one, those in later stages of kidney disease (usually stage 4 or greater), or those who otherwise have a contraindication to taking one.

2. Make female patients of childbearing age aware of the risk of ACEi and ARBs in pregnancy and have them use birth control, and stop the ACEi or ARB immediately if they become pregnant

3. Titrate patients to the maximum tolerable dose of an ACEi or ARB, unless otherwise contraindicated.

4. In cases of ACEi- or ARB-induced hyperkalemia, unless contraindicated, treat patients with CKD with a potassium binder to allow continued use of these medications.

5. Monitor patients with CKD and DM taking insulin for excessive blood glucose control. As CKD progresses, the amount of insulin needed to reduce blood glucose levels can decline.

6. Providers should be aware that the stage of CKD can impact the accuracy of HbA_{1c} measurements, with it more likely to run artificially low in later stages of CKD.

7. Reduce metformin dose by half once patients with CKD with DM reach an eGFR between 30 and 44, and completely stop the medication once they reach an eGFR of less than 30 to reduce the risk of lactic acidosis.

8. In patients with CKD and type 2 DM, SGLT2i is the preferential treatment over other diabetes medications when not contraindicated.

9. Owing to the increased risk of infection, avoid SGLT2i use in patients on immunosuppressive therapy.

DISCLOSURE

The author has nothing to disclose.

REFERENCES

1. Kidney Disease: Improving Global Outcomes (KDIGO) Diabetes Work group. KDIGO 2020 Clinical Practice Guideline for Diabetes Management in Chronic Kidney Disease. Kid Int 2020;98(4S):S1–115.

2. World Health Organization (WHO). fact sheet, Diabetes. Available at: https://www.who.int/news-room/fact-sheets/detail/diabetes. Accessed July 23 2021.

3. Fu H, Liu S, Bastacky SI, et al. Diabetic kidney diseases revisited: A new perspective for a new era. Mol Metab 2019;30:250–63.

4. Cheng HT, Xu X, Lim PS, et al. Worldwide Epidemiology of Diabetes-Related End-Stage Renal Disease, 2000-2015. Diabetes Care 2021;44(1):89–97.

5. Levey AS, Eckardt KU, Tsukamoto Y, et al. Definition and classification of chronic kidney disease: a position statement from Kidney Disease: Improving Global Outcomes (KDIGO). Kidney Int 2005;67(6):2089–100.

6. Papadakis M, McPhee S, with associate authors. Current medical diagnosis and treatment 2013. 52nd ed. Copyright: The McGraw-Hill Companies; 2013.

7. Persson F, Rossing P. Diagnosis of diabetic kidney disease: state of the art and future perspective. Kidney Int Suppl (2011) 2018;8(1):2–7.

8. Cañadas-Garre M, Anderson K, Cappa R, et al. Genetic Susceptibility to Chronic Kidney Disease - Some More Pieces for the Heritability Puzzle. Front Genet 2019; 10:453.

9. Satko SG, Sedor JR, Iyengar SK, et al. Familial clustering of chronic kidney disease. Semin Dial 2007;20(3):229–36.

10. Duru OK, Middleton T, Tewari MK, et al. The Landscape of Diabetic Kidney Disease in the United States. Curr Diab Rep 2018;18(3):14.

11. Centers for Disease Control and Prevention. National Diabetes Statistics Report, 2020. Centers for Disease Control and Prevention. 2020. Available at: https://www.cdc.gov/diabetes/data/statistics-report/index.html. Accessed July 2 2021.

12. Tabák AG, Herder C, Rathmann W, et al. Prediabetes: a high-risk state for diabetes development. Lancet 2012;379(9833):2279–90.

13. Eberly LA, Yang L, Eneanya ND, et al. Association of Race/Ethnicity, Gender, and Socioeconomic Status With Sodium-Glucose Cotransporter 2 Inhibitor Use Among Patients With Diabetes in the US. JAMA Netw Open 2021;4(4):e216139.

14. Bonventre JV. Can we target tubular damage to prevent renal function decline in diabetes? Semin Nephrol 2012;32(5):452–62.

15. Adhikari R, Blaha M. New Insights into Prescribing of SGLT2 Inhibitors and GLP-1 Receptor Agonists by Cardiologists in 2020: Major Barriers Limiting Role. 2021. Available at: https://www.acc.org/Latest-in-Cardiology/Articles/2021/01/19/14/27/New-Insights-into-Prescribing-of-SGLT2-Inhibitors-and-GLP-1-Receptor-Agonists-in-2020. Accessed May 22 2021.

16. Cision PR Newswire. Nephrologists Are Hesitant to Fully Embrace Janssen's INVOKANA Despite Being the First and Only SGLT2 Inhibitor with an FDA Indication to Treat Diabetic Kidney Disease. Cision PR Newswire 2020. Available at: https://www.prnewswire.com/news-releases/nephrologists-are-hesitant-to-fully-embrace-janssens-invokana-despite-being-the-first-and-only-sglt2-inhibitor-with-an-fda-indication-to-treat-diabetic-kidney-disease-301079788.html. Accessed May 22 2021.

17. Food and Drug Administration. FDA Approves Treatment for Chronic Kidney Disease. 2021. Available at: https://www.fda.gov/news-events/press-announcements/fda-approves-treatment-chronic-kidney-disease. Accessed May 1 2021.

18. Kato M, Natarajan R. Epigenetics and epigenomics in diabetic kidney disease and metabolic memory. Nat Rev Nephrol 2019;15(6):327–45.

19. Bakris G, Oshima M, Mahaffey KW, et al. Effects of Canagliflozin in Patients with Baseline eGFR <30 ml/min per 1.73 m2: Subgroup Analysis of the Randomized CREDENCE Trial. Clin J Am Soc Nephrol 2020;15(12):1705–14.

20. Fernandez-Fernandez B, Sarafidis P, Kanbay M, et al. SGLT2 inhibitors for non-diabetic kidney disease: drugs to treat CKD that also improve glycaemia. Clin Kidney J 2020;13(5):728–33.

Hypertension and Chronic Kidney Disease – An Unhappy Marriage

Harvey A. Feldman, MD, FACP, FASN

KEYWORDS

- Hypertension phenotype • Aldosteronism • Obstructive sleep apnea • Obesity
- CKD hypertension Guidelines

KEY POINTS

- Hypertension and chronic kidney disease contribute to each other, and both are major risk factors for cardiovascular morbidity and mortality.
- Hypertension phenotypes more prevalent in chronic kidney disease are masked, nocturnal, and resistant hypertension. All phenotypes require both in and out-of-office measurements to diagnose.
- Aldosterone is a central contributor to both hypertension and chronic kidney disease as well as to important comorbidities, including sleep apnea, obesity, and insulin resistance.
- First-line medications for hypertension in chronic kidney disease are diuretics, renin–angiotensin blockers, and calcium channel blockers. Aldosterone inhibitors are the best add-on drugs for resistant hypertension.

INTRODUCTION

Hypertension is the most common primary diagnosis in adult general practice in the United States (US).[1] Using the 2017 American College of Cardiology/American Heart Association (ACC/AHA) blood pressure (BP) classification, 47.3% of adults ages 18 years and older have hypertension.[2,3] It is also the second most common comorbidity associated with chronic kidney disease (CKD) after diabetes and the leading contributor to cardiovascular morbidity and mortality worldwide.[4,5] Importantly, although these consequences of hypertension are preventable with appropriate treatment, BP control is suboptimal and declining.[6] A major contributor to this downward trend is undertreatment by clinicians.[7] In the US, nearly 37 million people (15% of the adult population) have CKD and the numbers are rising.[4] CKD is an independent risk factor for cardiovascular disease (CVD) morbidity and mortality.[4] Like hypertension, CKD is often suboptimally managed in primary care.[8] To assist in combating this bidirectional unhappy marriage between hypertension and CKD, this review will focus on

Physician Assistant Program, Nova Southeastern University, 3200 S. University Drive, Terry Building 1258, Ft. Lauderdale, FL 33328-2018, USA
E-mail address: hfeldman@nova.edu

Physician Assist Clin 7 (2022) 273–293
https://doi.org/10.1016/j.cpha.2021.11.003
2405-7991/22/© 2021 Elsevier Inc. All rights reserved.

physicianassistant.theclinics.com

its underlying pathophysiology, the hypertension phenotypes commonly seen in CKD, and current guideline recommendations for the management of hypertension in adult patients with pre-end stage kidney disease (ESKD).

PATHOPHYSIOLOGIC RELATIONSHIPS

Hypertension and CKD share a bidirectional pathophysiologic relationship, and both are risk factors for CVD. Hypertension contributes to kidney impairment that can be gradual or rapid depending on its duration and severity. Conversely, CKD is commonly associated with worsening BP control that is directly proportionate to the severity of kidney failure.[9] In both directions, the mechanisms are complex and controversies exist.

Hypertension as a Cause of Kidney Disease

Acute severe elevation of BP, as seen in hypertensive crisis, causes acute kidney injury (AKI), histologically termed malignant nephrosclerosis. Clinically, patients can have hematuria, proteinuria, microangiopathic hemolytic anemia, and rapid decline in kidney function. Histologically, one sees fibrinoid necrosis and thrombosis in the renal microvasculature.[10] In contrast, the histologic lesion known as benign nephrosclerosis consists of scarring of the preglomerular microvasculature, glomeruli, and interstitium.[10] Clinically, it is characterized by slowly rising serum creatinine with little or no proteinuria. For decades, benign nephrosclerosis has been attributed to longstanding mild to moderate hypertension and has been labeled "hypertensive nephrosclerosis," thereby implying causality. Hypertension is listed as the primary etiology in about 25% of patients with ESKD.[4] Yet, despite evidence supporting a graded risk of ESKD with increasing levels of BP, mild to moderate hypertension *very infrequently* progresses to ESKD.[11,12] Explanations for this paradox include:

- Hypertension is so common that even the small percentage of patients at risk of ESKD constitutes a large number[12]
- Because kidney biopsies are rarely performed, many patients diagnosed with hypertensive nephrosclerosis may have a different cause of CKD[11,12]
- African Americans, who have the highest prevalence of ESKD attributable to hypertensive nephrosclerosis, have a genetic variant in the apolipoprotein L1 gene (APOL1) that causes glomerulosclerosis. In these patients, hypertension may be the consequence rather than the cause of kidney disease[11]
- The clinical phenotype associated with hypertensive nephrosclerosis has a low diagnostic accuracy[11,12]
- The pathologic changes on biopsy are not specific to hypertensive renal injury; they are also observed in normotensive individuals, with normal aging, in other causes of intrinsic renal parenchymal disease, and ischemic nephropathy from renal artery stenosis[11]

Thus, the true prevalence of hypertension-induced CKD, and especially ESKD, is uncertain and probably overestimated.

Despite these uncertainties, there are 2 mutually compatible postulated mechanisms through which chronic hypertension could cause renal injury.[13] Both involve the disruption of normal autoregulation of renal blood flow and glomerular filtration rate (GFR) that protect the kidney from changes in BP (**Fig. 1**).

Chronic Kidney Disease as a Cause of Hypertension

There is no controversy regarding CKD as a cause of secondary hypertension whose prevalence correlates with the following factors:

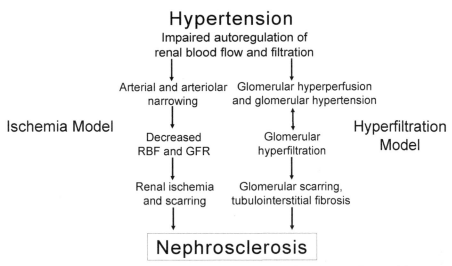

Fig. 1. Pathophysiologic mechanisms for hypertensive nephrosclerosis. (Derived from Meyrier A. Nephrosclerosis: update on a centenarian. Nephrol Dial Transplant 2015;30:1833 to 41.)

- Severity of kidney impairment, reaching ≥85% in late-stage CKD[14]
- Etiology of kidney disease (ischemic and diabetic nephropathy have the highest prevalence rates of hypertension)[14]
- Albuminuria – This is one of the strongest risk factors for hypertension in CKD and correlates with poorer BP control[15]
- Race – Self-identified Blacks and Hispanics with CKD have a higher prevalence and severity of hypertension than Caucasians and are more likely to progress to ESKD[4]
- Male sex – Compared to females, male sex increases the risk for both hypertension and CKD[4]
- Age – Older age increases the risk for both hypertension and CKD[4]

The pathophysiologic mechanisms of hypertension in CKD are complex but involve factors that lead to both sodium retention and vasoconstriction.[14,16] (**Box 1**)

HYPERTENSION PHENOTYPES IN CHRONIC KIDNEY DISEASE

The ACC/AHA hypertension guideline stresses the importance of obtaining out-of-office BP readings which are better predictors of adverse clinical outcomes.[2] The use of home blood pressure monitoring (HBPM) and ambulatory blood pressure monitoring (ABPM) devices can identify hypertension phenotypes that cannot be determined by office BP measurements alone.[2,17] (**Table 1**) Clinic BP provides a potentially misleading assessment of BP, especially in the CKD population. A meta-analysis showed that 40% of patients with CKD who were thought to be normotensive or adequately treated based on office BP, had hypertension at home (ie, masked hypertension). Conversely, 30% of patients who were thought to have hypertension based on office BPs were normotensive at home (ie, white coat hypertension).[18] In the recent analysis of ABPM data from the Chronic Renal Insufficiency Cohort (CRIC) study consisting of patients with CKD aged 21 to 74 years with estimated GFR (eGFR) between 20 and 70 mL/min/1.73 m², 24-h ABPM systolic BP (SBP), but

---

Box 1
Pathogenesis of hypertension in chronic kidney disease

Renal sodium retention

- Decreased GFR
- Impaired natriuresis
- Extracellular volume expansion
- Increased angiotensin II
- Arterial stiffness

Increased peripheral vascular resistance

- Activation of the renin–angiotensin system
- Activation of the sympathetic nervous system
- Increased endothelin

Impaired vasodilation

- Decreased prostaglandins or bradykinin
- Decreased nitric oxide

Secondary hyperparathyroidism

- Arterial calcification

Data from Refs.[14,16]

---

not clinic SBP, was associated with cardiovascular and kidney failure outcomes and mortality.[19] Sustained hypertension is common in CKD. However, due to marked perturbations in 24-h BP profile in CKD, other phenotypes are also more common than in the general population. Their relative impact on target organ damage is shown in **Fig. 2**.[19]

White Coat Hypertension

The reported prevalence of white coat hypertension (WCH) in the general population based on clinic BP measurements varies widely, ranging between 11% per the JNC 7 hypertensive threshold to 35% per the lower ACC/AHA threshold.[2,20] The prevalence of WCH in patients with CKD is even harder to determine as most patients with CKD take antihypertensive medications and therefore fall into the category of *treated* WCH, known as *white coat effect* (WCE). Prevalence rates range widely from 4% to 5% in Asian countries and the US to 22% to 28% in Europe.[21,22] These disparate rates reflect differences in population characteristics, definitions of BP thresholds, methods of measurement, level of kidney dysfunction, and duration of follow-up. In the general population, the prognosis of WCH has been inconsistent with some studies showing no cardiovascular risk or mortality and others showing increased risk compared with normotension.[23] A recent meta-analysis of 27 studies found that *untreated* WCH increased the risk of adverse outcomes in older persons and those at increased CVD risk, but *treated* WCH (ie, WCE) was *not* associated with these outcomes.[24] Studies in patients with CKD also report mixed results. ABPM data from the CRIC study showed no association of WCE with cardiovascular or kidney outcomes or mortality, but the small number of patients with WCE (4%) limited the power to detect these associations.[19] In contrast, 3 studies from Japan and the United States have shown adverse effects of WCE in CKD.[9,21,25] Thus,

Table 1
Hypertension phenotypes identifiable by out-of-office blood pressure monitoring

Phenotype	Definition
Sustained hypertension	Hypertension in office/clinic and at home or by ABPM
White coat hypertension[a]	Hypertension in office/clinic; no hypertension at home or by ABPM not on antihypertensive medication
White coat effect (aka treated white coat hypertension or white coat uncontrolled hypertension)[a]	Hypertension in office/clinic; no hypertension at home or by ABPM on antihypertensive medication
Masked hypertension[a]	No hypertension in office/clinic; hypertension at home or by ABPM not on antihypertensive medication
Masked uncontrolled hypertension[a]	No hypertension in office/clinic; hypertension at home or by ABPM on antihypertensive medication
Nocturnal hypertension[a] Nondipping nocturnal BP Reverse-dipping nocturnal BP	Nighttime ABP above the hypertensive threshold Failure of nocturnal BP to fall by at least 10%: Night to day ratio 0.9–1.0, with or without antihypertensive medication Paradoxic rise in nocturnal BP: Night to day ratio >1.0, with or without antihypertensive medication
Resistant hypertension	BP that remains above goal despite optimal doses of three or more antihypertensive medications of different classes including a diuretic if tolerated or that is controlled with four or more medications.

Abbreviation: ABPM, ambulatory blood pressure monitoring.
  [a] Using 2017 ACC/AHA BP classification, the corresponding threshold hypertensive BP values are: Office/Clinic, 130/80; Home, 130/80; Daytime ABP, 130/80; Nighttime ABP, 110/65; 24-h ABP, 125/75. Using the JNC 7 BP classification, the corresponding threshold hypertensive BP values are: Office/Clinic, 140/90, Home, 135/85; Daytime ABP, 135/85, Nighttime ABP, 120/70, 24-h ABP, 130/80.
  Data from Refs.[2,17]

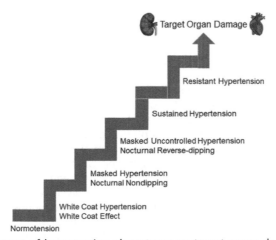

Fig. 2. Relative impact of hypertension phenotypes on target organ damage. (*Data from multiple sources.*)

WCH/WCE likely carries a greater risk of adverse outcomes in patients with CKD than in the non-CKD population, but further research is needed. Of note is the tendency for patients with WCH and WCE to progress to sustained hypertension which may account for their poorer prognosis compared with normotensive subjects.[2,26]

Masked Hypertension

The prevalence of masked hypertension (MH) in the general population ranges between 8% and 20% in untreated patients and up to 50% in treated patients with masked uncontrolled hypertension (MUCH).[27] In CKD, the prevalence rates of MH and MUCH are higher than in the general population, especially among African Americans in whom the rates reach 50% to 70%.[28,29] The prevalence of MUCH increases in proportion to clinic BP. At a clinic BP of 120 to 129 mm Hg, the prevalence is 34%; at 130 to 139 mm Hg, it rises to 66%.[30] MH and MUCH are especially dangerous because they are missed if only office BP is checked. In diverse non-CKD populations, these 2 phenotypes are associate with increased cardiovascular morbidity, all-cause mortality, and incident CKD.[29,31,32] In patients with CKD, MH and MUCH consistently carry a cardiovascular, kidney, and mortality risk approaching or equaling sustained hypertension.[19,28,33] These adverse outcomes include left ventricular hypertrophy, heart failure, elevated pulse wave velocity (an indicator of vascular stiffness), ischemic heart disease, stroke, peripheral vascular disease, proteinuria, decline in kidney function, ESKD, and mortality. In addition, like WCH, MH tends to progress to sustained hypertension with its heightened risks for adverse outcomes.[34]

Nocturnal Hypertension, Nondipping, and Reverse Dipping

These 3 hypertensive phenotypes are categories of MH that result from disruption of the normal diurnal pattern of BP regulation seen in normotensive individuals. The phenotypes include 3 abnormal patterns, all of which are more prevalent in patients with CKD than in the general population and are often the dominant component of MUCH.[28,35]

- Failure to fall below the nocturnal hypertensive threshold (nocturnal, or asleep hypertension)
- Failure to fall less than 10% below daytime levels (nondipping)
- Paradoxic rise during sleep (reverse dipping)

In the largest and most recent US study, 22.7% of adults (53.7 million) had masked asleep hypertension and 13.3% (31.5 million) had isolated masked asleep hypertension (ie, without high awake BP) using the 2017 ACC/AHA guideline BP criteria.[36] In patients with CKD, dysregulation of nocturnal BP is very prevalent, especially in African Americans among whom 80% were found to be nondippers or reverse dippers.[28] Studies in other populations confirm high prevalence rates of nondipping and reverse dipping in CKD.[37,38] Abnormal nocturnal BP has been linked to adverse cardiovascular and kidney and mortality in non-CKD populations independent of average 24-h or daytime BP.[31,39] Similar results have been reported in CKD populations. In the CRIC study, nondipping and especially reverse dipping predicted increased risk for renal function decline, stroke, and peripheral vascular disease even after adjustment for 24-h ABPM.[19] Correlates of both MH and nocturnal hypertension include diabetes/metabolic syndrome, obesity, obstructive sleep apnea, old age, male gender, African American race, angina, heart failure, proteinuria, and advanced renal dysfunction.[36,40]

Resistant Hypertension

Resistant hypertension (RH) must be distinguished from uncontrolled hypertension. Whereas about 56% of hypertensive patients have uncontrolled hypertension, only a small fraction of that population is uncontrolled on ≥ 3 medications or require ≥ 4 medications for control. These patients either have true RH (tRH) or pseudo-RH due to one or more of 4 confounding factors.[34] (**Table 2**) The term apparent RH (aRH) is sometimes used because it is rarely possible to exclude every factor that can cause pseudo-RH. The prevalence of aRH in patients with CKD is high and increases with worsening kidney function.[41,42] In a study of more than 30,000 Black and White adults in the US, the prevalence of aRH rose from 15.8% with eGFR ≥ 60 to 33.4% at less than 45 mL/min/1.73 m².[41] In the CRIC study, the prevalence of aRH was 22.3% at eGFR greater than 60 and 54.2% at less than 30 mL/min per 1.73 m².[42] The underlying pathogenesis of RH involves the activation of the renin-angiotensin-aldosterone system resulting in volume expansion, activation of the sympathetic nervous system, endothelial dysfunction, and arterial stiffness.[43] Among over 470,000 hypertensive patients in the Kaiser Permanente Southern California health system, CKD was the strongest risk factor for RH with an adjusted odds ratio of 1.84, followed by Black race, obesity and diabetes.[44] Risk factors for RH in patients with CKD include Black race, higher BMI, diabetes mellitus, older age, male sex, history of myocardial infarction or stroke, statin use, lower estimated eGFR, and higher albumin-to-creatinine ratio.[41,42] In both the CKD and non-CKD populations, uncontrolled RH is associated with a higher risk of adverse cardiovascular and renal outcomes than non-RH.[42,45]

EVALUATION OF HYPERTENSION IN CHRONIC KIDNEY DISEASE

The initial evaluation of hypertension in CKD follows the same path as for patients without CKD. A detailed discussion of this topic can be found in the 2017 ACC/AHA guideline.[2] The key points are summarized here and in the accompanying Boxes.

Table 2 Pseudo-resistant hypertension (apparent resistant hypertension)		
Causes	Frequency (%)	Diagnosis
Incorrect auscultatory BP measurement due to poor technique	33	Follow ACC/AHA Hypertension Guidelines for proper manual BP technique or preferably, use an automated office BP monitor unattended by staff or clinician
White coat effect	38	Compare office BP with a 24-h ABPM
Inadequate treatment (clinician inertia)	50	Compare treatment with recommendations in the ACC/AHA Hypertension Guidelines
Nonadherence to treatment	31 (3–86)[a]	Patient self-report Pill counts Electronic pill monitoring Prescription refill rates Directly observed pill administration Direct measurement of drug and/or drug metabolites in blood or urine

[a] The wide frequency range reflects differences in the sensitivity of methods for detecting nonadherence, ranging from under 10% for patient self-reports and pill counts to over 80% for measurement of drug and/or drug metabolites in urine.

Data from Calhoun DA, Grassi G. True versus pseudoresistant hypertension. J Hypertens 2017;35:2367 to 68.

- Confirm hypertension severity and phenotype with **both office and out-of-office BP measurements.** Use **standardized** manual auscultatory technique, or preferably an automated office BP monitor combined with HBPM or ABPM.[2,46] (**Box 2**)
- Obtain a detailed focused history[2,5] (**Box 3**)
- Perform a detailed focused physical examination[2,5] (**Box 4**)
- Perform guideline-recommended screening tests[2,5] (**Box 5**)
- Evaluate for secondary hypertension if the history, physical examination, and/or severity or trajectory of hypertension suggests a cause other than CKD itself

Note that severe or RH and/or a nondipping or reverse dipping nocturnal BP pattern is characteristic of CKD and should also raise suspicion of secondary hypertension that, in turn, could cause or accelerate CKD.[47]

SECONDARY HYPERTENSION

Detailed discussions of the detection, evaluation, and treatment of secondary hypertension can be found elsewhere.[5,47] Although kidney disease itself is a leading cause

---

Box 2
Standardized blood pressure measurement: key points

Patient and equipment preparation

- Abstinence from caffeine, exercise, and smoking for $\geq$30 min
- Empty bladder
- Feet on floor, legs uncrossed, arm and back supported
- Keep quiet and relaxed for $\geq$5 min (no talking by patient or to patient)
- Correct cuff size (bladder length 80% and width 40% of arm circumference)
- Validated and calibrated equipment
- Patient's arm supported at heart level (mid-sternum)
- Position bottom of cuff 1 cm above antecubital fossa

For auscultatory blood pressure measurements

- Use a palpated estimate of radial pulse obliteration pressure to estimate SBP
- Inflate the cuff 20–30 mm Hg above this level to initiate auscultation
- Deflate the cuff at 2 mm Hg per second and listen for Korotkoff sounds
- Record systolic and diastolic BP as the onset of the first Korotkoff sound and disappearance of all Korotkoff sounds, using the nearest even number.
- Use an average of $\geq$2 readings obtained on $\geq$2 occasions to estimate the patient's level of BP
- At the first visit, record BP in both arms. Use the arm with the higher reading for subsequent measurements

For automated office BP device

- Follow same preparation as noted above
- If the device will self-initiate readings, leave patient alone in room for 5 min before initiation of readings
- Set device to take at least 3 consecutive readings 1-min apart and use the average of the 3 readings

Data from Refs.[2,46]

Box 3
Medical history: Four key points in evaluating the hypertensive patient with CKD

Assess genetic and lifestyle factors

- Family history of hypertension, CVD, renal disease, diabetes, gout
- Excess alcohol, high salt diet
- Work or other related stress
- Socioeconomic status, education level

Cardiovascular risk factors

- Smoking
- Dyslipidemia
- Obesity, metabolic syndrome, diabetes
- Physical inactivity

Evaluate for secondary causes of hypertension

- Drugs and herbal products
- Renal artery stenosis, renal parenchymal disease
- Endocrine disorders
- Obstructive sleep apnea

Identify target organ damage

- CVD – angina, claudication, heart failure (edema, dyspnea on exertion)
- CNS – TIA, stroke
- Eye – blurred vision, loss of vision
- Renal – nocturia; h/o UTIs, stones, trauma, or glomerulonephritis

Data from Refs.[2,5]

---

of secondary hypertension, two other common causes are pertinent to this review: **primary aldosteronism (PA)** and **obstructive sleep apnea (OSA)**. Like kidney disease, they are often associated with stage 2 hypertension, RH, and obesity-related metabolic disorders. Together they can impact the course and treatment of hypertension in patients with CKD.

Clinically important relationships exist between increased aldosterone levels, RH, CKD, OSA, and obesity-related disorders (**Fig. 3**).

PA is the most prevalent endocrine cause of hypertension. Although its reported prevalence in the general hypertensive population is 5% to 10%, recent research indicates that PA is more common, underdiagnosed, and undertreated in primary care practice.[48] Screening for PA is usually performed only in patients with severe or resistant hypertension. However, Brown and colleagues recently reported a graded increase in renin-independent aldosterone production across the entire spectrum of BP levels from normotension to RH.[49] The prevalence of PA in RH is at least 20% and plasma aldosterone levels increase with the difficulty of controlling BP.[49]

Aldosterone promotes inflammation, oxidative stress, fibrosis, and endothelial dysfunction in multiple organs.[50,51] As a result, patients with PA have higher rates of cardiovascular and cerebrovascular morbidity and mortality and greater risk of CKD than patients with essential (primary) hypertension matched for age, sex and BP.[51]

Box 4
Physical examination: Six key areas to examine in the hypertensive patient with CKD

General appearance

- Height, weight, BMI (obese ≥30)

- Body habitus and physical features (clues to endocrine disorders)

Take BP bilaterally in 3 positions on the first visit

- Primary hypertension: diastolic rise from supine to standing

- Pheochromocytoma: BP may fall from supine to standing

- If coarctation of aorta is proximal to left subclavian artery, left arm BP will be lower than right arm. Even if coarctation is absent, always use the higher arm BP if a consistent significant difference exists

Careful funduscopic examination

- Important clue to duration, severity, and prognosis of hypertension

Cardiopulmonary examination

- Check for signs of left ventricular hypertrophy (lift, S4 gallop)

- Check for signs of heart failure (rales, S3 gallop, edema, jugular vein distention)

- Check for extracardiac murmurs and intercostal pulsations in a patient <30 yo; clues to coarctation of aorta

Peripheral vascular examination

- Palpate and auscultate carotid arteries for bruits; clue to atherosclerosis and possible renal artery stenosis

- Palpate abdominal aorta for aneurysm

- Check for signs of coarctations of aorta
  ○ weak or delayed femoral pulse compared to radial pulse
  ○ thigh BP less than upper limb, usually by > 30 mm Hg

- Auscultate renal arteries (bruit present in 40%–50% of cases of renal artery stenosis)

Neurologic examination

- Check for cranial nerve abnormalities, motor deficits, or speech or gait abnormalities that would indicate a prior stroke

Data from Refs.[2,5]

Conversely, CKD can promote excessive aldosterone production through the activation of the renin–angiotensin system (see **Box 1**).

Aldosterone is also linked to OSA and obesity-related disorders (insulin resistance, metabolic syndrome, and diabetes):

- A recent cross-sectional multiethnic study reported a 67% prevalence of OSA in PA which supports testing for OSA in patients with PA, but not vice versa.[52]
- Adipocytes in visceral fat produce cytokines that stimulate adrenal production of aldosterone.[51]
- Aldosterone promotes insulin resistance and destroys pancreatic beta-cells resulting in metabolic syndrome and diabetes.[51]
- Patients with PA have a 33% increased risk of diabetes and a 53% increased risk of metabolic syndrome compared with patients with essential hypertension. They also have substantially higher risks of coronary artery disease, stroke, atrial fibrillation, left ventricular hypertrophy, and heart failure.[49]

Box 5
Screening tests: Key tests to perform in the hypertensive patient with CKD

Basic tests (perform on all hypertensive patients with or without CKD)

- Complete metabolic profile, with special attention to:
  - Blood glucose (fasting)
  - Serum creatinine with estimated glomerular filtration rate (eGFR)
  - Serum sodium, potassium, and calcium

- Complete blood count

- Urinalysis

- Urine albumin to creatinine ratio (CKD only)

- Lipid profile

- Thyroid-stimulating hormone (not universally recommended in guidelines)

- Electrocardiogram

Optional tests (if indicated based on history, physical examination, severity of hypertension)

- Echocardiogram

- Chest X-ray

- Uric acid

- Doppler ultrasound or magnetic resonance angiogram for renal artery stenosis

- Plasma aldosterone to renin ratio for primary aldosteronism

- Polysomnography for obstructive sleep apnea

- 24-h urine for metanephrines for pheochromocytoma

- Dexamethasone suppression test for Cushing's syndrome

Data from Refs.[2,5]

OSA is the most common secondary cause of RH with prevalence ranging from ~60 to 80%.[53] OSA-induced RH is accompanied by nondipping and nocturnal hypertension that correlate with the severity of OSA.[53]

OSA is also linked to obesity-related disorders and CKD:

- The prevalence of OSA increases with higher BMI, larger waist-to-hip ratio, and increased neck circumference. Neck adiposity and upper airway fat contribute to the development of OSA.[54,55]

- Independent of obesity, OSA is a major risk factor for insulin resistance and type 2 diabetes.[54] The prevalence of diabetes in patients with OSA ranges from 15% to 30%, and conversely, the prevalence of OSA in patients with obesity-induced type 2 diabetes ranges from 58% to 86%.[54]

- OSA and obesity share common mechanisms such as inflammatory activation, oxidative stress, and increased sympathetic activity, all of which contribute to CKD.[55] However, the association of OSA with incident CKD is most likely mediated through obesity.[56]

Visceral (central) obesity causes hypertension and renal dysfunction through multiple mechanisms among which are:[57]

- Impaired sodium excretion due to compression by fat accumulation in and around the kidneys

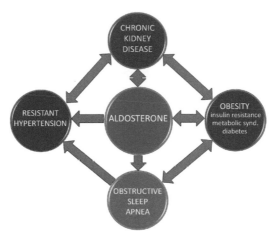

Fig. 3. Interrelationships between aldosterone, obstructive sleep apnea, hypertension, chronic kidney disease, and obesity-related metabolic disorders. (*Data from* multiple sources.)

- Insulin resistance
- Sympathetic nervous system hyperactivity
- Renin–angiotensin–aldosterone system activation
- Release of inflammatory cytokines from adipose tissue
- Visceral obesity directly causes structural renal injury by causing glomerulomegaly with hyperfiltration and proteinuria that then induce endothelial dysfunction, glomerulosclerosis, and tubulointerstitial fibrosis

Aldosterone excess, RH, OSA, and obesity-related disorders commonly coexist. These multiple interrelationships describe a viscous cycle in which each component contributes to the others that ultimately lead to adverse consequences affecting the cardiovascular and renal systems.

NONPHARMACOLOGIC MANAGEMENT OF HYPERTENSION IN CHRONIC KIDNEY DISEASE

Lifestyle modifications are the first line of therapy for every hypertensive patient with or without CKD.[2] (**Table 3**) Two modifications merit comment because, in addition to lowering BP, they have the greatest impact on CKD: weight loss and dietary modification.

Weight Loss

Evidence is sparce, but 2 recent observational studies have shown reversing obesity through surgical means can have beneficial effects on renal function.

- A Swedish nationwide cohort study of obese patients with type 2 diabetes compared 5000 patients undergoing gastric bypass surgery (GBS) with 5000 matched controls followed over a mean of 4.7 years. GBS reduced the incidence or progression of CKD by 44%, including in individuals with eGFR less than 30 mL/min[58]
- A US cohort of 2144 patients undergoing GBS overwhelmingly showed improvement in CKD risk over 7 years in patients at moderate to high baseline risk.[59]

Table 3
Effect of lifestyle modifications on reductions in systolic BP and CKD

Intervention	Description	Approximate Reductions in Systolic BP and Incident or Worsening CKD
Weight loss	Expect ~1 mm Hg reduction for every 1-kg reduction in body weight	SBP: 5–20 mm Hg/10 kg wt. loss CKD: 44% to ≥90%[a]
DASH diet[b] Mediterranean diet[b,c]	**Rich in:** fruits, vegetables, low-fat dairy, whole grains, legumes, poultry, fish, and nuts **Low in:** red/processed meats, sweets, sugar-containing drinks, alcohol, and saturated fats	SBP (DASH): 8–14 mm Hg SBP (↑ potassium): 4–5 mm Hg CKD: ↑ vegetables: 21% ↑ potassium: 22%
Sodium intake[d]	Aim for 2300 mg/d or at least a 1000 mg/d reduction	SBP: 2–8 mm Hg CKD: 18%
Moderate alcohol intake (for patients who drink)	Men: ≤2 drinks per day Women: ≤1 drink per day	SBP: 2–4 mm Hg CKD: 14%
Physical activity	150 min of moderate aerobic exercise per week	SBP: 4–9 mm Hg CKD: 18%

[a] Refers to Roux-en-Y gastric bypass surgery. Wide range is due to differences in outcomes assessment between studies.
[b] May not be appropriate for patients with advanced CKD or with hyporeninemic hypoaldosteronism due to the risk of hyperkalemia.
[c] Mediterranean diet promotes more fish and less dairy versus DASH, plus olive oil and moderate red wine consumption.
[d] KIDGO 2021 recommends less than 2000 mg/d (<5g NaCl/d); ACC/AHA 2017 recommends optimal less than 1500 mg/d.
Data from Refs.[2,58–60,65]

Dietary Modification

Plant-based diets such as the Mediterranean diet, the DASH diet (see **Table 3**), and similar "heart healthy" diets, reduce the risk of albuminuria, incident CKD, and progression and mortality in patients with moderate CKD.[60–62] Conversely, diets high in animal protein from red meat, processed meat, and animal fat worsen kidney function. Benefits of plant-based diets in CKD include:[61]

- Lower acid load compared with animal protein sources which counters metabolic acidosis
- Lower blood pressure due to a favorable sodium:potassium ratio (lower sodium, higher potassium content)
- Lower serum phosphorus due to dietary phosphate binding to nonabsorbable phytate
- Enhanced fecal excretion of uremic toxins due to a favorable gut microbiome created by high dietary fiber
- Decreased insulin resistance, glucose intolerance, dyslipidemia, and inflammation

Concern about hyperkalemia from plant-based diets in CKD may be inflated. Prospective observational studies and cross-sectional data indicate little to no correlation between serum potassium and dietary potassium in patients with CKD, including those on hemodialysis.[61,63] Reasons for this paradox include:

- Fiber in plant-based diets increases intestinal motility and excretion of potassium
- The GI tract increases excretion of potassium 3-fold in kidney failure
- The alkalinizing effect of carbohydrates in plant-based foods and their stimulation of insulin secretion drive potassium into cells. In contrast, meat that is low in carbohydrates causes a greater increase in serum potassium.

Importantly, the newer potassium-binding agents, patiromer and sodium zirconium cyclosilicate, may enable patients with advanced CKD to take advantage of the beneficial nutrients in plant-based diets without the risk of hyperkalemia.[64] Nonetheless, caution must be exercised, and serum potassium carefully monitored if potassium intake is liberalized, and those with advanced CKD should avoid liberal potassium intake.

PHARMACOLOGIC MANAGEMENT OF HYPERTENSION IN CHRONIC KIDNEY DISEASE
Blood Pressure Targets and Initial Therapy

Globally, there are many hypertension guidelines. However, the 2017 ACC/AHA and 2021 Kidney Disease Improving Global Outcomes (KDIGO) guidelines are the most pertinent to the adult US CKD population.[2,65] Both were strongly influenced by the Systolic Pressure Intervention Trial (SPRINT) in which targeting an SBP less than 120 mm Hg versus less than 140 mm Hg significantly reduced adverse cardiovascular endpoints and all-cause mortality in patients with and without CKD.[2,65,66] The 2 guidelines share some recommendations in common:

- Emphasis on standardized office BP measurements (see **Box 2**)
- Importance of lifestyle modifications (see **Table 3**)
- Individualization of BP targets and shared decision-making with patients

However, they also differ in certain key respects. The most noteworthy of these are the more aggressive SBP target of less than 120 mm Hg in KDIGO versus less than 130 mm Hg in the ACC/AHA guideline, and the lack of a DBP target in KDIGO versus less than 80 mm Hg in the ACC/AHA guideline.[2,65] **(Table 4)**

Two additional important points must be made with respect to intensive BP lowering in CKD.

- Intensive therapy reduces CVD events and mortality but does not seem to reduce the rate of CKD progression, except perhaps in patients with severe proteinuria.[65,67]
- In SPRINT, intensive BP lowering resulted in more frequent episodes of AKI than standard therapy in patients with CKD and the incidence of CKD in participants without CKD at baseline.[68,69] However, most cases of AKI were mild and reversible, and in participants with incident CKD, biomarkers of structural kidney damage decreased over 1 year with intensive BP lowering.[68,70] These findings suggest that eGFR reductions from intensive BP lowering are mostly hemodynamic due to decreased intraglomerular pressure. Nonetheless, the long-term effects of intensive SBP lowering on CKD progression need further study. In the meantime, caution should be exercised when aggressively lowering BP in patients with or at high risk of CKD.[67]

An excellent detailed synopsis of the KDIGO guideline is available.[71]

Table 4
Differences between the AHA/ACC and KDIGO hypertension guidelines for patients with chronic kidney disease

	ACC/AHA 2017	KDIGO 2021
Definition of hypertension	≥130/≥80 [a]	"High BP" is defined as a BP above target.
BP threshold for drug intervention	130/80 (with lifestyle modifications)	BP above target (with lifestyle modifications)
BP target	<130/<80[b] Deviates from SPRINT SBP <120 to prevent hypotension if casual BP measurements are used	SBP <120[b,c] (no DBP target)[d] Adheres strictly to SPRINT based on the obligatory use of standardized BP measurements
Out of office BP (HBPM or ABPM)[e]	Strong recommendation to confirm the diagnosis of hypertension and for titration of BP-lowering medication	Weaker recommendation: use HBPM or ABPM to "complement standardized office BP readings for the management of high BP"
Initial drug therapy	Monotherapy for <140/90; SPCT for ≥140/90 Algorithm for add-on therapy	RAS inhibitor (RASi)[f] No formal recommendations given for add-on therapy

Abbreviations: ACR, urine; albumin, creatinine ratio (mg/g); see, text for others; SPCT, single-pill combination therapy.

[a] All numbers refer to blood pressure values in mm Hg.

[b] BP targets refer to standardized office BP measurements.

[c] Because of exclusion criteria in SPRINT, there is uncertainty of potential benefit versus harm of an SBP target less than 120 in these subgroups: diabetes, advanced CKD (eGFR <30 mL/min), proteinuria greater than 1 g/d, baseline SBP 120 to 129 mm Hg, WCH, very low DBP, advanced age, frailty, age less than 50 with low CVD risk.

[d] KDIGO: No DBP target because outcomes data are scarce and the wide pulse pressure commonly present in patients with CKD will usually result in a DBP less than 70 mm Hg when targeting an SBP less than 120 mm Hg. Exception: For young patients with diastolic hypertension, it is reasonable to target a DBP less than 80 mm Hg.

[e] KDIGO rationale: No outcome-based trial has used ABPM or HBPM targets to guide treatment.

[f] Recommendations for RASi: Without diabetes: If ACR greater than 300 (strong); if ACR 30 to 300 (weak). With diabetes: If ACR greater than 30 (strong). With or without diabetes and ACR less than 30: RAS blockade is reasonable, but other first-line agents are acceptable.

Data from Refs.[2,65]

Choice of Antihypertensive Medication in CKD

First-line antihypertensive medications appropriate for patients with and without CKD include:

- Renin–angiotensin system blockers (RAS) – angiotensin-converting enzyme inhibitors (ACEIs) and angiotensin receptor blockers (ARBs)
- Thiazide (eg, hydrochlorothiazide) or thiazide-like diuretics (eg, chlorthalidone, indapamide)
- Calcium channel blockers (CCBs) (eg, amlodipine, felodipine)

Although a detailed discussion of these medications is beyond the scope of this review, a few key points of clinical importance are worth mentioning in each class.

ACEIs and ARBs

- These 2 classes should not be combined with one another or with the direct renin inhibitor, aliskiren, due to the risk of hyperkalemia and acute kidney injury.[2,65]
- Kidney function (eGFR) and potassium should be checked within 2 to 4 weeks after initiating or titrating up these medications.
- Be especially vigilant for hyperkalemia if the patient is on other potassium-raising drugs or has moderately advanced CKD, especially diabetic nephropathy.
- Expect up to a 20-30% increase in serum creatinine within the first month after starting these drugs due to their hemodynamic effect of lowering intraglomerular pressure. If the increase is greater than this, look for renal artery stenosis, volume contraction, or a nephrotoxic agent as the cause.[2]

Diuretics

- Because a significant driving factor for hypertension in CKD is sodium retention, diuretics are especially important for BP control.[14]
- Thiazide-like diuretics are favored over hydrochlorothiazide because of their greater potency, longer duration of action, and proven efficacy in reducing CVD in clinical trials.[2,72] These include chlorthalidone and indapamide.
- In advanced CKD (eGFR <30 mL/min), a loop diuretic is preferred but limited data suggest some efficacy of thiazides in advanced CKD.[73,74]
- Torsemide has a longer duration of action and greater bioavailability than furosemide. Thus, it can be taken once daily.
- Diuretic-induced hyperuricemia is common in CKD, so a uric acid-lowering agent will often be needed to prevent gout.
- If signs of volume expansion and hypertension persist, check a 24-h urine for sodium excretion to ascertain adherence to a low sodium diet.

Calcium channel blockers

- Dihydropyridine CCBs are more commonly used because they are more potent vasodilators than the nondihydropyridine CCBs (verapamil, diltiazem) and have fewer drug interactions.[73]
- Although nondihydropyridine CCBs have the additional benefit of reducing proteinuria, they should not be routinely used with beta-blockers because of the increased risk of bradycardia and heart block.[2]

Beyond First-Line Therapy: Treating Resistant Hypertension

If BP is not lowered to goal with a combination of the 3 first-line drug classes, the patient has apparent RH. First, verify adherence to medication and lifestyle modifications. If this is satisfactory, capitalize on the central roles of aldosterone and sodium retention in RH. Based on clinical trial evidence, a mineralocorticoid receptor antagonist (MRA) should be the fourth agent for RH. However, the risk of hyperkalemia increases with the severity of CKD and concomitant use of RAS blockers and other potassium-raising drugs. In a meta-analysis of 19 trials of patients with CKD, the addition of spironolactone to RAS blockers reduced proteinuria but caused a threefold increase in withdrawal due to hyperkalemia.[75] Hyperkalemia has been the major limiting factor in using RAS blockers and MRAs in patients with CKD. However, 2 recent additions to our pharmacologic armamentarium are offering hope of achieving the cardiovascular and kidney benefits of these medications without causing unacceptable risk of hyperkalemia. First, finerenone, a nonsteroidal MRA has shown less tendency to cause hyperkalemia. In the recently reported FIDELIO-DKD trial, finerenone, now

FDA-approved, lowered the risk of CKD progression and cardiovascular events in patients with proteinuric diabetic nephropathy and eGFR as low as 25 mL/min while causing hyperkalemia in only 2.3% versus/0.9% for placebo.[76] Second, patiromer and sodium-zirconium cyclosilicate have shown efficacy in preventing hyperkalemia in CKD patients taking RAS blockers and/or MRAs.[77] Nonetheless, caution and careful monitoring of serum potassium must be exercised when using MRAs and RAS blockers in patients with CKD, especially those with advanced disease.

SUMMARY

Hypertension and CKD form a toxic synergistic partnership that greatly increases the risk of cardiovascular morbidity and mortality. Essential to the evaluation of hypertension in CKD is the accurate diagnosis of hypertension phenotypes that are prevalent in CKD: masked, nocturnal with nondipping, and resistant. Clinicians must obtain guideline-directed standardized BP measurements in the office. Combining them with outside readings either by HBPM or ABPM will prevent missing the most dangerous hypertension phenotypes and overtreating patients based on casual office readings that often overestimate BP. Careful search for comorbidities and secondary causes of hypertension are also essential elements in evaluating patients with CKD before prescribing antihypertensive medication. Treatment should always include lifestyle modifications and guideline-based pharmacologic interventions.

DISCLOSURE

The authors have nothing to disclose.

REFERENCES

1. Rui P, Okeyode T. National Ambulatory Medical Care Survey: 2016 National Summary, Tables 15 and 19. Available at: https://www.cdc.gov/nchs/data/ahcd/namcs_summary/2016_namcs_web_tables.pdf. Accessed December 17, 2021.
2. Whelton PK, Carey RM, Aronow WS, et al. 2017 ACC/AHA/AAPA/ABC/ACPM/AGS/APhA/ASH/ASPC/NMA/PCNA guideline for the prevention, detection, evaluation, and management of high blood pressure in adults: a report of the American College of Cardiology/American Heart Association Task Force on Clinical Practice Guidelines. Hypertens 2018;71:e13–115.
3. CDC. Hypertension Cascade: Hypertension Prevalence, Treatment and Control Estimates Among US Adults Aged 18 Years and Older—NHANES 2015–2018. Atlanta, GA: US Department of Health and Human Services; 2021. Available at: https://millionhearts.hhs.gov/data-reports/hypertension-prevalence.html. Accessed December 17, 2021.
4. Johansen KL, Chertow GM, Foley RN, et al. US Renal Data System 2020 Annual Data Report: epidemiology of kidney disease in the United States. Am J Kidney Dis 2021;77 (4)(suppl 1):Svii-Sviii, S1-S597. Available at: https://www.usrds.org/media/2371/2019-executive-summary.pdf. Accessed December 17, 2021.
5. Elliott WJ, Peixoto AJ, Bakris GL. Primary and Secondary Hypertension. In: Yu ASL, Chertow GM, Luyckx VA, et al, editors. Brenner and Rector's The Kidney. 11th edition, Chapter 46. Philadelphia: Elsevier; 2020. p. 1536–79.
6. Muntner P, Hardy ST, Fine LJ, et al. Trends in blood pressure control among US adults with hypertension, 1999-2000 to 2017-2018. JAMA 2020;324(12):1190–200.

7. Derington CG, King JB, Herrick JS, et al. Trends In antihypertensive medication monotherapy and combination use among US adults. National Health and Nutrition Examination Survey 2005-2016. Hypertens 2020;75(4):973–81.

8. Van Gelder VA, Scherpbier-de Haan N, DeGrauw WJC, et al. Quality of chronic kidney disease management In primary care: a retrospective study. Scand J Prim Health Care 2016;34(1):73–80.

9. Ku E, Lee BJ, Wie J, et al. Hypertension in CKD: Core Curriculum 2019. Am J Kidney Dis 2019;74(1):20–31.

10. Amin MS, Bonsib SM. Nonneoplastic Diseases of the Kidney. In: Cheng L, MacLennan GT, Bostwick DG, editors. Urologic Surgical Pathology. 4th ed. Philadelphia: Elsevier; 2020. p. 47–8. Available at: https://play.google.com/books/reader?id=WeaGDwAAQBAJ&hl=en_US&pg=GBS. Accessed December 17, 2021.

11. Freedman BI, Cohen AH. Hypertension-attributed nephropathy: what's In a name? Nat Rev Nephrol 2016;12(1):27–36.

12. Hallan SI, Øvrehus MA, Bjømeklett R, et al. Hypertensive nephrosclerosis: wider kidney biopsy indications may be needed to Improve diagnostics. J Intern Med 2020. https://doi.org/10.1111/joim.13146.

13. Meyrier A. Nephrosclerosis: update on a centenarian. Nephrol Dial Transplant 2015;30:1833–41.

14. Tedla FM, Brar A, Browne R. Hypertension In chronic kidney disease: navigating the evidence. Int J Hypertens 2011;2011:132405.

15. Agarwal R, Andersen MJ. Correlates of systolic hypertension in patients with chronic kidney disease. Hypertens 2005;46:514–20.

16. Phan O, Burnier M, Wuerzner G. Hypertension in chronic kidney disease – role of arterial calcification and impact on treatment. Eur Cardiol 2014;9(2):115–9.

17. Chobanian AV, Bakris GL, Black HR, et al. The Seventh Report of the Joint National Committee on Prevention, Detection, Evaluation, and Treatment of High Blood Pressure: the JNC 7 report. J Am Med Assoc 2003;289:2560–72.

18. Bangash F, Agarwal R. Masked hypertension and white-coat hypertension in chronic kidney disease: a meta-analysis. Clin J Am Soc Nephrol 2009;4:656–64.

19. Rahman M, Wang X, Bundy JD, et al. Prognostic significance of ambulatory BP monitoring in CKD: a report from the Chronic Renal Insufficiency Cohort (CRIC) Study. J Am Soc Nephrol 2020;31:2609–21.

20. Poudel B, Booth JN II, Sakhuja S, et al. Prevalence of ambulatory blood pressure phenotypes using the 2017 American College of Cardiology/American Heart Association blood pressure guideline thresholds: data from the Coronary Artery Risk Development in Young Adults study. J Hypertens 2019;37:1401–10.

21. Wang Q, Wang Y, Wang J, et al. White-coat hypertension and incident end-stage renal disease in patients with non-dialysis chronic kidney disease: results from the C_STRIDE Study. J Transl Med 2020;18:238.

22. Drawz PE, Brown R, De Nicola L, et al. Variations in 24-hour profiles in cohorts of patients with kidney disease around the world. Clin J Am Soc Nephrol 2018;13:1348–57.

23. Paroti G, Ochoa JE, Bilo G. White coat and masked hypertension in chronic kidney disease: importance of the difference between office and out-of-office blood pressure measurements. J Am Heart Assoc 2019;8:e012299.

24. Cohen JB, Lotito MJ, Trivedi UK, et al. Cardiovascular events and mortality in white coat hypertension: a systematic review and meta-analysis. Ann Intern Med 2019;170:853–62.

25. Kanno A, Metoki H, Kikuya M, et al. Usefulness of assessing masked and white coat hypertension by ambulatory blood pressure monitoring for determining prevalent risk of chronic kidney disease: the Ohasama study. Hypertens Res 2010;33:1192–8.
26. Fujiwara T, Matsumoto C, Asayama K, et al. Are the cardiovascular outcomes of participants with white-coat hypertension poor compared to those of participants with normotension? A systemic review and meta-analysis. Hypertens Res 2019; 42:825–33.
27. Bobrie G, Clerson P, Menard J, et al. Masked hypertension: a systematic review. J Hypertens 2008;26:1715–25.
28. Pogue V, Rahman M, Lipkowitz M, et al. Disparate estimates of hypertension control from ambulatory and clinic blood pressure measurements in hypertensive kidney disease. Hypertens 2009;53:20–7.
29. Mwasongwe S, Min Y-I, Boot JN III, et al. Masked hypertension and kidney function decline: the Jackson Heart Study. J Hypertens 2018;36:1524–32.
30. Agarwal R, Pappas MK, Sinha AD. Masked uncontrolled hypertension in CKD. J Am Soc Nephrol 2016;27:924–32.
31. Aung K, Htay T. Relationship between outpatient clinic and ambulatory blood pressure measurements and mortality. Curr Cardiol Rep 2019;21:28–35.
32. Pierdomenico SD, Pierdomenico AM, Coccina F, et al. Prognostic value of masked uncontrolled hypertension. Systematic review and meta-analysis. Hypertens 2018;72:862–9.
33. Babu M, Drawz P. Masked hypertension in CKD: increased prevalence and risk for cardiovascular and renal events. Curr Cardiol Rep 2019;21:58–62.
34. Calhoun DA, Grassi G. True versus pseudoresistant hypertension. J Hypertens 2017;35:2367–8.
35. Banegas JR, Ruilope LM, de la Sierra A, et al. High prevalence of masked uncontrolled hypertension in people with treated hypertension. Eur Heart J 2014;35: 3304–12.
36. Li S, Schwartz JE, Shimbo D, et al. Estimated Prevalence of Masked Asleep Hypertension in US Adults. J Am Med Assoc Cardiol 2020. https://doi.org/10.1001/jamacardio.2020.5212.
37. Minutolo R, Agarwal R, Borrelli S, et al. Prognostic role of ambulatory blood pressure measurement in patients with nondialysis chronic kidney disease. Arch Intern Med 2011;171(12):1090–8.
38. Mojon A, Ayala DE, Pineiro L, et al. Comparison of ambulatory blood pressure parameters of hypertensive patients with and without chronic kidney disease. Chronobiol Int 2013;30(1–2):145–58.
39. Kanno A, Kikuya M, Asayama K, et al. Night-time blood pressure is associated with the development of chronic kidney disease in a general population: the Ohasama Study. J Hypertens 2013;31:2410–7.
40. Franklin SS, O'Brien, Staessen JA. Masked hypertension: understanding its complexity. Eur Heart J 2017;38:1112–8.
41. Tanner RM, Calhoun DA, Bell EK, et al. Prevalence of apparent treatment-resistant hypertension among individuals with CKD. Clin J Am Soc Nephrol 2013;8:1583–90.
42. Thomas G, Xie D, Chen H-Y, et al. Prevalence and prognostic significance of apparent treatment resistant hypertension in chronic kidney disease. Hypertension 2016;67:387–96.
43. Townsend RR. Pathogenesis of drug-resistant hypertension. Semin Nephrol 2014; 34:506–13.

44. Sim JJ, Bhandari SK, Shi J, et al. Characteristics of resistant hypertension in a large, ethnically diverse hypertension population of an integrated health system. Mayo Clin Proc 2013;88(10):1099–107.

45. Sim JJ, Bhandari SK, Shi J, et al. Comparative risk of renal, cardiovascular, and mortality outcomes in controlled, uncontrolled resistant, and nonresistant hypertension. Kidney Int 2015;88:622–32.

46. Muntner P, Shimbo D, Carey RM, et al. Measurement of blood pressure in humans. A scientific statement from the American Heart Association. Hypertens 2019;73:e35–66.

47. Hegde S, Aeddula NR. Secondary hypertension [Updated 2020 Dec 1]. In: StatPearls [Internet]. Treasure Island (FL). StatPearls Publishing; 2020. Available at: https://www.ncbi.nlm.nih.gov/books/NBK544305/. Accessed December 17, 2021.

48. Cohen JB, Cohen DL, Herman DS, et al. Testing for primary aldosteronism and mineralocorticoid receptor antagonist use among U.S. veterans. A retrospective cohort study. Ann Intern Med 2021;174:289–97.

49. Brown JM, Siddiqui M, Calhoun DA, et al. The unrecognized prevalence of primary aldosteronism. Ann Intern Med 2020;173:10–20.

50. Monticone S, D'Ascenzo F, Moretti C, et al. Cardiovascular events and target organ damage in primary aldosteronism compared with essential hypertension: a systematic review and meta-analysis. Lancet Diabetes Endocrinol 2018;6:41–50.

51. Sowers JR, Whaley-Connell A, Epstein M. Narrative review: the emerging clinical implications of the role of aldosterone in the metabolic syndrome and resistant hypertension. Ann Intern Med 2009;150:776–83.

52. Buffolo F, Li Q, Monticone S, et al. Primary aldosteronism and obstructive sleep apnea. A cross-sectional multi-ethnic study. Hypertens 2019;74:1532–40.

53. Muxfeldt ES, Margallo VS, Guimaraes GM, et al. Prevalence and associated factors of obstructive sleep apnea in patients with resistant hypertension. Am J Hypertens 2014;27(8):1069–78.

54. Reutrakul S, van Cauter E. Interactions between sleep, circadian function, and glucose metabolism: implications for risk and severity of diabetes. Ann N Y Acad Sci 2014;1311:151–73.

55. Bonsignore MR, McNicholas, Montserrat JM, et al. Adipose tissue in obesity and obstructive sleep apnoea. Erur Respir J 2012;39(3):746–67.

56. Full KM, Jackson CL, Rebholz CM, et al. Obstructive Sleep Apnea, Other Sleep Characteristics, and Risk of CKD in the Atherosclerosis Risk in Communities Sleep Heart Health Study. J Am Soc Nephrol 2020;31:1859–69.

57. Whaley-Connell A, Sowers JR. Obesity and kidney disease: from population to basic science and the search for new therapeutic targets. Kidney Int 2017;92:313–23.

58. Liakopoulos V, Franzen S, Svensson A-M, et al. Renal and cardiovascular outcomes after weight loss from gastric bypass surgery in type 2 diabetes: cardiorenal risk reductions exceed atherosclerotic benefits. Diabetes Care 2020;43(6):1276–84.

59. Friedman AN, Wahed AS, Wang J, et al. Effect of bariatric surgery on CKD risk. J Am Soc Nephrol 2018;29:1289–300.

60. Kelly JT, Su G, Zhang L, et al. Modifiable lifestyle factors for primary prevention of CKD: A systematic review and meta-analysis. J Am Soc Nephrol 2021;32:239–53.

61. Joshi S, McMacken M, Kalantar-Zadeh K. Plant-based diets for kidney disease: a guide for clinicians. Am J Kidney Dis 2020. https://doi.org/10.1053/j.ajkd.2020.10.003.

62. Hu EA, Coresh J, Anderson CAM, et al. Adherence to healthy dietary patterns and risk of CKD progression and all-cause mortality: findings from the CRIC study. Am J Kidney Dis 2020. https://doi.org/10.1053/j.ajkd.2020.04.019.
63. Clegg DJ, Headley SA, Germain MJ. Impact of dietary potassium restrictions in CKD on clinical outcomes: benefits of a plant-based diet. Kidney Med 2020; 2(4):476–87.
64. Palmer BF. Potassium binders for hyperkalemia in chronic kidney disease – diet, renin-angiotensin-aldosterone inhibitor therapy, and hemodialysis. Mayo Clin Proc 2020;95:339–54.
65. Kidney Disease: Improving Global Outcomes (KDIGO) Blood Pressure Work Group. KDIGO 2021 Clinical Practice Guideline for the Management of Blood Pressure in Chronic Kidney Disease. Kidney Int 2021;99(3S):S1–87.
66. SPRINT Research Group, et al.. A Randomized Trial of Intensive versus Standard Blood-Pressure Control. N Engl J Med 2015;373(22):2103–16.
67. Wells R, Rahman M. SPRINT and the kidney: what have we learned? Curr Hypertens Rep 2018;20:95–8.
68. Rocco MV, Sink KM, Lovato LC, et al. Effects of intensive blood pressure treatment on acute kidney injury events in the SPRINT trial. Am J Kidney Dis 2017; 71(3):352–61.
69. Beddhu S, Rocco MV, Toto R, et al. Effects of intensive systolic blood pressure control on kidney and cardiovascular outcomes in persons without kidney disease. A secondary analysis of a randomized trial. Ann Intern Med 2017;167: 375–83.
70. Zhang WR, Craven TE, Malhotra R, et al. Kidney damage biomarkers and incident chronic kidney disease during blood pressure reduction. A case-control study. Ann Intern Med 2018;169:610–8.
71. Tomson CRV, Cheung AK, Mann JFE, et al. Management of blood pressure in patients with chronic kidney disease not receiving dialysis: Synopsis of the 2021 KDIGO Clinical Practice Guideline. Ann Intern Med 2021. https://doi.org/10.7326/M21-0834.
72. Burnier M, Bakris G, Williams B. Redefining diuretics use in hypertension: why select a thiazide-like diuretic? J Hypertens 2019;37:1574–86.
73. Sinha AD, Agarwal R. Clinical pharmacology of antihypertensive therapy for the treatment of hypertension in CKD. Clin J Am Soc Nephrol 2019;14:757–64.
74. Agarwal R, Sinha AD, Cramer AE, et al. Chlorthalidone for Hypertension in Advanced Chronic Kidney Disease. New Engl J Med 2021. https://doi.org/10.1056/NEJMoa2110730. Accessed December 17, 2021.
75. Currie G, Taylor AHM, Fujita T, et al. Effect of mineralocorticoid receptor antagonists on proteinuria and progression of chronic kidney disease: a systematic review and meta-analysis. BMC Nephrol 2016;17:127–40.
76. Bakris GL, Agarwal R, Anker SD, et al. Effect of finerenone on chronic kidney disease outcomes in type 2 diabetes. N Engl J Med 2020;383:2219029.
77. Kassem H, Chatila K. Mineralocorticoid receptor antagonists in heart failure patients with chronic kidney disease: why, when, and how? Curr Opin Nephrol Hypertens 2020;29:258–63.

It's Not Just for Kids

Molly E. Band, MHS, PA-C

KEYWORDS

- Pediatric • Children • Daytime urinary incontinence • Nocturnal enuresis
- Chronic kidney disease • Prematurity • Nephron mass

KEY POINTS

- There are key differences in children and adults regarding the evaluation and diagnosis of common nephrological and disorders of the urinary system.
- Many disorders will follow the pediatric patient into adulthood.
- Prematurity can be a risk factor for chronic kidney disease.

INTRODUCTION
Daytime Urinary Incontinence and Nocturnal Enuresis

Daytime urinary incontinence

Daytime urinary incontinence (DUI) has been defined by the International Children's Continence Society (ICCS) as intermittent urinary leakage during the day that is involuntary, occurring in children ages 5 and older and occurring more than once a month for a duration of over 3 months. DUI can be complex first one must rule out structural or neurogenic etiologies.[1]

While evaluating a pediatric patient with DUI, the patient's obstetric history (fetal distress, birth trauma, prenatal hydronephrosis, and amniotic fluid levels), developmental history (age of toilet training, gross motor milestones, etc.), urologic history (urinary tract infections), and medical history (congenital abnormalities, prior relevant surgeries) are important.[2]

It is helpful to obtain a voiding diary that includes fluid intake, voiding frequency, voided volumes, and episodes of incontinence. Bowel movements should also be noted in the voiding diary; taking note of frequency, caliber, and consistency using the Bristol stool scale.[3] It is preferable to have a minimum of 3 days.[2]

A thorough pediatric physical examination is essential. It will be important to note whether stool is palpable in the abdomen. A genitourinary examination looks for any abnormalities, IE: labial adhesions. A spinal examination is crucial, noting the presence or absence of a sacral dimple, hair tuft, or other signs of occult spinal cord abnormalities. A lower extremity examination is also important, looking for muscle

---

Pediatric Urology, Yale New Haven Hospital, 1 Park Street, New Haven, CT 06510, USA
E-mail address: Molly.band@ynhh.org

Physician Assist Clin 7 (2022) 295–303
https://doi.org/10.1016/j.cpha.2021.11.004
2405-7991/22/© 2021 Elsevier Inc. All rights reserved.

physicianassistant.theclinics.com

atrophy, foot deformities IE: foot drop, asymmetry of the buttocks, or abnormal gait that can lead toward a diagnosis of an underlying neuropathological condition.[2]

Additional noninvasive modalities for evaluation include an ultrasound, noting pre- and postvoid bladder volumes, bladder wall thickness, detecting structural abnormalities of the genitourinary tract. A urinalysis is a quick test to rule out urinary tract infection, proteinuria, or glucosuria. Another ideal noninvasive evaluation is a uroflowmetry which can reveal voiding disorders by measuring urinary stream and quantifying voided volume.[2]

DUI is often associated with comorbidities, estimated at 20% to 40%, including constipation or fecal incontinence, nocturnal enuresis, urinary tract infections, and/or psychiatric disorders. If present, constipation and fecal incontinence must be addressed before the treatment of DUI can be pursued. The theories as to why constipation and fecal incontinence worsen DUI include rectal distension distorting normal bladder contour leading to detrusor overactivity, shared nerve innervation, and pelvic floor overactivity resulting in bladder outlet resistance.[1]

The majority of psychiatric disorders considered externalizing disorders include the attention-deficit/hyperactivity disorder (ADHD), oppositional defiant disorder (ODD), and conduct disorder (CD). Internalizing disorders, also seen in patients with DUI, include social anxiety and separation anxiety disorders (SAD).[1]

The treatment of DUI should be patient-specific with the goal to achieve daytime continence. Successful treatment must include treatment of the specific condition while addressing comorbid conditions. Treatment, especially with children must be patient-centered and family-friendly. This can include nonpharmacological treatment (urotherapy), pharmacologic treatment, surgical treatment of structural/anatomic abnormalities, or a combination of these.[1]

The ICCS has outlined a treatment algorithm focusing on children greater than 5 years old who are neurologically and anatomically intact with intermittent functional DUI.[1] For patients with continuous DUI, an anatomic abnormality is likely and a referral for evaluation/treatment by a surgical specialist is warranted. Otherwise, initial treatment should begin with noninvasive urotherapy, stepping up to pharmacologic therapy when indicated. Even when pharmacologic treatment is initiated, urotherapy should be continued. Some of the pharmacologic treatments are FDA approved for use in pediatric patients, however many of the pharmacologic treatments are used off-label.[1] (**Tables 1** and **2**).

Nocturnal enuresis

Nocturnal enuresis is common in childhood, affecting an estimated 10% of 5 to 7 year olds.[4,5] It is defined as wetting occurring in children the age of 5 and older, occurring at least twice per week for at $\geq$ 3 months and not due to a substance or general medical condition. It occurs more commonly in males than in females.[4]

Nocturnal enuresis can be divided into 4 different categories based on the onset and presence/absence of other symptoms (**Table 3**).

A thorough history should be obtained, detailing both day and night symptoms and the onset of nocturnal enuresis. Evaluation, treatment, and success rates for continence vary based on the category. The greater majority of children, estimated at 75%, with nocturnal enuresis will have primary nocturnal enuresis.[5] The presentation for secondary nocturnal enuresis is similar to that of primary nocturnal enuresis apart from the time frame in which it has been occurring. One major difference is that children with secondary nocturnal enuresis are more likely to have other comorbid conditions.

Children with monosymptomatic nocturnal enuresis (MNE) tend to achieve continence more easily than those with nonmonosymptomatic nocturnal enuresis

Table 1 Nonpharmacologic treatment of DUI[1,3]	

Standard Urotherapy
• To be used 1st line
• Has a high success rate, estimated around 40%
	• Patient and caregiver education
	• 3-d bladder diary
	• Behavioral modifications:
	  ○ Timed voiding, utilizing timer assistance (vibrating watch, alarm)
	  ○ Discussion on voiding posture (seated with feet supported)
	  ○ Avoidance of withholding maneuvers
	• Life-style modifications:
	  ○ Balanced diet
	  ○ Adequate fluid intake
	  ○ Reduce caffeine and other bladder irritants
	  ○ Regular bowel and bladder emptying
	• Regular follow-up

Specific Urotherapy	Biofeedback: to be used only for dysfunctional voiding) • Helps to train pelvic floor muscle relaxation • Uses visual and auditory signals to train Neuromodulation: can be used to treat overactive bladder and neurogenic bladder dysfunction • Application modes: transcutaneous, intravesical, endoanal, an-genital, posterior tibial nerve, sacral nerve • Transcutaneous electrical nerve stimulation (TENS): shown to reduce incontinence and urgency Cognitive therapy: increases motivation and decreases stress • Self-monitoring: observing and registering • Labeling: using positive suggestive statements • Activity scheduling: organizing activities Psychotherapy: address comorbid conditions affection DUI • Full child psychological or psychiatric assessment • Clinically relevant psychotherapy and/or pharmacotherapy

Abbreviation: DUI, daytime urinary incontinence.

(NMNE). NMNE accounts for 30% of patients with nocturnal enuresis and these children are often incontinent during the day as well.

There are several comorbidities and risk factors for nocturnal enuresis (**Table 4**).

Identifying the secondary diagnosis will allow for more patient-specific treatment. The evaluation of children with nocturnal enuresis may differ based on the type and comorbidities. A basic evaluation should include a thorough history including birth history, psychological comorbidities, history of urinary tract infections, and family history. A voiding diary can be useful in determining if there are any concerns for daytime urinary symptoms as well as identifying constipation. A full physical examination should be performed, taking note of the presence/absence of stool on palpation of the abdomen as well as and sacral or spinal abnormalities. The initial evaluation should also include a urinalysis to rule out glycosuria, UTI, and/or proteinuria. A bladder scan can be helpful to ensure complete bladder emptying as well as measuring rectal diameter as a tool to screen for constipation. Additional evaluation is warranted if there are concerns for neurogenic bladder, severe lower urinary tract symptoms, or other relevant comorbid conditions.[5]

The treatment of nocturnal enuresis is based on the presence or absence of a subtype of enuresis (ie MNE or NMNE) as well as the patient and family's level of motivation to achieve nighttime continence. Treatment initially begins with a bowel regimen and addressing constipation and/or fecal incontinence. In addition, nonpharmacological

Table 2
Pharmacologic treatment for DUI[1,3]

Pharmacologic Class	Mechanism of Action	Selected Side Effects	Counseling for Families
Anticholinergic agents	• Blockage of M2/M3 receptors in the bladder • Suppresses bladder contractility	• Dry mouth • Facial flushing • Blurred vision • Tachycardia • Constipation	• Typically used as first line • Oxybutynin is the only FDA-approved agent • Others including tolterodine, solifenacin, and darifenacin are seeking approval
Alpha-blockers (alpha-adrenergic antagonists)	• Blockage of α adrenergic receptors in the bladder neck • Reduces bladder outlet resistance • Facilitates bladder emptying	• Hypotension • Fatigue • Muscle weakness	• Off-label • Can help to ameliorate symptoms of urgency and urge incontinence
Tricyclic antidepressants	• Has effects on both muscarinic receptors and on α adrenergic receptors	• Postural hypotension • Cardiac conduction abnormalities	• Useful in treating urge incontinence, nocturnal enuresis, and giggle incontinence • Must be administered by parent or guardian due to concern for overdose
SSRIs and SNRIs	• Modulates voiding and storage reflexes	• Diarrhea • Nausea • Dizziness	• Off-label • Useful in treatment-refractory incontinence • Most effective in patients with known or subclinical neuropsychiatric disorders
B-adrenergic agonists	• Smooth muscle relaxation, increasing detrusor stability • Increases bladder capacity without increasing voiding pressure or postvoid residual	• Hypertension	• Approved in adults and recently approved in children >3 y

Abbreviations: M2, M3, muscarinic; SSRI, selective serotonin reuptake inhibitor; SNRI- serotonin and norepinephrine reuptake inhibitor.

Table 3	
Categories of nocturnal enuresis[4,5]	
Category	**Definition**
Primary nocturnal enuresis (PNE)	Occurring in children age >5 y that have never achieved urinary continence overnight for >6 mo
Secondary nocturnal enuresis (SNE)	Occurring in children that have previously achieved urinary continence overnight for >6 mo
Monosymptomatic nocturnal enuresis (MNE)	Occurring without the presence of any other bladder dysfunction symptoms
Nonmonosymptomatic nocturnal enuresis (NMNE)	Occurring associated with other symptoms of bladder dysfunction: • Daytime incontinence • Urinary urgency • Urinary frequency • Urinary withholding

counseling can be provided to the family, including limiting fluids in the evening, bladder diaries with positive reinforcement, and timed voiding during the day.[5]

If nocturnal enuresis persists despite the above measures, a bed alarm can be recommended. The benefits of this therapy include that it is nonpharmacologic and has the highest long-term success rate, up to about 78%.[4] The downsides of this therapy include that it can be burdensome for the parents if the child does not wake with the alarm. It is recommended for use up to 10 to 12 weeks with the lowest percentage of relapse.[4,5]

Alternatively, pharmacologic therapy can be prescribed including desmopressin, imipramine, or anticholinergic drugs (**Table 5**).

Chronic Kidney Disease and End-Stage Kidney Disease in Children

The kidney disease: Improving Global Outcomes (KDIGO) defines CKD as any abnormality in kidney structure or function that has been present for more than 3 months with implications to health.[6] CKD can occur at any age, but the etiologies and complications of CKD in a pediatric patient are far different than those in an adult.[6,7]

While there is an abundance of data on the epidemiology of CKD in adulthood, there is less known in the pediatric population. The incidence of pediatric CKD began to rise in the 1980s, peaking in 2003, and has slowly declined since 2008.[7] In pediatric kidney disease, there has been an increased survival rate due to more advanced knowledge and treatment.[7] Thus, more of these children will transition to the adult CKD population.

As mentioned above, the etiologies of CKD in children are vastly different than that of adult. Congenital disorders account for the primary cause of CKD in children, including congenital anomalies of the kidney and urinary tract (CAKUT). This includes vesicoureteral reflux (VUR), genitourinary tract obstruction, urinary tract infections, and hereditary nephropathies including Alport syndrome. Glomerulonephritis is another prevalent cause of CKD in the pediatric population, including Lupus nephritis and steroid-resistant nephrotic syndrome.[7] Less common causes of CKD in the pediatric population include thrombotic microangiopathies (hemolytic uremic syndrome, etc.), nephrolithiasis, nephrocalcinosis, and Wilms tumor. Newer diagnoses include pediatric obesity and prematurity, which will be discussed later in discussion.[6]

| Table 4 | |
| Comorbidities and risk factors for nocturnal enuresis[5] | |
Comorbidities/Risk Factor for Nocturnal Enuresis	Additional Information
Family history of nocturnal enuresis	• Autosomal dominant inheritance with high penetrance • 44% risk in children with one affected parent • 77% in children with 2 affected parents
Psychological externalizing and/or internalizing disorders	• Examples: • ADD/ADHD • Present in 20%–30% of all children with nocturnal enuresis • SNE can occur in the setting of stressful events (change in home life, school, etc.)
Constipation	• Nocturnal enuresis has a high-resolution rate with successful treatment of constipation

Abbreviations: ADD, attention deficient disorder; ADHD, attention deficit hyperactivity disorder; SNE, secondary nocturnal enuresis.

Other implications to the etiologies of CKD in children include age, gender, and race. In younger children, CAKUT and hereditary nephropathies are more common; whereas glomerulonephritis is more common in children over the age of 12 years.[7] There is a higher prevalence of CKD among men versus women. In North America, the incidence rate of CKD is 2 to 3 times higher in African American children than Caucasian children.[7]

With improving technologies, there have been genetic advances in specific causes of pediatric CKD. There are more than 200 genes that have been identified as causative for the most common etiologies of CKD in children, including CAKUT, steroid-resistant nephrotic syndrome, glomerulonephritis, and ciliopathies. The most widely known gene is represented by APOL1. APOL1 leads to a significantly higher risk of developing focal segmental glomerulosclerosis (FSGS). With these advancements, there is the potential to avoid ineffective treatments, and to provide prenatal testing, and genetic counseling to families.[6]

The complications of pediatric CKD have some similarities to those of adulthood, but with certain specific differences as it relates to growth and development. A common complication of CKD in the pediatric patient is growth impairment, particularly if the child is diagnosed with CKD as an infant or young child before puberty. It is also the most outwardly visible complication lending toward psychosocial complications. The cause of growth impairment is multifactorial, including poor nutrition/appetite,

Table 5 Pharmacologic treatment of nocturnal enuresis[4,5]			
Pharmacologic Agent	**Side Effects**	**Success Rates**	**Counseling for Families**
Desmopressin – synthetic analog of arginine vasopressin	• Hyponatremia, which can result in seizure • Headache • Nausea/vomiting	• 50%–70%	• Take within 30–60 min of sleep • Evening fluid restriction is imperative given the risk of hyponatremia • Can be used intermittently for special occasions • Structured withdrawal is recommended to maintain highest success rates
Imipramine – tricyclic antidepressant	• Dry mouth • Mood changes • Cardiotoxicity	• 20%–40%	• Can be used intermittently for special occasions
Oxybutynin – anticholinergic agent	• Dry mouth • Constipation • Urinary retention • Tachycardia • Blurry vision • Mood changes	• Not reported	• Useful in patients that have NMNE or signs of overactive bladder • Can be used in combination with desmopressin

Abbreviations: NMNE, nonmonosymptomatic nocturnal enuresis.

metabolic acidosis, bone and mineral disorder (CKD-BMD), growth abnormalities, and disturbances in growth hormone metabolism.[6,7]

Anemia is common in patients with CKD; however for children, it has a significant impact on neurocognitive abilities. The goal of treatment of anemia with iron and re-combinant human erythropoiesis-stimulating agents includes decreasing cardiovascular risks, improvement in growth and nutrition, as well as improvement in cognitive function and scholastic performance.[6,7]

Cardiovascular disease mortality is much higher in pediatric patients with CKD and ESKD than the general pediatric population. Hypertension can be present from earlier stages of CKD and must be aggressively managed. The ESCAPE trial showed the benefit of treating hypertension in children with the goal of blood pressure less than 50th percentile. This is in comparison to the general population whereby the goal is between the 50th and 90th percentile.[6]

The transition of a patient with CKD from pediatric care providers to adult care providers can be challenging. Adolescents are in a stage of development known to be at higher risk for noncompliance, particularly during the time of transition. Using an integrated transition clinic for adolescents and young adults with CKD should be considered as this will allow for more seamless transfer. It also allows for education regarding ongoing care, higher education, employment, and social development. The goal of a transition clinic is to decrease the rate of CKD progression and/or transplant rejection for those patients who have undergone organ transplantation.[7]

OB/GYN and Nephron Mass

There has been a larger focus on the effects of premature birth, low birth weight, and nephron development in the recent past, particularly with more than 95% of children born prematurely surviving into adulthood. With higher survival for preterm births and extremely preterm birth (<28 weeks gestation) infants, it is critical that this population have long-term follow-up. Monitoring and prevention are needed to decrease risks for the development of CKD.[8]

The normal development and maturation of the kidney (nephronogenesis) begins around 15 weeks gestation and continues up through 34 to 36 gestational weeks, with more than 60% of nephrons formed in the third trimester of pregnancy.[9,10] The pathophysiology of this is postulated that with a reduced number of functioning nephrons in these at-risk infants, there is a resultant compensatory glomerular hyperperfusion causing glomerular and tubulointerstitial damange.[9,10] There has also been more recent evidence that prematurity and perinatal stress also results in podocyte damage and vasculogensis.[9]

If a child is born before completing 34 to 36 weeks of gestational age, or if there are other neonatal stressors, there is a much higher risk of negative outcomes. These can include an increased risk of CKD developing in childhood to mid-adulthood. One study by Crump and colleagues estimated a two times higher risk of development of CKD in premature infants, and a three times higher risk of CKD in extremely premature infants when compared with full-term births.[8] A pre-term birth is a risk factor for neonatal acute kidney injury.[8] Other risk factors for the development of CKD include intrauterine growth restriction (IUGR) and chorioamnionitis.

SUMMARY

There are many conditions that arise during childhood that can carry into adulthood, including kidney disease. It is important for both pediatric and adult providers to be aware of pediatric-specific disorders as with more the advancement in technology, children with complex diseases are living longer. These children will eventually transition into adulthood and require ongoing care that likely differs from that of patients with adult-specific disorders.

CLINICS CARE POINTS

- CAKUT is the most common cause of CKD in children
- Nephronogenesis occurs in the last weeks of pregnancy
- Pediatric survival is increasing and so a large number of these children will transition to adult nephrology

DISCLOSURE

Some treatment modalities discussed in this article include off-label usage of medications.

REFERENCES

1. Chang SJ, Van Laecke E, Bauer SB, et al. Treatment of daytime urinary incontinence: a standardization document from the international children's continence society. Neurol Urodynamics 2017;36:43–50.
2. Hoebeke P, Bower W, Combs A, et al. Diagnostic evaluation of children with daytime incontinence. Urol J 2010;183:699–703.
3. Franco I. Overactive bladder in children. Nature 2016;13:520–32.

4. Brown ML, Pope AW, Brown EJ. Treatment of primary nocturnal enuresis in children: a review. Child Care Health Dev 2010;37:153–60.
5. Kuwertz-Broking E, von Gontard A. Clinical management of nocturnal enuresis. Pediatr Nephrol 2018;33:1145–54.
6. Becherucci F, Roperto RM, Materassi M, et al. Chronic kidney disease in children. Clin Kidney J 2016;9:583–91.
7. Band ME, D'Alessandri-Silva C. Pediatrics: the forgotten stepchild of nephrology. Physician Assit Clin 2016;1:175–85.
8. Crump C, Sundquist J, Winkleby M, et al. Preterm birth and risk of chronic kidney disease from childhood into mid-adulthood: national cohort study. BMJ 2019; 365:1–10.
9. Hoogenboom LA, Wolds TGAM, Hutten MC, et al. Prematurity, perinatal inflammatory stress, and the predisposition to develop chronic kidney disease beyond oligonephropathy. Pediatr Nephrol 2021;36(7):1673–81.
10. Mendez-Castro C, Nitz D, Cordasic N, et al. Neonatal nephron loss during active nephrogenesis – detrimental impact with long-term renal consequences. Scientific Rep 2018;8:1–11.

Everything Else

Marlene Shaw-Gallagher, MS, PA-C[a,b,*], Flor A. Rangel, DMD, PA-S[a],
Kelly A. Sweeney, PA-S[a], Jyothi Digambaranath, PhD, PA-S[a], Faraaz Siddiqui, PA-S[a],
Megan McKay, PA-S[a], Kimberly Gadulka, MA, CCC-SLP, PA-S[a], Jane S. Davis, DNP[c]

KEYWORDS

- CKD • Proteinuria • Acute kidney injury • Urinalysis • eGFR • Race

KEY POINTS

- Kidney disease is associated with a variety of medical conditions and can be overlooked in the primary care setting
- Identification and close monitoring are key to slowing the progression of CKD in these patients
- The use of race in eGFR calculations has led to a completely new calculator in an attempt to promptly diagnose CKD in African American patients

INTRODUCTION

The incidence of chronic kidney disease (CKD) continues to increase currently impacting 15% of the US population.[1] Patients with diabetes and hypertension (HTN) tend to be monitored closely for CKD but signs in patients with less common causes of CKD often are missed. This article will review some of these other causes of kidney disease. Multiple autoimmune disorders can lead to the progression of kidney disease and we will outline the etiology, presentation, and potential treatments for these disorders. We will review the criteria for the diagnosis of pre-eclampsia and the importance of early identification. Acute kidney injury (AKI) is a serious complication of rhabdomyolysis and close monitoring of these patients is essential to determine which patients are most at risk. HIV-associated nephropathy (HIVAN) is becoming more common as HIV patients are living longer because of more effective treatments. We will look at the genetic components that put HIV patients at higher risk of HIVAN and the recommended monitoring. Central American nephropathy (CAN) has only recently been identified and is not well understood. We review current treatment options although none have proven effective for this often-terminal disease. Finally, we will address

[a] University of Detroit Mercy, 4001 West McNichols Road, Detroit, MI 48221-3038, USA;
[b] Nephrology Division, University of Michigan, 1500 East Medical Center Drive, Ann Arbor, MI 48109, USA; [c] Division of Nephrology, University of Alabama at Birmingham, 3605 Oakdale Road, Birmingham, AL 35223, USA
* Corresponding author. University of Detroit Mercy, 4001 West McNichols Road, Detroit, MI 48221-3038.
E-mail address: marleneg@med.umich.edu
Twitter: @mshawgal (M.S.-G.)

Physician Assist Clin 7 (2022) 305–317
https://doi.org/10.1016/j.cpha.2021.11.016
2405-7991/22/© 2021 Elsevier Inc. All rights reserved.

the recent controversy around the use of race in estimated glomerular filtration rate (eGFR) calculation, the decision to remove the race variable, and the potential impact this may have on CKD diagnosis in African American patients.

AUTOIMMUNE NEPHROPATHY

Autoimmune diseases can damage the kidney in multiple ways at the level of small blood vessels through the immune system or from the reaction of kidneys to autoantigens (proteins). The involvement may be at the glomerular, tubular, and/or vascular level.[2] Cellular injury provokes a loss of resistance to both intracellular and extracellular protein, which in turn targets autoantigens causing tissue injury. Autoimmune antigens are circulating in the blood and when they lodge in the glomeruli, they cause inflammation and damage at the cellular level.[2] On kidney biopsy, this presents as vasculitis or glomerulonephritis (GN). The most common autoimmune processes that affect the kidney are as follows:

- Lupus
- GN
- Scleroderma
- Sjögren syndrome (SS)
- Granulomatosis with polyangiitis (GPA, previously *Wegener disease*)
- Monoclonal gammopathy of undetermined significance (MGUS)/Myeloma
- IgA

Systemic Lupus Erythematosus

Lupus (systemic lupus erythematosus [SLE]) is a chronic autoimmune disease of unknown etiology that can affect virtually any organ of the body and leads to an array of clinical manifestations.[3] Immunologic abnormalities, especially the production of several antinuclear antibodies (ANAs), are a prominent feature and an ANA serum level is used for diagnosis.[3] Patients with SLE can have kidney involvement, which often progresses to end-stage kidney disease (ESKD). Diffuse proliferative glomerulonephritis is the most serious complication of lupus nephropathy and occurs in 35% to 60% of patients. It is thought that the glomerular structures' binding mechanism induces inflammatory reactions responsible for the GN.

Several autoantibodies are generated in lupus patients: ANAs and anti–double-stranded DNA antibodies (dsDNA).[2,3] The diagnosis of SLE is generally based on clinical and laboratory findings after excluding alternative diagnoses. The clinical presentation is highly variable, ranging from asymptomatic hematuria and/or proteinuria to nephrotic syndrome and rapidly progressive GN with loss of kidney function. Several forms of GN can occur and kidney biopsy is useful to define the type and extent of kidney involvement.[3] Treatment, directed by biopsy, is standard of care. SLE can be treated with hydroxychloroquine, corticosteroids, and/or immunosuppressive drugs. For special circumstances, the use of eculizumab to inhibit complement and/or angiotensin-converting enzyme inhibitors (ACEi) and angiotensin receptor blockers (ARBs) to control blood pressure (BP) are recommended.[4]

Scleroderma

Scleroderma is a rare multisystem immune disease, which involves vasculopathies and autoimmune antibody activation. Scleroderma patients are categorized depending on the amount of skin involved. Kidney damage occurs in approximately 50% of scleroderma patients and although associated with other blood vessel diseases, it rarely progresses to ESKD.[5] That said, a scleroderma renal crisis (SRC) is one of the most commonly associated complications and remains an important cause of morbidity and mortality in scleroderma. Causes of crisis include nephrotoxic medications and/or dehydration. SRC presents with malignant HTN, hyperreninemia, azotemia, microangiopathic hemolytic anemia, and kidney failure.[6] Diagnosis is made by urinalysis (UA; bland sediments on micro), complete blood count (CBC) with microangiopathic hemolytic anemia, an elevated blood urea nitrogen (BUN)/serum creatinine (SCr), high renin blood test, and low platelet count. Treatment for SRC consists of aggressive HTN management with an ACEi/ARBs and other medications as needed.[5,6]

Sjögren Syndrome

SS is a heterogeneous autoimmune disease that presents with dry eyes, dry mouth, and commonly occurs with other autoimmune disorders (such as rheumatoid arthritis and lupus).[7] It is more common in women and in the fourth decade of life. Kidney involvement occurs at the tubular level with renal tubular acidosis or GN. Atypical autoantibodies—anti-SSA (Ro) or anti-SSB (La)—are believed to be the cause of kidney involvement.[8,9] Presentation can be nonspecific although edema and nephrotic syndrome are usually present. Microscopic UA shows proteinuria, hematuria, and red blood cell casts. A kidney biopsy is highly recommended and treatment with a combination of rituximab, steroids, and plasma exchange is usually prescribed.[7]

Granulomatosis with Polyangiitis (Previously Known Wegener Disease)

Granulomatosis presents with a rapidly progressive GN with macroscopic or microscopic hematuria, proteinuria, edema, decreased urine output, and a rapid deterioration of kidney function.[7,10] Most frequently there is involvement in the upper/lower respiratory tract developing into a systemic vasculitis affecting the kidneys. As the cause of GPA is a vasculitis of blood vessels, there can be and often is oral and/or uveal bleeding and hemoptysis. The kidney involvement may be insidious with a mild or moderate kidney damage.[7,10] Clinical or morphologic evidence of kidney involvement has been found in about 80% of patients with GPA. GPA is considered the most common antineutrophil cytoplasmic antibodies (ANCA)-associated vasculitis. Diagnosis is made with standard indirect immunofluorescence microscopy, ANCA test, and erythrocyte sedimentation rate. Untreated GPA will lead to ESKD. Treatment is pulse corticosteroids followed by intravenous immunosuppressive drugs (rituximab) along with plasma exchange.[11]

MGUS/Myeloma

The earliest stage of myeloma is a benign condition with an overproduction of plasma cells referred to as MGUS.[7] This asymptomatic plasma cell dyscrasia is found in more than 3% of the general white population older than 50 years. The overproduction of plasma cells can be either light or heavy chain (light chain disease, heavy chain disease).[7] The progression of MGUS to multiple myeloma (MM) occurs more often in light chain disease with up to 70% converting to medium-risk myeloma at 5 years.[12]

MM is a malignant neoplasm of plasma cells in the bone marrow associated with an overproduction of monoclonal (M) protein causing characteristic osteolytic lesions, anemia, kidney failure, and hypercalcemia.[12] There are several mechanisms that can contribute to kidney involvement, including nephrotoxic monoclonal immunoglobulin chains, which are deposited in the tubules and/or the glomeruli and cause irreversible damage.[13]

Clinically, presentation includes weight loss, malaise, fatigue, bone pain, hypercalcemia, and/or proteinuria.[13] MM is diagnosed with a serum and urine electrophoresis that includes a free chain assay. Treatment includes systemic therapy with a proteasome inhibitor and/or stem cell transplantation.[13]

IgA

IgA nephropathy (IgAN) is the most common GN in the world and thus a common cause of CKD and kidney failure.[14] Pathogenesis of IgAN is due to activation of the complement system leading to local inflammation, cellular proliferation, and fibrosis.[14] The 2 most common clinical presentations are asymptomatic hematuria and/or progressive CKD with proteinuria.[14] Biopsy with immunofluorescence will show positive staining of the IgA (**Fig. 1**). Treatment is usually conservative with ACEi/ARBs. If and when progression occurs, as documented by proteinuria, the next level of treatment is started: corticosteroids and/or immunosuppressive agents.[14]

Pre-eclampsia/eclampsia

Pre-eclampsia/eclampsia is a leading complication of pregnancy affecting approximately 5% of pregnancies and globally causes 60,000 maternal deaths annually.[15,16] Pre-eclampsia is characterized by HTN and proteinuria.[16–18] Risk assessment involves patient history, clinical signs, and angiogenic biomarkers.[16,19] Management of pre-eclampsia includes low-dose aspirin, calcium supplementation, intravenous labetalol (if hospitalized), oral nifedipine (for outpatient treatment), BP monitoring, preconception counseling, timely delivery of the fetus, and postpartum surveillance.[16,18]

Pre-eclampsia is indicated by proteinuria and new-onset HTN at ≥20 weeks' gestation.[15,16] This multiorgan syndrome is associated with increased preterm births, heightened maternal and fetal morbidity and mortality, and long-term cardiovascular disease in the mother.[16] Genetic predisposition/family history, maternal smoking, maternal age, use of in vitro fertilization, and pre-existing diseases (diabetes, obesity, CKD, and chronic HTN) increase the incidence.[16,20] Additional symptoms include headache, visual impairments, right upper quadrant abdominal pain, edema, and oliguria.[16] If pre-eclampsia is not treated, it can lead to more serious conditions: eclampsia, intracranial hemorrhage, HELLP (hemolysis, elevated liver enzymes, and low platelets) syndrome, kidney failure, pulmonary edema, and/or respiratory distress syndrome.[20]

Diagnosing pre-eclampsia remains a challenge because of variable clinical presentation and asymptomatic cases.[15,19] HTN in pregnancy is defined as systolic BP > 140 mm Hg and/or diastolic BP > 90 mm Hg taken over 2 separate

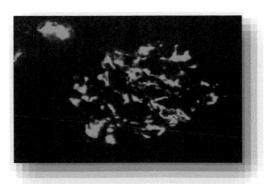

Fig. 1. IgA biopsy. IgA fluorescence under electron microscope

measurements, 15 minutes apart.[21] Measuring BP and checking for proteinuria during each antenatal visit is imperative.[21] To manage pre-eclampsia, home BP should be checked 4 times daily. Serum blood tests for kidney function, bilirubin, CBC, fasting blood glucose, and transaminases are paramount.[21]

Angiogenic biomarkers such as placental growth factor (PGIF) and vascular endothelial growth factor are important for the function of placental development and endothelial cells.[17] PGIF is a protein associated with placental angiogenesis, and PGIF concentration should increase and peak at 26 to 30 weeks.[19] However, PGIF levels which do not rise accordingly indicate placental dysfunction.[20]

Triage PGIF-based tests and Elecsys immunoassay sFlt-1/PIGF ratio laboratory tests are using such biomarkers to diagnose suspected pre-eclampsia.[19,22] Current evidence suggests that administering low dose aspirin along with daily calcium supplementation before 16 weeks' gestation can significantly reduce the risk of pre-eclampsia.[15,20,21] For severe cases of pre-eclampsia, intravenous labetalol or oral nifedipine are used to manage HTN.[18] However, the only definitive treatment for pre-eclampsia is the timely delivery of the fetus.[16,22]

NATURAL DISASTER/TRAUMA-INDUCED RHABDOMYOLYSIS

In adults, the most common cause of rhabdomyolysis (rhabdo), the destruction of muscle tissue, is trauma.[23,24] Any traumatic injury can cause skeletal muscle breakdown with the concurrent release of these contents into the bloodstream. The most serious sequela of rhabdo is AKI.[7]

Rhabdo is characterized by leakage of cell contents into the bloodstream and interstitium. Studies report rhabdo in 85% of patients with traumatic injury with 10% to 40% of these patients developing AKI.[23,25,26] Traumatic injury may result from the following:[23]

- A fall
- Crush injury
- Trapped under collapsed building
- Motor vehicle accidents
- Earthquakes
- Electric shock
- Lightning injuries
- Prolonged immobilization
- Taser injuries
- Third-degree burns

Nontraumatic causes of rhabdo include the following:[24]

- Infection
- Drugs
- Toxins
- Ischemia
- Cocaine use
- Genetic defects
- Strenuous exercise in previously untrained individuals
- Surgery
- Hyperthermia
- Medication-induced
- Metabolic
- Endocrine

- Autoimmune disorders
- Prolonged immobility

Nontraumatic causes will not be reviewed in this article.[24] Risk factors for trauma-induced rhabdo include a high body mass index more than 35 kg/m^2, being of African American heritage, and/or having CKD.[27]

Myoglobin released during muscle injury forms obstructive intratubular casts in the presence of acidic urine leading to AKI; AKI is characterized by a reduced eGFR and an increase in SCr. Although AKI is the life-threatening complication of rhabdo, other potentially serious complications include kidney failure, compartment syndrome, and disseminated intravascular coagulation.[23,28]

Patient history is the key to timely diagnosis of trauma-related rhabdo. However, when the massive trauma patient is extricated from a trauma scene, the diagnosis is very straightforward. In those with less massive trauma, the diagnosis may be more subtle. Patients with rhabdo may present with myalgia, muscle weakness dark urine, or be asymptomatic. Only about 10% of patients present with a classic triad of myalgia, muscle weakness, and dark/reddish-brown urine.[28] Most rhabdo patients are asymptomatic or simply present with myoglobinuria.[24]

Diagnosis can be confirmed through blood creatine kinase (CK) levels, muscle enzymes, electrocardiogram (ECG), UA, and/or electrolytes. The physical examination may be normal in regards to vital signs and lack of muscle cramps. A CK level 5× normal level (45–260U/L) is used to establish the rhabdo diagnosis. A CK level greater than 5000 IU/L indicates kidney injury.

Myoglobin is a less reliable indicator because of its short half-life (2-3 hours) and rapid kidney clearance. Electrolyte imbalances include early hypocalcemia, hypophosphatemia, hyperkalemia (usually the fatal issue in crush injuries), late hypercalcemia, and/or hyperuricemia. An ECG can diagnose cardiac issues related to hyperkalemia. BUN and SCr levels assess the extent of kidney injury. Muscle damage occurs with intercompartment pressure greater than 30 mm Hg causing an increase in CK levels in compartment syndrome. McMahon score ≥6 may aid in predicting AKI risk or mortality in patients with rhabdo (**Table 1**).[23,28,29]

Treatment of rhabdo is supportive with aggressive fluid resuscitation to increase urine flow to 200 to 300 mL/h. This should prevent complications in trauma-induced rhabdo.[26,28] Fluid replacement therapy is also effective in patients with rhabdo-induced AKI or other complications.[23] Nephrotoxic medications should be discontinued and caution used with radiocontrast. Use of osmotic or loop diuretics or urine alkalinization with bicarbonate are still considered second line.[28,30]

HIV-ASSOCIATED NEPHROPATHY

HIVAN, first described in 1984, is a collapsing form of focal segmental glomerulosclerosis (FSGS) and is the most aggressive kidney disease in HIV-infected patients.[7,31] HIVAN is predominantly a late manifestation of HIV infection when low CD4 cell counts and high viral loads are present. The patient population predominantly affected by HIVAN are of African ancestry, noted in both the United States and Western Europe. It is relatively rare in the white population, and thus the belief that HIVAN is due to a 2-hit theory.[32] Genetics has shown that the APOL1 gene is carried in those of African ancestry.[33] APOL1 can increase the risk for kidney failure, and thus both the APOL1 gene and HIV can lead to HIVAN in the high-risk genetic population. A recent publication showed that using the race adjustment in eGFR calculators compared with measured glomerular filtration rate (GFR) via iohexol had poor accuracy in black patients with HIV.[32]

Table 1
McMahon risk score for prediction of AKI[29]

Variable	Score (in points)
Age, y	
>50 to ≤70	1.5
>70 to ≤80	2.5
>80	3
Sex—female	1
Initial creatinine, mg/dL	
1.4–2.2	1.5
>2.2	3
Initial calcium <7.5 mg/dL	2
Initial CPK >40,000 U/L	2
Origin—not seizures, syncope, exercise, statins, or myositis	3
Initial PO₄	
4.0–5.4	1.5
>5.4	3
Initial bicarbonate <19 mEq/L	2

A score of ≥6 indicates high risk for AKI/mortality.

Gender or comorbidities do not play a significant role but the use of highly active antiretroviral therapy (HAART) can cause HIVAN. With an increased use of HAART, survival with HIV has increased to the point where chronic nephrotoxic medications increase the incidence of HIVAN.[31] Essentially, the success of HAART medications and the increased survival of the HIV patient are now causing HIVAN.

The diagnosis of HIVAN is not made by a single parameter but rather by looking at a variety of factors. Clinically, this disease presents with nephrotic-range proteinuria, kidney dysfunction, collapsing FSGS, interstitial inflammation, and/or microcystic tubular dilation. Typically, proteinuria is more than 3 g/24 h and SCr more than 2 mg/dL.[31]

Clinical criteria alone cannot diagnose HIVAN. A kidney biopsy provides the indicator and should be performed as soon as the patient meets clinical criteria. Kidney echogenicity has also been shown to be increased significantly in patients with HIVAN when compared with HIV-infected patients with other kidney diseases.[31]

HIV patients, in general, have an increased risk of CKD. As a result, the HIV Medicine Association of the Infectious Diseases Society of America recommends annual kidney screening to include both urine protein:creatinine ratio and urine albumin:creatinine ratio. Other annual screening laboratories include BP, SCr, and eGFR. For those patients on tenofovir, screening for proximal tubular disease must be included. The recommendation for referral to nephrology is aggressive when the eGFR decreases by greater than 25% from baseline or when GFR is less than 60 mL/min/1.73 m.[34,35]

The progression of HIVAN to ESKD occurs quickly without HIV treatment. Although HAART medications can be nephrotoxic, the disease state of HIV is also nephrotoxic. A true chicken and egg conundrum. No randomized controlled trials have been conducted to determine the best treatment of HIVAN but retrospective studies have shown HAART to be the best management approach. Aggressive management of the HIV disease will slow kidney damage although these medications may be nephrotoxic in the long run (many years of treatment). The guidelines of the Infectious Diseases Society of America state HAART should be started on all patients presenting with HIV-associated kidney disease.[34] If no kidney function improvement is noted in these patients, then ACEi and ARBs and/or prednisone can be added.[31]

No randomized trial has been done on the effectiveness of ACEi or ARBs for the treatment of HIVAN. The theory behind the use of these medications is from the data gathered from the treatment of other glomerular diseases. The standard suggestions for any CKD patient are also true for the HIVAN patient: BP less than 110/70 mm Hg, control of bicarbonate and serum urate, smoking cessation, weight loss in obese patients, and avoiding nephrotoxins.[36]

CENTRAL AMERICAN NEPHROPATHY

CAN, also referred to as Mesoamerican Endemic Nephropathy (MeN), is chronic kidney injury without traditional risk factors that affect residents in the coastal Pacific Ocean regions of southern Mexico and Central America.[37,38] Before 2013, CAN was not recognized as a disease. Evidence dating back to the 1970s points to CKD with unknown cause in young males occurred frequently in this region.[37]

The etiology is unknown, but there are many hypotheses with the primary belief that CAN is due to repeated heat stress and dehydration associated with low altitude environmental conditions.[37,38] Strenuous manual labor in areas with high heat and poor working protections support this theory. Manual labor is the primary and often only source of employment for workers in regions of Mexico and Central America where CAN is described. Low socioeconomic status plays a role in diagnosing and treating CAN because of the decreased ability for detection and treatment among a population with less access to medical care.[37,38]

A second hypothesis is that work and living conditions allow exposure to pesticides, heavy metals, and nephrotoxic substances, all of which can contribute to CAN. This theory is supported through long-standing issues with silica, a known kidney toxin that is released in the ash during burning of sugar cane. Lastly, there is anecdotal evidence of a family CAN history as well as a family history of CKD with known risk factors to developing CAN.

Symptoms at presentation depend on the stage of disease when identified. Owing to increased awareness of CAN, community and employer screenings are now in place. Kidney biopsy is definitive for diagnosis; although, few patients obtain this because of cost and availability.[37,38] To keep from delaying treatment, diagnosis is made on the constellation of patient history, symptoms, blood work, and, if possible, imaging. Symptoms can include lower urinary tract discomfort, urinary urgency, cramps/muscular weakness, feverish-sensation, and AKI on laboratory work.[37,38] On physical examination, patients are normotensive with no signs of fluid overload, whereas in later stages, they can be hypertensive.[37] Laboratory work shows a decreased eGFR (<60 mL/min/1.73 m^2), albuminuria (>30 mg/g), proteinuria (non-nephrotic levels >150 mg/g but less than 2 g/g), and/or electrolyte disturbances (hypokalemia and hyperuricemia).[37,38] Ultrasound shows small echogenic kidneys.[38]

CAN is often a terminal diagnosis because of the late stage at which it is found, high cost of kidney replacement therapy, and poor working conditions that exacerbate the issue.[37,38]

Primary treatment is prevention[37]:

- Identification of disease by clinicians
- Community and employment screening
- Better working environments

- Hydration stations
- Shaded areas for rest spots

Medical treatment does not change the clinical course; therefore, no standard treatment exists. However, clinicians prescribe medications including allopurinol, potassium supplements, potassium-sparing diuretics, and bicarbonate to decrease hypokalemic events. ACEi and corticosteroids are not readily available.[37]

CAN is now recognized as an endemic issue with rates of deaths due to CKD as much as 30× higher than CKD deaths in the United States.[37] There are multiple hypotheses for CAN; however, because of the low socioeconomic status of the region, conditions likely will not change because of the patients' need to work. Symptoms of CAN vary on identification and presentation of the disease. Pharmacologic treatment is expensive and does not change patient outcomes, so focus on prevention with improved working environments, screenings, and awareness is slowly being implemented.

USE OF RACE IN THE eGFR CALCULATION

Accurate assessment of kidney function is crucial in the detection and treatment of kidney disease; however, creating a test that delivers accurate results in a relatively noninvasive, inexpensive, and timely manner has been a challenge.

SCr was the standard for assessment of kidney function in the mid-1900s primarily because it forms at a relatively constant rate by the muscles, is freely filtered by the glomerulus, and is not reabsorbed by the tubules.[39] Although creatinine is secreted at a constant rate, that rate can vary depending on several independent and personal factors such as muscle mass, diet, age, gender, and medications.[39] Researchers attempted to solve this dilemma by creating mathematical formulas that took into account age, sex, and body weight when determining the GFR.

GFR is defined as how much blood is filtered through the glomeruli per minute and is used to estimate the relative health and functioning of the kidney. Formulas that calculate GFR rather than directly measure it are referred to as estimated GFR or eGFR. The first formula was the Cockcroft-Gault (CG). Created in 1973, it used age, weight, gender, and SCr to estimate GFR.[40] As the CG formula was developed using measured GFR from 249 hospitalized white males, the formula tended to overestimate GFR and there was confusion as to how to handle bodyweight. This was especially true for patients with ascites, morbid obesity, limb amputation, or other conditions.[39] In addition, the CG formula did not address creatinine clearance in women or nonwhite patients.[41] Despite the limitations, CG was the standard to measure eGFR and therefore kidney function for almost 20 years.

In 1999, the Modification of Diet in Renal Disease (MDRD) study yielded a new equation to address the issues with the CG equation.[41] Weight was removed but a correction factor for race, specifically African American race, was added. Black patients enrolled in MDRD had a higher measured GFR than whites with the same SCr levels. Therefore a 1.6X modifier was added.[41] The authors stated that this difference in SCr was due to increased muscle mass found in black cohort enrollees.[41] Assumptions of muscle mass were taken from 3 older studies that had not measured muscle mass directly but instead relied on densitometry and visual determination.[42–44] In these previous studies, race was assigned by the researchers while the MDRD researchers allowed patients to define race.[42–44] The inclusion of this correction factor in the MDRD equation served to increase the eGFR value for black patients. So, with a similar SCr, black patients appeared to have better kidney function than white patients.

Differences in race-based eGFRs are believed to have contributed to delays in diagnosis, evaluation, treatment, and transplant listing for the African American population.[45] An update of the MDRD formula occurred in 2005 decreasing the race correction factor by 5% but the racial adjustment was left in the formula.[46]

In 2009, inclusion of multiple large data sets available through the National Institutes of Health (NIH) led to a revision of the MDRD formula. The chronic kidney disease epidemiology collaboration (CKD-EPI) equation had a larger participant pool with more African Americans, inclusion of healthy people (from the National Health and Nutrition Examination Survey [NHANES]), and individuals with conditions such as mild kidney disease, diabetes, and transplants. The data pool was still lacking significant numbers of Asian, Hispanic, or multiracial groups.[47] The CKD-EPI equation continued to use the race correction factor, but it was again adjusted downwards to 1.16.[47]

The discussion of race versus eGFR has many ramifications: from trials (NIH and drug trials) that are already in progress to laboratories that need to standardize testing to the FDA which uses eGFR to recommend medication dosages. Initial calculations of measured versus estimated GFR may have been affected by the inclusion of more "blue-collar" black workers versus "white collar" white workers. This would have meant that muscle mass was the difference in measured creatinine and not due to race.[48] In multiethnic populations, the measured GFR is closer to the uncorrected CKD-EPI equation.[49]

As more serum markers are discovered, cystatin C, beta-2-microglobulin (B2M), beta-trace protein (BTP), that are not dependent on muscle mass, as is the SCr, new eGFR calculators are being developed.[50,51] The National Kidney Foundation (NKF) and the American Society of Nephrology (ASN) created a task force in August 2020.[52] NKF-ASN stated that race will be removed from the eGFR calculators.[53] The initial report of the task force noted that simply removing race and using the old formulas will not be scientifically sound.[54] To allow all stakeholders to be heard, including patients for whom this can be life-changing, the task force spent over a year on this process.[54] In September 2021, the task force introduced a refitted CKD-EPI formula that not only removes race, but also developed an adjusted mathematical formula that includes diversity.[55] This CKD-EPI refit does not disproportionally affect any one group and can be introduced into laboratories nationwide immediately. The task force refers to this new formula as CKD-EPI (2021). Although the task force feels that the cystatin C eGFR formula should be used for confirmation of CKD and slowly introduced as a permanent replacement for creatinine, they realize that cost constraints do not allow widespread use of cystatin C at this time.

SUMMARY

As the rate of CKD shows no signs of slowing, increased provider education of the less common causes of kidney failure will be key. This article reviews some of these disorders to aid the primary care provider in identifying patients who require close monitoring of kidney function.

DISCLOSURE

Dr J. Davis is on the Amgen and Bayer Speakers Bureau. All authors were responsible for the research, development, and writing of the article.

REFERENCES

1. Centers for Disease Control and Prevention. Chronic kidney disease in the United States, 2021. Atlanta (GA): US Department of Health and Human Services, Centers

for Disease Control and Prevention; 2021. Available at: https://www.cdc.gov/kidneydisease/publications-resources/ckd-national-facts.html. Accessed May 5, 2021.

2. Gorenjak M. 4. Kidneys and Autoimmune Disease. EJIFCC 2009;20(1):28–32.
3. Cojocaru M, Cojocaru IM, Silosi I, et al. Manifestations of systemic lupus erythematosus. Maedica (Bucur) 2011;6(4):330–6.
4. Justiz Vaillant AA, Goyal A, Bansal P, et al. Systemic lupus erythematosus. In: StatPearls. Treasure Island (FL): StatPearls Publishing; 2021. Available at: https://www.ncbi.nlm.nih.gov/books/NBK535405/. Accessed May 5, 2021.
5. Shanmugam VK, Steen VD. Renal disease in scleroderma: an update on evaluation, risk stratification, pathogenesis and management. Curr Opin Rheumatol 2012;24(6):669–76.
6. Mouthon L, Bérezné A, Bussone G, et al. Scleroderma renal crisis: a rare but severe complication of systemic sclerosis. Clin Rev Allergy Immunol 2011;40(2):84–91.
7. Weiner D, Gilbert S, editors. National kidney foundation primer on kidney diseases. 7th edition. Philadelphia: Elsevier; 2017.
8. Jung SW, Park EJ, Kim JS, et al. Renal tubular acidosis in patients with primary Sjögren's syndrome. Electrolyte Blood Press 2017;15(1):17–22.
9. Ramos-Casals M, Nardi N, Brito-Zerón P, et al. Atypical autoantibodies in patients with primary Sjögren syndrome: clinical characteristics and follow-up of 82 cases. Semin Arthritis Rheum 2006;35(5):312–21.
10. Renaudineau Y, Le Meur Y. Renal involvement in Wegener's granulomatosis. Clin Rev Allergy Immunol 2008;35(1–2):22–9.
11. Geetha D, Kallenberg C, Stone JH, et al. Current therapy of granulomatosis with polyangiitis and microscopic polyangiitis: the role of rituximab. J Nephrol 2015; 28(1):17–27.
12. Landgren O, Hofmann JN, McShane CM, et al. Association of immune marker changes with progression of monoclonal gammopathy of undetermined significance to multiple myeloma. JAMA Oncol 2019;5(9):1293–301.
13. Heher EC, Rennke HG, Laubach JP, et al. Kidney disease and multiple myeloma. Clin J Am Soc Nephrol 2013;8(11):2007–17.
14. Rodrigues JC, Haas M, Reich HN. IgA Nephropathy. Clin J Am Soc Nephrol 2017; 12(4):677–86.
15. Duhig KE, Chappell LC, Shennan AH. How placental growth factor detection might improve diagnosis and management of pre-eclampsia. Expert Rev Mol Diagn 2014;14(4):403–6.
16. Phipps EA, Thadhani R, Benzing T, et al. Pre-eclampsia: pathogenesis, novel diagnostics and therapies. Nat Rev Nephrol 2019;15(5):275–89.
17. Chaiworapongsa T, Romero R, Kim YM, et al. Plasma soluble vascular endothelial growth factor receptor-1 concentration is elevated prior to the clinical diagnosis of pre-eclampsia. J Matern Fetal Neonatal Med 2005;17(1):3–18.
18. Shi DD, Yang FZ, Zhou L, et al. Oral nifedipine vs. intravenous labetalol for treatment of pregnancy-induced severe pre-eclampsia. J Clin Pharm Ther 2016;41(6):657–61.
19. Hurrell A, Beardmore-Gray A, Duhig K, et al. Placental growth factor in suspected preterm pre-eclampsia: a review of the evidence and practicalities of implementation. BJOG 2020;127(13):1590–7.
20. Poon LC, Shennan A, Hyett JA, et al. The International Federation of Gynecology and Obstetrics (FIGO) initiative on pre-eclampsia: a pragmatic guide for first-

trimester screening and prevention. Int J Gynaecol Obstet 2019;145(Suppl 1):1–33.

21. Magee LA, Pels A, Helewa M, et al. Canadian Hypertensive Disorders of Pregnancy (HDP) Working Group. Diagnosis, evaluation, and management of the hypertensive disorders of pregnancy. Pregnancy Hypertens 2014;4(2):105–45.

22. Chau K, Hennessy A, Makris A. Placental growth factor and pre-eclampsia. J Hum Hypertens 2017;31(12):782–6.

23. Bosch X, Poch E, Grau JM. Rhabdomyolysis and acute kidney injury. N Engl J Med 2009;361(1):62–72.

24. Huerta-Alardín AL, Varon J, Marik PE. Bench-to-bedside review: Rhabdomyolysis – an overview for clinicians. Crit Care 2005;9(2):158–69.

25. Hoste EAJ, Kellum JA, Selby NM, et al. Global epidemiology and outcomes of acute kidney injury. Nat Rev Nephrol 2018;14(10):607–25.

26. Esposito P, Estienne L, Serpieri N, et al. Rhabdomyolysis-associated acute kidney injury. Am J Kidney Dis 2018;71(6):A12–4.

27. Grigorian A, Gabriel V, Nguyen NT, et al. Black race and body mass index are risk factors for rhabdomyolysis and acute kidney injury in trauma. J Invest Surg 2020;33(3):283–90.

28. Torres PA, Helmstetter JA, Kaye AM, et al. Rhabdomyolysis: Pathogenesis, diagnosis, and treatment. Ochsner J 2015;15(1):58–69.

29. McMahon GM, Zeng X, Waikar SS. A risk prediction score for kidney failure or mortality in rhabdomyolysis. JAMA Intern Med 2013;173(19):1821–8.

30. Nielsen JS, Sally M, Mullins RJ, et al. Bicarbonate and mannitol treatment for traumatic rhabdomyolysis revisited. Am J Surg 2017;213(1):73–9.

31. Atta MG, Lucas GM, Fine DM. HIV-associated nephropathy: epidemiology, pathogenesis, diagnosis and management. Expert Rev Anti Infect Ther 2008;6(3):365–71.

32. Atta M, Zook K, Brown T, et al. Racial adjustment adversely affects glomerular filtration estimates in African Americans Living with HIV. J Am Soc Nephrol 2021;32(9):2143–7.

33. Lan X, Rao TK, Chander PN, et al. Apolipoprotein L1 (APOL1) Variants (Vs) a possible link between Heroin-associated Nephropathy (HAN) and HIV-associated Nephropathy (HIVAN). Front Microbiol 2015;6:571.

34. Thompson MA, Horberg MA, Agwu AL, et al. Primary care guidance for persons with human immunodeficiency virus: 2020 Update by the HIV Medicine Association of the Infectious Diseases Society of America. Clin Infect Dis 2020;73(11):e3572–605, ciaa1391.

35. Rosenberg AZ, Naicker S, Winkler CA, et al. HIV-associated nephropathies: epidemiology, pathology, mechanisms and treatment. Nat Rev Nephrol 2015;11(3):150–60.

36. Palau L, Menez S, Rodriguez-Sanchez J, et al. HIV-associated nephropathy: links, risks and management. HIV AIDS (Auckl) 2018;10:73–81.

37. Sanchez Polo V, Garcia-Trabanino R, Rodriguez G, et al. Mesoamerican Nephropathy (MeN): what we know so far. Int J Nephrol Renovasc Dis 2020;13:261–72.

38. Weiner DE, McClean MD, Kaufman JS, et al. The Central American epidemic of CKD. Clin J Am Soc Nephrol 2013;8(3):504–11.

39. Ferguson MA, Waikar SS. Established and emerging markers of kidney function. Clin Chem 2012;58(4):680–9.

40. National Kidney Foundation. Frequently asked questions about GFR. 2020. Available at: https://www.kidney.org/professionals/KDOQI/gfr. Accessed December 12, 2020.

41. Levey AS, Bosch JP, Lewis JB, et al. A more accurate method to estimate glomerular filtration rate from serum creatinine: a new prediction equation. Modification of Diet in Renal Disease Study Group. Ann Intern Med 1999;130(6):461–70.

42. Cohn SH, Abesamis C, Zanzi I, et al. Body elemental composition comparison between Black and White adults. Am J Physiol 1977;232(4):419–22.

43. Harsha DW, Frerichs RR, Berenson GS. Densitometry and anthropometry of Black and White Children. Hum Biol 1978;50(3):261–80.

44. Worrall JG, Phongsathorn V, Hooper RJ, et al. Racial variation in serum creatine kinase unrelated to lean body mass. Br J Rheumatol 1990;29(5):371–3.

45. Ahmed S, Nutt CT, Eneanya ND, et al. Examining the potential impact of race multiplier utilization in estimated glomerular filtration rate calculation on African American Care Outcomes. J Gen Intern Med 2020. https://doi.org/10.1007/s11606-020-06280-5.

46. Levey AS, Coresh J, Greene T, et al. Using standardized serum creatinine values in the modification of diet in renal disease study equation for estimating glomerular filtration rate. Ann Intern Med 2006;145(4):247–54 [Erratum appears in Ann Intern Med 2008;149(7):519].

47. Levey AS, Stevens LA, Schmid CH, et al. A new equation to estimate glomerular filtration rate. Ann Intern Med 2009;150(9):604–12 [Erratum appears in Ann Intern Med 2011;155(6):408].

48. Hsu J, Johansen KL, Hsu C, et al. Higher serum creatinine concentrations in black patients with Chronic Kidney Disease: beyond nutritional status and body composition. Clin J Am Soc Nephrol 2008;3(4):992–7.

49. Zanocco JA, Nishida SK, Passos MT, et al. Race adjustment for estimating glomerular filtration rate is not always necessary. Nephron Extra 2012;2(1):293–302.

50. Ferguson MA, Waikar SS. Established and emerging markers of kidney function. Clin Chem 2012;58(4):680–9.

51. Inker LA, Couture SJ, Tighiouart H, et al. on behalf of the CKD-EPI GFR Collaborators, A New Panel Estimated GFR, Including β2-Microglobulin and β-Trace Protein and Not Including Race, Developed in a Diverse Population. Am J Kidney Dis 2021;77(5):673–83.e1.

52. National Kidney Foundation. NKF and ASN form joint task force to focus on use of race in eGFR. Available at: https://www.kidney.org/newsletter/nkf-and-asn-form-joint-task-force-to-focus-use-race-egfr. Accessed December 26, 2020.

53. National Kidney Foundation. Removing race from kidney disease. Available at: https://www.kidney.org/news/removing-race-estimates-kidney-function. Accessed May 23, 2021.

54. Feldman HI, Briggs JP. Race and the Estimation of GFR: Getting it Right. J Am Soc Nephrol 2021;32(6):1269–70.

55. Delgado C, Baweja M, Crews D, et al. Unifying approach for GFR estimation: recommendations of the NKF-ASN task force on reassessing the inclusion of race in diagnosing kidney disease. J Am Soc Nephrol 2021;32(12):2994–3015.

The Failed Kidney
Beyond Redemption

Kara-Ann Valentine, MMS, PA-C[a], Amy Mosman, MMS, PA-C[b],*

KEYWORDS

- Kidney failure • Hemodialysis • Peritoneal dialysis • Kidney transplant
- Conservative management • Kidney replacement therapy

KEY POINTS

- Kidney failure ensues once the majority of function is lost and kidney replacement therapy is required to sustain life.
- The decision to initiate kidney replacement therapy is a shared decision between the practitioner and the patient-family unit and is not based solely on eGFR but rather on the presence of clinical manifestations of kidney failure.
- Hemodialysis is the most commonly used kidney replacement therapy modality; however, home therapies such as peritoneal dialysis are becoming more popular.
- Kidney transplant is the ultimate goal for eligible patients for the best prognosis.
- Conservative management may be appropriate for some patients based on frailty, comorbid conditions, impaired function, or patient preference.

INTRODUCTION

The kidneys are complex organs that play a role in various organ systems. They are primarily responsible for removing extra fluid, waste products, and bioactive substances from the blood, but are also involved in regulating blood pressure (BP), producing erythropoietin for red blood cell production, and converting vitamin D into its active form.[1] The interruption or failure of kidney function impacts these essential physiologic functions and places an individual at risk for shortened life expectancy. Kidney failure can occur abruptly as in acute kidney injury (AKI) or gradually from progressive chronic kidney disease (CKD). Regardless of speed, failure results in the accumulation of waste products and bioactive substances along with the inability to balance and control fluid, hormones, and electrolytes by the kidneys.[2]

[a] Barry University Physician Assistant Program, 11300 Northeast 2nd Avenue, Miami Shores, FL 33161, USA; [b] Division of Nephrology, Saint Louis University, 1008 S Spring Street, Saint Louis, MO 63110, USA
* Corresponding author.
E-mail address: Amy.mosman@health.slu.edu

Physician Assist Clin 7 (2022) 319–330
https://doi.org/10.1016/j.cpha.2021.11.005
2405-7991/22/© 2021 Elsevier Inc. All rights reserved.
physicianassistant.theclinics.com

CKD is defined as abnormal kidney findings, whether functional or structural, for more than 3 months and is categorized by stages I-V (**Fig. 1**).[3]

Some examples of abnormal kidney findings include:

- An estimated glomerular filtration rate (eGFR) less than 60 mL/min/1.73 m^2
- The presence of albumin in the urine or other urinary sediments
- Atrophic kidneys on diagnostic imaging.[2]

Kidney failure or end-stage kidney disease (ESKD) occurs with CKD stage V when kidney replacement therapy (KRT) is needed to sustain life. KRT is initiated when a patient either develops clinical manifestations of kidney failure, loss of volume and BP control, nutritional deprivation unresponsive to dietary intervention, and/or cognitive impairment (**Box 1**).[2]

There are 3 modalities for KRT: hemodialysis (HD), peritoneal dialysis (PD), and kidney transplant. A kidney transplant can potentially restore function, whereas HD, PD, and conservative kidney management (CKM) only compensate to a certain degree and for a limited amount of time. The purpose of this article is to discuss the initiation of KRT and CKM and to discuss how each modality is used in the management of ESKD.

Fast Facts

- The Center for Disease Control and Prevention (CDC) states that approximately 37 million American adults likely have CKD and alarmingly most of them are unaware of their diagnosis, with 40% of this group having severe CKD[4]

Prognosis of CKD by GFR and Albuminuria Categories: KDIGO 2012			Persistent albuminuria categories Description and range		
			A1	A2	A3
			Normal to mildly increased	Moderately increased	Severely increased
			<30 mg/g <3 mg/mmol	30-300 mg/g 3-30 mg/mmol	>300 mg/g >30 mg/mmol
GFR categories (ml/min/ 1.73 m²) Description and range	G1	Normal or high	≥90		
	G2	Mildly decreased	60-89		
	G3a	Mildly to moderately decreased	45-59		
	G3b	Moderately to severely decreased	30-44		
	G4	Severely decreased	15-29		
	G5	Kidney failure	<15		

Fig. 1. Heat map illustrating the stages of kidney disease. GFR, glomerular filtration rate.[3] (*From* Inker LA, Astor BC, Fox CH, et al. KDOQI US commentary on the 2012 KDIGO clinical practice guideline for the evaluation and management of CKD. Am J Kidney Dis. 2014 May;63(5):713-35.)

Box 1
Clinical manifestations of kidney failure[2]

- Anorexia, nausea, and vomiting
- Acid-base disorder (eg, metabolic acidosis)
- Electrolyte imbalance (eg, hyperkalemia)
- Pruritus
- Serositis

- The leading causes of ESKD in the United States are diabetes mellitus and hypertension, 75% of new cases[4]
- Kidney disease is the 10th leading cause of death in the United States
- The cost to treat patients with ESKD, not including prescription medications, was $36 billion in 2018[4]
- The CDC reports that 360 people start dialysis daily[4]
- According to the United States Renal Data System (USRDS), in 2018, more than 554,000 patients were on dialysis and more than 229,000 with a functioning kidney transplant[5]

COVID-19 AND KIDNEY DISEASE

The CDC reports CKD as one of the several underlying conditions associated with a higher risk for severe COVID-19 illness (ie, requiring intensive care unit [ICU] or similar unit admission, invasive mechanical ventilation, and death).[6] Hospitalized COVID-19 patients are at substantial risk for AKI, which correlates to severe illness, need for dialysis, and increased mortality. For patients who needed dialysis during the initial COVID crisis, hospitals and ICUs were often overwhelmed by a need for HD machines and experienced staff. Several New York hospitals moved to use PD in their ICUs to manage patients with good results.[7] Many patients who recover from COVID-19–related AKI continue to have decreased kidney function and are now at higher risk of developing CKD and ESKD.[8]

Patients with ESKD are at a higher risk for severe disease and mortality with COVID-19 and a congregate setting such as a dialysis center could potentially increase the risk of contracting COVID-19. This has led to an uptick in the interest in home therapies. Transmission within the dialysis unit, however, has been low, overall thanks to a comprehensive and widespread infection control response. This response includes universal masking in the center; social distancing in units and waiting rooms; and diligent screening, testing, and isolating protocols.[9]

GUIDELINES FOR INITIATION OF DIALYSIS

The Kidney Disease Improving Global outcomes (KDIGO) guidelines recommend that patients with progressive CKD and greater than 10% to 20% chance for ESKD within 1 year be referred to kidney specialists for planning of KRT in advance of initiation.[3] Although not all patients will progress to ESKD, it is still crucial to discuss plans for ESKD. A physician (or provider)-patient relationship must be formed to establish a rapport for shared decision-making. The provider should fully educate patients on their diagnosis, specific prognosis, and available treatment options. Then the provider-patient team can implement an advanced care plan as patients recognize their goals for care and start to make decisions for their future health care, including if dialysis should be started and under what circumstances it should be discontinued.[10]

Previous studies had suggested that early initiation of dialysis with a higher eGFR could improve patient outcomes. However, the Initiating Dialysis Early and Late (IDEAL) study gave pause to this as it showed no improvement in survival or patient-centered outcome with strategic early initiation of dialysis versus later. The findings were impactful for several reasons; the early initiation of dialysis was associated with an increase in overall cost with no benefit of improved patient outcomes.[11] The trend of a later start in the use of dialysis after the IDEAL study has not shown any worsening of patient outcomes.[6] All current global guidelines, except for the Canada Association of Nephrology's 2014 clinical practice guidelines, now avoid the recommendation of dialysis initiation based on eGFR in the absence of uremic symptoms allowing for a more patient-centered approach.[12]

HEMODIALYSIS

HD is the most common form of KRT used in the United States.[6] In HD, blood runs along a circuit opposite a dialysate solution to filter water; excess electrolytes such as potassium, sodium, and phosphorus; and toxins including urea across a semipermeable membrane (the "dialyzer"). The 2 main principles behind traditional HD are hemofiltration and diffusion, which are used conjointly for most outpatient treatments. Diffusion removes solutes via a countercurrent circuit across the semipermeable membrane. Hemofiltration refers to solute removal via convection or solvent drag, which occurs as water is forced through the membrane from high to low pressure to produce an ultrafiltrate. When combined, these processes are known as hemodiafiltration. Dialysate solution generally contains a low potassium and magnesium concentration, normal glucose concentration, and varying calcium and bicarbonate concentrations to properly balance the patient's accumulating electrolytes and acid load between treatments.[13]

Typical outpatient, in-center HD treatments require an average of 4 hours thrice weekly to adequately support the patient and safely remove excess/toxic solutes and fluid. For those with close adherence to care plans and significant residual kidney function, these sessions can sometimes be reduced in frequency or duration. Some patients choose nocturnal dialysis, where treatments may still be in-center but are administered slower and over a longer duration (6–8 hours per night). A third option is home HD, which can be done with a variety of prescriptions for time and number of days, including short daily or nocturnal, according to patient preferences and treatment dose requirements.[13] **Tables 1–3** list pros and cons for these HD options.

Adequate vascular access is crucial to successful HD treatment and the long-term prognosis of the patient. The following 3 main access types exist: arteriovenous fistula (AVF), arteriovenous graft (AVG: an arterial-venous connection via prosthetic or bovine conduit), and central venous catheter (CVC). The choice among these options depends on the patient's anatomy, long-term dialysis expectations, and time to HD initiation. Although a *"fistula first"* approach has been traditionally followed in the United States, the latest KDOQI guidelines stress individualization to allow for *"the right access in the right patient at the right time for the right reasons."* CVCs, however, remain least desirable because of their higher risk of infection, hospitalization rate and mortality, and damage to central vessels. CVC use is limited to patients who:

- Are not surgical candidates
- Have an imminent kidney transplant planned

Table 1
Pros and cons of traditional in-center hemodialysis[14,15]

Pros	Cons
• Continuous nursing/technician care and monitoring during treatment • Little patient responsibility for treatment administration • Camaraderie/socialization with fellow patients	• Reliance on health care providers/less individual control of treatments • Regular transportation time and costs • Regimented schedule demands • Requires adequate vascular access and needle cannulation • Higher rates of treatment side effects • Strict diet and fluid requirements

- Must start HD before an AV fistula or graft is placed/useable.

Planning vascular access early is crucial to have a viable AVF or AVG when HD is initiated. Therefore, it is recommended to start the process when a patient's eGFR is around 15 to 20 mL/min/1.72 m^2.[16] Starting treatment with an AVF or AVG remains difficult to achieve, as 80.8% of HD patients in the United States still start HD via CVC as of 2018.[6]

HD comes with a variety of complications and demands, both in and out of treatment. Some complications can lead to larger issues and worsen mortality risk. Intradialytic hypotension, for example, can induce myocardial stunning, dysrhythmias, kidney ischemia (and loss of residual function), seizures, and/or loss of consciousness.

Other complications include:

- Cramping with fluid/osmolality shifts
- Fatigue
- Pruritus
- Dysrhythmias/sudden cardiac death irrespective of BP
- Bacteremia/access infections
- Allergic reactions to dialyzer.[17]

Many of these issues are reduced/improved by longer and/or more frequent dialysis.[15,17–19] Beyond the demands of HD treatment, patients must also manage a diet low in phosphorus, sodium, and potassium and fluids restricted to account for interdialytic accumulation and higher in protein to account for losses from various sources including inflammation, uremia, and the catabolic effects of HD.[20] Again, these dietary considerations are usually liberalized with longer or more frequent HD and residual kidney function.[15,18,19]

Table 2
Pros and cons of in-center nocturnal hemodialysis[14,15]

Pros	Cons
Continuous nursing/technician care and monitoring during treatment • Little patient responsibility for treatment administration • Commonly: ○ Liberalized diet/fluid restrictions ○ Lower side effects of treatment ○ Lower medication requirements	• Reliance on health care providers/less individual control of treatments • Regular transportation time and costs • Regimented schedule demands • Requires adequate vascular access and needle cannulation

Table 3
Pros and cons of home hemodialysis[18,19]?

Pros	Cons
• Liberalized schedule	• Full treatment responsibility on patient
• No transportation demands	• Requires adequate vascular access and self-cannulation
• Commonly:	• May require a care partner for emergencies
○ Liberalized diet/fluid restrictions	• Utility costs and home space, storage, and cleanliness needed for setup
○ Lower side effects of treatment	
○ Lower medication requirements	

PERITONEAL DIALYSIS

PD uses the peritoneum for diffusion and ultrafiltration rather than the extracorporeal system of HD. Dialysate solution fills the peritoneal cavity and waste products are drained by an indwelling catheter, which can be placed surgically or by radiologic intervention. The 2 to 3 L bags of PD dialysate or *"PD solution"* consists of sodium chloride, calcium, magnesium, lactate for bicarbonate, and glucose for ultrafiltration. Bags of PD dialysate come in varying glucose concentrations depending on the amount of fluid removal needed per treatment.[21]

PD requires multiple solution exchanges to adequately dialyze the patient each day. This can be completed by 2 different strategies: continuous ambulatory peritoneal dialysis (CAPD) or continuous cycling peritoneal dialysis (CCPD, also referred to as automated PD or APD). CAPD is completed by the patient manually instilling and draining bags of solution throughout the day. Usually, 4 cycles are needed over 24 hours. In CCPD, a machine or "cycler" automatically fills and drains solution according to a programmed prescription overnight, completed over 8 to 10 hours. Some patients on CCPD also retain some dialysate in daytime hours for additional treatment. Prescriptions for PD vary by time and number of fluid exchanges based on the patient's body size, residual kidney function, and peritoneal membrane qualities. The last of these is assessed by a peritoneal equilibration test, which evaluates how quickly diffusion and ultrafiltration peak with fresh peritoneal dialysate.[21]

PD is the preferred kidney replacement option for pediatric patients and is strongly encouraged for most capable patients.[21] A PD catheter has a lower infection rate than a CVC and is known for being a gentler, softer form of dialysis than HD, and its aforementioned side effects.[21–23] PD also has financial advantages for the patient, with Medicare eligibility starting immediately instead of the 3-month wait for those started on HD.[24] Despite its advantages, most patients still start on HD as previously noted.[6] **Table 4** lists the pros and cons of PD.

Preparations for PD include placement of a peritoneal catheter and training for the patient and/or treatment partner if used. Ideally, training and use of the peritoneal catheter is done 14 days after insertion; however, urgent start PD can be done at experienced centers, usually started 2 to 3 days after catheter insertion. Low dialysate volumes are used initially, patients are often required to lie flat during the procedure and there is a higher risk initially for fluid leaks around the exit site and catheter malfunction. Despite risks, this strategy is effective to avoid even brief stints on HD, as many patients who start on HD fail to convert to PD.[22]

Several complications and considerations exist for PD. For diabetics, the dialysate glucose may complicate serum glucose and weight control.[21,25]

Table 4
Pros and cons of peritoneal dialysis[21,25]

Pros	Cons
• Completed at home	• Patient fully responsible for performing treatments
• Flexible schedule for patient	• Requires extended time in one location for treatments
• Travel flexibility	(CCPD)
• Preserves residual renal function	• Requires room at home for supplies and a clean, secluded space for sterile PD steps
• No vascular access needs	• Must be performed every day
• Commonly:	
○ Liberalized diet/fluid restrictions	
○ Lower side effects of treatment	
○ Lower medication requirements	

Other complications include:

- Infections
- Fluid leaks
- Catheter migration/dysfunction
- Hernias
- Peritoneal membrane failure (unable to reach adequacy/ultrafiltration goals)
- Dyslipidemia and metabolic syndrome.[26]

Infections (peritonitis or exit site) are the most common issue, with 0.28 episodes/patient-year. Training on sterile techniques and frequent refreshers by the PD nurse help to minimize infection episodes. Also, bowel regimens are closely followed to avoid catheter malfunction and peritonitis risk.[26]

COMORBID CONDITIONS IN ESKD

Conditions present in almost all patients with ESKD include:

- Secondary renal hyperparathyroidism/mineral-bone disease (MBD)—This develops as the eGFR declines and causes abnormalities in calcium, phosphorus, parathyroid hormone (PTH), and vitamin D. Treatment is multifactorial including oral binders to lower serum phosphorus toward normal, balancing of serum calcium, and use of vitamin D and calcimimetics to lower PTH.[27]
- Anemia—Main contributors include reduced erythropoietin production from the failing kidneys and iron deficiency. Treatment includes iron replacement (orally or IV), erythropoietin stimulating agents along with screening for exacerbating factors such as inflammation, chronic blood losses, and so forth.[28]
- Hypertension and fluid overload—These intertwined issues require treatment in tandem, with fluid removal, antihypertensives, and dietary salt/fluid restrictions to reach goal BP. Mortality in patients with ESKD is predominantly cardiovascular in nature. In relation to BP, this mortality risk is U-shaped in that patients with extreme lows or elevations in BP are at the highest risk.[29,30]

DIALYSIS AND THE INTERDISCIPLINARY TEAM

Given the challenges and burdens of ESKD and dialysis, a multidisciplinary team is crucial for success. Each dialysis unit includes such a team for patients of all modalities. This includes a dietician and social worker in addition to the nephrologist (and PA/NP) and nursing staff. Registered dieticians assist patients with fluid and food restrictions as well as assessing for protein wasting, food insecurities, and oral health. They also work on MBD closely with the nephrology providers. Social workers assist with connecting patients to community resources, evaluating mental health and quality of life, and monitoring all psychosocial needs.[31]

KIDNEY TRANSPLANT

Dialysis is ideally a bridge to the ultimate goal of kidney transplantation. Kidney transplant allows for kidney replacement leading to the longest life span opportunity.[32] Kidneys can come from deceased or living donors, the latter being particularly important given the shortage of deceased donor kidneys available compared with the number of patients in need. Living donors can be related or unrelated. Exchanged kidney donations, also referred to as "paired" or "domino" exchange, can maximize the number of patients transplanted.[33]

The United Network for Organ Sharing (UNOS) modified the kidney allocation system in 2014 to better match the health of a donor kidney to the health—and thus expected life span—of the recipient. Instead of distributing purely on waitlist time, the donor organ is assigned an index value (Kidney Donor Profile Index or KDPI) based on various health factors. This is matched to a patient with the most equivalent estimated post-transplant survival. Patients can be listed before dialysis (pre-emptive transplant, eGFR <20 mL/min/1.72 m^2) or after dialysis initiation.[32] Those listed after starting dialysis are credited waitlist time starting from their date of the first dialysis, another change made by UNOS to address system disparities.[34]

Transplant candidacy criteria vary from center to center. Evaluation is extensive, including but not limited to:

- Cardiopulmonary health: Focused on coronary artery disease, congestive heart failure, peripheral vessel disease (for transplant perfusion), pulmonary hypertension, and chronic lung diseases
- Urologic function: Voiding and retention capabilities, infection risks, and so forth
- Malignancy screening
- Autoimmune and hematologic/hypercoagulable conditions
- Infectious disease/bloodborne pathogen screening: HIV+ and hepatitis C+ patients may still receive kidneys, including those with matching viral infection
- Alcohol, tobacco, and illicit substance use: Smoking cessation is often required pretransplant; marijuana policies vary
- Control of metabolic conditions such as diabetes and obesity
- Compliance with dialysis and treatment plan
- Psychosocial health and social support
- Age: Advanced age may require a living donor for eligibility.[35]

Time waiting for a kidney varies across the country; however, the average wait is 3 to 5 years.[32]

CONSERVATIVE KIDNEY MANAGEMENT

This option is also referred to as comprehensive conservative care, comfort care, or active medical management without dialysis. A choice of CKM indicates a shared decision has been made to continue management of ESKD without dialysis or transplant.[36] This can be the result of patient preference or by medical advice.[37] The goal of CKM is to optimize quality of life and symptom control.[36] It involves intervention to protect remaining kidney function, limit adverse events, decrease uremic symptoms, and maintain fluid balance and nutritional status.[37–39] Some tools for this include:

- dietary protein, fluid, and food restrictions
- loop diuretics
- potassium and phosphorus binders
- calcium regulatory agents and vitamin D supplements
- hypertension and anemia pharmacologic agents.

A choice of CKM can be made during initial planning for KRT or anytime into their management via dialysis. One reason for deciding to forgo dialysis initially or discontinue dialysis is when the patient has a poor prognosis or dialysis cannot be safely delivered. This is the case with patients with impaired functional status and multiple comorbidities.[10,39] Nephrology should recommend palliative care if not already a part of management as patients report a high symptom burden with CKM.[38,39] A systematic review by O'Connor and colleagues reported a patient median survival range of 6 to 23 months with CKM, whereas imminent death occurs for those who withdraw from dialysis to start CKM.[39]

Traditionally, patients who are already on dialysis must cease dialysis treatments to be eligible for hospice services. However, a Washington state program has started the first palliative care program housed in a dialysis center in the country. The Seattle-based dialysis center program provides palliative care to ESKD patients on HD and then matches patients with hospice care through a partnering company. This allows the patient to continue HD along with traditional hospice services. This concept may become a precedent in coming years.[40]

SUMMARY

KRT is used when kidney failure is too severe to sustain life. Current guidelines emphasize the need for planning of KRT well before it is initiated. Nephrology and the patient-family unit share in the planning and the decision-making process. Important decisions include choosing the modality of KRT including discussion of CKM along with the timing of initiation if dialysis is chosen. Initiation of dialysis should be based on clinical manifestations, which often coincide with an eGFR between 5 and 10 mL/min/1.73 m^2. The modality with the best 10-year survival is kidney transplant but this option is limited by patient health and number of available kidneys. HD and PD are more accessible but have their own drawbacks. Conservative kidney management allows for some semblance of quality of life without placing patients at risk for dialysis-related complications. There is much to be researched to enhance the current practices in the management of kidney failure and more to be done in the education of patients with kidney disease and the global nephrology community.

CLINICS CARE POINTS

- Management of kidney failure begins well before the patient needs renal replacement therapy. Patient education and counseling should occur during CKD stage 4.

- The ideal choice for renal replacement therapy is kidney transplant but due to limited availability, dialysis is the more prevalent modality. Both forms of dialysis come with advantages and disadvantages.

- Conservative kidney management is a practical option for a select group of patients who have a treatment goal of highest quality of life available versus lifespan extension.

- COVID-19 is a risk factor for CKD and ESKD in those with a history of COVID-19–related AKI. Patients with ESKD are also at a higher risk for severe disease and mortality with COVID-19 infection.

DISCLOSURE

The authors have nothing to disclose.

REFERENCES

1. How your kidneys work. National Kidney Foundation. Available at: https://www. kidney.org/kidneydisease/howkidneyswrk. September 9, 2021.
2. Kidney Disease: Improving Global Outcomes (KDIGO) CKD Work Group. KDIGO 2012 Clinical Practice Guideline for the Evaluation and Management of Chronic Kidney Disease. Kidney Int 2013;3:1–150.
3. Inker LA, Astor BC, Fox CH, et al. KDOQI US commentary on the 2012 KDIGO clinical practice guideline for the evaluation and management of CKD. Am J Kidney Dis 2014;63(5):713–35.
4. Chronic Kidney Disease Basics. Centers for Disease Control and Prevention. Available at: https://www.cdc.gov/kidneydisease/basics.html. [Accessed 7 September 2021].
5. United States Renal Data System. 2020 USRDS Annual Data report: Epidemiology of kidney disease in the United States. Bethesda, MD: National Institutes of Health, National Institute of Diabetes and Digestive and Kidney Diseases; 2020.
6. Kompaniyets L, Pennington AF, Goodman AB, et al. Underlying Medical Conditions and Severe Illness Among 540,667 Adults Hospitalized With COVID-19, March 2020–March 2021. Prev Chronic Dis 2021;18:210123.
7. Sourial MY, Sourial MH, Dalsan R, et al. Urgent Peritoneal Dialysis in Patients With COVID-19 and Acute Kidney Injury: A Single-Center Experience in a Time of Crisis in the United States. Am J Kidney Dis 2020;76(3):401–6.
8. Kidney disease & COVID-19. National Kidney Foundation. Available at: https://www. kidney.org/coronavirus/kidney-disease-covid-19. [Accessed 7 September 2021].
9. Hsu CM, Weiner DE, Aweh G, et al. COVID-19 among US dialysis patients: risk factors and outcomes from a national dialysis provider. Am J Kidney Dis 2021; 77(5):748–56.
10. Shared Decision-Making in the Appropriate Initiation of and Withdrawal from Dialysis, RPA clinical practice guideline. 2nd ed. Available at:https://connect.aahpm. org/HigherLogic/System/DownloadDocumentFile.ashx?DocumentFileKey=6ec 5a73d-ecab-44f9-b3ee-7e99702e67b5. [Accessed 15 September 2021].
11. Cooper BA, Branley P, Bulfone L, et al. for the IDEAL Study. A randomized controlled trial of early versus late initiation of dialysis. N Engl J Med 2010; 363(7):609–19.
12. Rivara MB, Mehrotra R. Timing of Dialysis Initiation – What Has Changed Since IDEAL? Semin Nephrol 2017;37(2):181–93.
13. Kotanko P, Kuhlmann MK, Chan C, et al. Hemodialysis: principles and techniques. In: Comprehensive clinical nephrology. 6th ed. Elsevier; 2019. p. 1073–81. Available at: https://www-clinicalkey-com.ezp.slu.edu/#!/content/book/3-s2.0-B9780323479097000937. [Accessed 25 August 2021].
14. In-center hemodialysis. Fresenius Kidney Care. Available at: https://www. freseniuskidneycare.com/treatment/in-center-hemodialysis. [Accessed 31 August 2021].
15. In-center treatment. Fresenius Kidney Care. Available at: https://www. freseniuskidneycare.com/treatment/in-center-hemodialysis/treatment-options. [Accessed 31 August 2021].

16. Lok CE, Huber TS, Lee T, et al. KDOQI Vascular Access Guideline Work Group. KDOQI clinical practice guideline for vascular access: 2019 update. Am J Kidney Dis 2020;75(4 suppl 2):S1–164.

17. Polkinghorne KR, Kerr PG. Acute complications during hemodialysis. In: Comprehensive clinical nephrology. 6th ed. Elsevier; 2019. p. 1090–102. Available at: https://www-clinicalkey-com.ezp.slu.edu/#!/content/book/3-s2.0-B97803 23479097000950?scrollTo=%23top. [Accessed 27 August 2021].

18. Home hemodialysis. National Kidney Foundation. 2020. Available at: https://www.kidney.org/atoz/content/homehemo. [Accessed 27 August 2021].

19. Home hemodialysis. Fresenius Kidney Care. Available at: https://www.freseniuskidneycare.com/treatment/home-hemodialysis. [Accessed 31 August 2021].

20. Ikizler TA, Deger SM. Nutritional management of hemodialysis patients. In: Handbook of dialysis therapy. 5th ed. Elsevier; 2017. p. 501–10.

21. Rippe B. Peritoneal dialysis: principles, techniques, and adequacy. In: Comprehensive clinical nephrology. 6th ed. Elsevier; 2019. p. 1103–13.

22. Blake PG, Jain AK. Urgent Start Peritoneal Dialysis: Defining What It Is and Why It Matters. Clin J Am Soc Nephrol 2018;13(8):1278–9.

23. Lok CE. Urgent peritoneal dialysis or hemodialysis catheter dialysis. J Vasc Access 2016;17(Suppl 1):S56–9.

24. Medicare Coverage of Kidney Dialysis and Kidney Transplant Services. Centers for Medicare and Medicaid Services. 2020. Available at: https://www.medicare.gov/Pubs/pdf/10128-Medicare-Coverage-ESRD.pdf. [Accessed 1 September 2021].

25. Home peritoneal dialysis. Fresenius Kidney Care. Available at: https://www.freseniuskidneycare.com/treatment/peritoneal-dialysis. [Accessed 1 September 2021].

26. Davies SJ, Wilkie ME. Complications of peritoneal dialysis. In: Comprehensive clinical nephrology. 6th ed. Elsevier; 2019. p. 1114–23.

27. Kidney Disease: Improving Global Outcomes (KDIGO) CKD-MBD Update Work Group. KDIGO 2017 clinical practice guideline update for the diagnosis, evaluation, prevention, and treatment of chronic kidney disease–mineral and bone disorder (CKD-MBD). Kidney Int Suppl 2017;7:1–59.

28. Kidney Disease: Improving Global Outcomes (KDIGO) Anemia Work Group. KDIGO clinical practice guideline for anemia in chronic kidney disease. *Kidney Int* Suppl 2012;2:279–335.

29. Agarwal R, Flynn J, Pogue V, et al. Assessment and management of hypertension in patients on dialysis. J Am Soc Nephrol 2014;25:1630–46.

30. Bansal N, McCulloch CE, Rahman M, et al. for the CRIC Study Investigators. Blood pressure and risk of all-cause mortality in advanced chronic kidney disease and hemodialysis: the chronic renal insufficiency cohort study. Hypertension 2015;65(1):93–100.

31. Your dialysis care team. National Kidney Foundation; 2016. Available at: https://www.kidney.org/atoz/content/dialcareteam. [Accessed 8 September 2021].

32. The kidney transplant waitlist: what you need to know, National Kidney Foundation. 2021. Available at: https://www.kidney.org/atoz/content/transplant-waitlist. [Accessed 8 September 2021].

33. Montgomery RA, Gentry SE, Marks WH, et al. Domino paired kidney donation: a strategy to make best use of live non-directed donation. Lancet 2006;368(9533):419–21.

34. Hart A, Gustafson SK, Skeans MA, et al. OPTN/SRTR 2015 Annual Data Report: Early effects of the new kidney allocation system. Am J Transplant 2017;17(Suppl 1):543–64.

35. Bunnapradist S, Danovitch GM. Evaluation of adult kidney transplant candidates. AJKD 2007;50(5):890–8.

36. Conservative management for kidney failure. National Institute of Diabetes and Digestive and Kidney Diseases. Available at: https://www.niddk.nih.gov/health-information/kidney-disease/kidney-failure/conservative-management#what. [Accessed 10 September 2021].

37. Harris DCH, Davies SJ, Finkelstein FO, et al. for the Working Groups of the International Society of Nephrology's 2nd Global Kidney Health Summit. Increasing access to integrated ESKD care as part of universal health coverage. Kidney Int 2019;95(4S):S1–33.

38. NKF KDOQI Guidelines. Clinical Practice Guidelines and Clinical Practice Recommendations. 2006 Updates: Hemodialysis Adequacy, Peritoneal Dialysis Adequacy, Vascular Access. Available at: http://kidneyfoundation.cachefly.net/professionals/KDOQI/guideline_upHD_PD_VA/hd_guide1.htm. [Accessed 1 September 2021].

39. O'Connor NR, Kumar P. Conservative management of end-stage renal disease without dialysis: a systematic review. J Palliat Med 2012;15(2):228–35.

40. Aleccia J. Innovative Washington state program provides palliative care to end-stage kidney patients. Kaiser Health News; 2021. Available at: https://www.oregonlive.com/pacific-northwest-news/2021/09/innovative-washington-state-program-provides-palliative-care-to-end-stage-kidney-patients.html. [Accessed 8 September 2021].

The Grocery Store Dilemma

Rebecca Grillo, PA-C, RD, LD/N[a],*, Ciara Mitchell, MA, RD, LD[b]

KEYWORDS

- Chronic kidney disease ● Nutrition fact label ● Fluid ● Sodium ● Protein
- Dietary supplements ● Education

KEY POINTS

- In the United States, two complications associated with obesity, diabetes, and hypertension, are on the rise causing an increase in the incidence of kidney disease.
- Dietary recommendations are based on the stage of kidney disease, comorbidities, and medications.
- Consumers are using nutrition tools but finding it difficult to identify healthy options, including the safety of nutrition supplements.
- Overall, there is not a one-size-fits-all solution to any dietary recommendation for patients living with kidney disease; therefore, a referral to nephrology, a dietitian, or nutrition professional may be imperative.

INTRODUCTION

Chronic kidney disease (CKD) is staged 1 to 5 depending on the severity[1–4] (**Fig. 1**). The patients stage of kidney disease as well as different types of medications and other comorbidities can alter dietary recommendations. In CKD, multiple medications are often used with opposite side-effect profiles. An example is spironolactone, which may increase serum potassium compared to furosemide, which may reduce serum potassium. Diet plays a key role in guiding patients to manage their kidney disease.

According to the US Department of Agriculture (USDA), Americans spend close to 10% of their disposable income on food expenditures, the largest part spent in full-service restaurants.[5] Overtime, the amount of disposable personal income spent on food has decreased, leading to negative implications on the diversity of dietary intake, food security, and food waste. Dietary energy requirements for day-to-day survival are more readily met by those at higher income levels, whereas lower income patient's budgets are spent on cheaper, more starchy foods (ie, rice, potatoes, and bread), leading to less nutritious, less diversified diets.[5]

The 2019 American Heart Association (AHA) food labeling survey reported 59% of participants always read labels on a packaged food before buying it the first time. Nearly all consumers surveyed stated they look for healthy options when grocery

[a] Renal Hypertension Center, 14134 Nephron Lane, Hudson, FL 34667, USA; [b] University of Alabama at Birmingham, 3276 Cahaba Manor Drive, Trussville, AL 35173, USA
* Corresponding author.
E-mail address: reba02@embarqmail.com

Physician Assist Clin 7 (2022) 331–345
https://doi.org/10.1016/j.cpha.2021.11.017   **physicianassistant.theclinics.com**

				Albuminuria categories		
				A1	**A2**	**A3**
				Normal to mildly increased	Moderately increased	Severely increased
				<30 mg/g <3 mg/mmol	30-299 mg/g 3-29 mg/mmol	≥300 mg/g ≥30 mg/mmol
GFR Stages	**G1**	Normal or high	≥90			
	G2	Mildly decreased	60-90			
	G3a	Mildly to moderately decreased	45-59			
	G3b	Moderately to severely decreased	30-44			
	G4	Severely decreased	15-29			
	G5	Kidney failure	<15			

Key to Figure:
Colors: Represents the risk for progression, morbidity and mortality by color from best to worst.
Green: Low Risk (if no other markers of kidney disease, no CKD)
Yellow: Moderately Increased Risk
Orange: High Risk
Red: Very High Risk
Deep Red: Highest Risk

Fig. 1. Stages of kidney disease (Estimated Glomerular Filtration Rate. National Kidney Foundation. www.kidney.org/atoz/content/gfr. Produced by the National Kidney Foundation, Inc. All rights reserved.)

shopping. This behavior was more common among younger, highly educated consumers. The survey concluded consumers usually read food packaging labels but found it difficult to identify healthy food options.[6]

SO, WHAT IS A FOOD LABEL?

In 2016, The *Nutrition Facts* label on packaged foods was revised to reflect updated scientific data including information about the link between diet and chronic diseases such as obesity (**Fig. 2**).[7] The updated label makes it easier for consumers to make healthier, more informed food choices and was expected to be implemented by all manufacturers by 2021. Changes to the label include a bolded, larger print for serving size and calories; an updated daily values section; a new line included for "added sugars;" and nutrients such as vitamin D, calcium, iron, and potassium with the actual amount per serving listed instead of simply the nutrients' percent daily value.[7] For

1. Serving Size

This section is the basis for determining the number of calories, amount of each nutrient, and percent Daily Value (%DV) of a food. Use it to compare a serving size to how much you actually eat. Serving sizes are given in familiar units, such as cups or pieces, followed by the metric amount, e.g., number of grams. The serving size reflects the amount people typically eat and drink today. It is not a recommendation of how much to eat.

2. Amount of Calories

If you want to manage your weight (lose, gain, or maintain), this section is especially helpful. The key is to balance how many calories you eat with how many calories your body uses.

3. Nutrients

You can use the label to support your personal dietary needs—look for foods that contain more of the nutrients you want to get more of and less of the nutrients you may want to limit.

• Nutrients to get more of: Dietary Fiber, Vitamin D, Calcium, Iron and Potassium. The recommended goal is to consume at least 100% Daily Value for each of these nutrients each day.

• Nutrients to get less of: Saturated fat, Sodium, and Added Sugars. The recommended goal is to stay below 100% Daily Value for each of these nutrients each day.

4. Percent Daily Value

This section tells you whether the nutrients (for example, saturated fat, sodium, dietary fiber, etc.) in one serving of food contribute a little or a lot to your total daily diet: 5%DV or less is low and 20%DV or more is high.

5. Footnote

The footnote explains that the %Daily Value (DV) tells you how much a nutrient in a serving of food contributes to a daily diet. 2,000 calories a day is used for general nutrition advice.

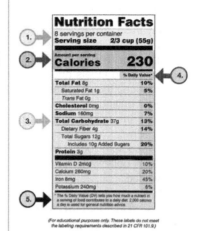

Fig. 2. Nutrition facts label.[8] (*From* United States Department of Agriculture. Nutrition Facts Labels for Download. Food and Drug Administration. Available at: www.fda.gov/food/food-labeling-nutrition/nutrition-facts-label-images-download. https://nam11.safelinks.protection. outlook.com/?url=http%3A%2F%2Fwww.fda.gov%2Ffood%2Ffood-labeling-nutrition% 2Fnutrition-facts-label-images-download&data=04%7C01%7CE.Bennitta%40elsevier.com% 7C753b6bffa82c4e947dac08d9ca10d8ba%7C9274ee3f94254109a27f9fb15c10675d.)

patients living with kidney disease, this can be especially important as the updated food label now includes milligrams of potassium per serving. Not only is potassium a concern, but as kidney function deteriorates, patients are faced with ongoing abnormal laboratory tests and adjustments for serum bicarbonate, calcium, phosphorus, parathyroid hormone, and vitamin D. With all of this in mind, what is a consumer living with kidney disease supposed to focus on when evaluating dietary intake or reading food labels? As stated in the 2019 AHA survey, consumers read food labels but find it difficult to identify healthy food options; this is much harder for patients with chronic disease, especially those with kidney disease. Herein lies the grocery store dilemma.

Fluid and Sodium Restrictions

Many issues arise when researching nutrition and kidney disease, as dietary recommendations are based on many different factors: stage of kidney disease, medications, and comorbidities. Reducing sodium intake benefits most patients, especially those with hypertension (HTN). The USDA Guidelines recommend less than 2300 mg of sodium a day.[9] The *Kidney Disease: Improving Global Outcomes (KDIGO)* guidelines suggest targeting a sodium intake less than 2000 mg of sodium per day in patients with HTN and/or CKD.[10] Consuming too much sodium puts a patient at increased risk for developing serious medical conditions including HTN, heart disease, and stroke. The typical American diet contains a daily average of more than 3400 mg, with greater than 70% of this sodium intake from processed foods and restaurant meals.[9] The health care provider needs to educate patients on using tools to reduce sodium intake.

Tips to Reduce Sodium in the Diet

At the grocery store

- Buy fresh, frozen, or canned vegetables with no salt or sauce added
- When available, choose packaged foods labeled "low sodium," "reduced sodium," or "no salt added"
- Read food labels and compare the amount of sodium (per serving) in different products; then choose the option with the lowest amounts
- When buying prepared meals, look for those with less than 600 mg of sodium per meal, the upper limit set by the FDA for a meal or main dish to be labeled "healthy"
- Low sodium foods are defined as 5% daily value/portion, whereas foods with ≥20% daily value/portion are considered high sodium and therefore should be avoided
- Check the amount of sodium per serving and do not forget to check the number of servings per container
- When possible, purchase fresh poultry, fish, pork, and lean meat rather than cured, salted, smoked, and other processed meats. For fresh items, check to see whether saline or salt solution has been added—if so, choose another brand
- Ask your grocer if a low sodium shopping list is available
- Ask to speak to the registered dietitian (RD) at your local grocery store, if one is available, to learn more about buying low-sodium products. An RD can provide valuable guidance on reducing sodium intake and managing blood pressure.[11]

At home

- When cooking, use alternatives to replace or reduce the amount of salt you use: garlic, citrus juice, salt-free seasonings, and/or spices
- Prepare rice, pasta, beans, and meats from their most basic forms (dry and fresh) when possible
- Eat more fresh fruits and vegetables
- Limit sauces, mixes, and "instant" products, including flavored rice and ready-made pasta[11]

Dining out

- Ask for nutrition information before you order and select a lower sodium meal. In some states, chain restaurants have the nutrition content listed on the menu. If not, look online for these data
- Ask that no salt be added to your meal
- Order vegetables with no salt added or fruit as a side item
- Split a meal with a friend or family member or have an appetizer as the main meal
- Keep takeout and fast food to an occasional treat[11]

Hydration

The kidneys play a key role in maintaining homeostasis in the body and can be affected by hydration status. The progression of kidney disease can lead to derangements of fluid, electrolytes, and acid-base balance. Reversing associated complications of fluid derangements is a goal of kidney disease treatment, that is, maintaining body fluid balance by using fluid resuscitation, diuretics, and/or dialysis.[12] The decision to initiate fluid resuscitation or restriction depends on multiple factors and is not always straightforward.

Acute kidney injury. Acute kidney injury (AKI) is a common complication in critically ill patients. The goal of fluid therapy in critical care medicine is to restore hemodynamic stability and vital organ perfusion while avoiding interstitial edema. Decisions regarding fluid management in critically ill patients with AKI are difficult, as these patients often have accompanying oliguria as well as body fluid overload. Both hypovolemia and volume overload are associated with increased morbidity and mortality in critically ill patients; therefore, accurate assessment of the intravascular volume status as well as the response to fluid replacement remains one of the most challenging and important issues for clinicians. In patients with established AKI who are unresponsive to fluid administration, fluid restriction is the treatment of choice. Volume management is an integral part of the care of critically ill patients with AKI and depends on each individual patient's needs and course of therapy.[13]

Cystic disease. One cause of kidney disease, not commonly highlighted, is polycystic kidney disease. Autosomal dominant polycystic kidney disease is characterized by the development of kidney cysts, HTN, and destruction of the kidney parenchyma. Studies suggest that lowering vasopressin concentrations plays an important role not only in the development of cystic disease but also in the progression of CKD in general. Therefore, lowering vasopressin concentration by increasing water intake is an intriguing treatment option. Patients who comply with moderate sodium and protein restrictions will have lower osmolar loads and therefore will need to drink less water.[14] This example reinforces how complicated fluid recommendations can be based on a patient's adherence to sodium and protein recommendations versus disease state.

Nephrotic syndrome. To further the great hydration debate, a cause/complication of CKD is nephrotic syndrome (NS).[15] Many underlying systemic conditions can cause NS including diabetes mellitus type 2. NS consists of peripheral edema, heavy proteinuria, and hypoalbuminemia, often with hyperlipidemia. Patients typically present with edema and fatigue without heart failure or severe liver disease. The diagnosis and other factors influence the treatment of NS. Often sodium and fluid restriction is needed for treatment.[15]

End-stage kidney disease. Most hemodialysis (HD) patients need to limit their fluid intake to 32 ounces per day.[16] Fluid is not just water; it means anything liquid at room temperature: coffee, Jell-O, sherbet, ice-cream, or soup. Also, many fruits contribute to fluid gain. The fluid intake for a peritoneal dialysis (PD) patient may be less strict than one for hemodialysis. Because PD is done every day, there is less time for wastes and extra fluids to build up between treatments.[17] Home hemodialysis is usually performed 5 to 6x/week with shorter but more frequent treatments, compared with a standard incenter HD schedule; this may allow for both a more liberalized diet and fluid intake.[17]

An ileostomy can be a common cause of dehydration that then causes kidney damage and in severe cases, ESKD. Appropriate strategies to decrease dehydration following ileostomy creation need to be monitored.[18] HD patients with ileostomies may require fluid replacement during dialysis treatments rather than fluid restriction.

HYDRATION SUMMARY

Management of hydration status in each patient with CKD/ESKD is diverse. Determining a fluid restriction for a patient can be complex and involves understanding lifestyle (construction worker vs office worker), residual kidney function, and multiple other factors. The key to fluid recommendations is to monitor closely and educate based the individual patient's needs.

Protein: to Restrict or Not to Restrict

In patients with CKD, an appropriate amount of protein is required to avoid both malnutrition and overnutrition. Protein-energy malnutrition in patients with CKD is a strong predictor of adverse outcomes. Malnutrition prevalence increases linearly with decreasing kidney function in nondialysis patients and may exceed 50% in those undergoing maintenance dialysis therapy.[19] Excess dietary protein leads to the accumulation of uremic toxins, whereas conversely insufficient protein intake may lead to loss of lean body mass and malnutrition. The role of dietary protein restriction in slowing the progression of CKD is controversial and in advanced CKD is associated with a protein wasting syndrome that directly correlates with morbidity and mortality. (Note that statements about reduction in dietary protein do not apply to pediatric populations, given issues related to growth and nutrition) There is some evidence to suggest that high protein diets with greater than the recommended daily intake may accelerate kidney function decline in people with early CKD. A high total protein intake, particularly high intake of animal protein, may accelerate kidney function decline in people with CKD and should be avoided[20]; this information is important to note based on the obesity epidemic and use of fad diets including high protein or keto diets.

Previously, the National Kidney Foundation (NKF) released the *Kidney Disease Outcomes Quality Initiative (KDOQI) Clinical Practice Guideline on Nutrition in Chronic Kidney Disease*, which reported a dietary protein restriction of less 0.8 gm/kg/d seem to offer no advantage.[20] Keep in mind, the recommended non-CKD adult dietary reference intake for protein intake is 0.8 gm/kg/d[21] Many adults in Western countries eat more than their minimum daily requirement (1.35 g protein/kg per day) as compared with their optimal daily needs of 0.8 gm/kg/d[22]

To further add to the protein controversy, in 2020, the NKF released a new version of guidelines on nutrition in the patient with CKD. *KDOQI*'s revised dietary protein recommendations[22] (as long as there is sufficient energy intake, ie, > 30 kcal/kg/d) are as follows:

CKD stages 3 to 5 adults, metabolically stable[a] not on dialysis and without diabetes:
- low protein diet
  - 0.55 to 0.60 gm/kg/d
- very low protein diet
  - 0.28 to 0.43 gm/kg/d with additional keto acid/amino acid analogues to meet the recommended low protein requirements (0.55–0.60 gm/kg/d)[22]

CKD stages 3 to 5 adults, [a]metabolically stable not on dialysis and with diabetes:
  - 0.6 to 0.8 gm/kg/d[22]

Maintenance hemodialysis and PD adults:
  - 1.0 to 1.2 gm/kg/d

For patients at risk of hyperglycemia and/or hypoglycemia, higher levels of dietary protein intake may need to be considered to maintain glycemic control.[22]

---

[a] Metabolically stable: indicates the absence of any active inflammatory or infectious diseases, no hospitalization within 2 weeks, absence of poorly controlled diabetes and consumptive diseases such as cancer, absence of antibiotic or immunosuppressive medication, and absence of significant short-term loss of body weight.[22]

Just as with the fluid recommendations, the aforementioned information shows how diverse each patient's protein recommendations are based on:

- Stage of kidney disease
- Laboratory values
- Age of the patient
- Type of treatment
- Comorbidities

High protein intake may accelerate the progression of kidney disease, whereas restricting too much protein may lead to malnutrition and increased morbidity. It is important to calculate, educate, and monitor patients for appropriate dietary protein intake.

PLANT-BASED DIETS

It has been long thought that vegetarianism and kidney disease would not be a healthy combination. Plant-based diets, despite containing low amounts of protein, are also rich in potassium and phosphorus and therefore were believed to be unsuitable for patients with CKD. However, evidence from clinical studies demonstrate that such diets can actually be very beneficial for CKD patients when they learn how to use them correctly.[19] Some trials suggest plant-based diets can delay the progression of CKD, protect endothelium, help to control HTN, and decrease proteinuria. A plant-based diet can provide adequate nutrition in addition to numerous beneficial effects. However, reports concerning the influence of a vegetarian diet on the progression of kidney failure are still conflicting. According to some studies, the consumption of a vegetarian diet slows down the progression of kidney injury, whereas others indicated that high protein intake is likely to accelerate CKD progression independently of the source of proteins (plant or animal). Therefore, a vegetarian diet may be beneficial due to the associated cardioprotective, antioxidant, and lipid-lowering properties; however, it must meet protein requirements to provide adequate nutrition in patients with CKD.[19] A plant-based diet can be acceptable for patients with CKD with the proper education, monitoring by a health care provider, and the guidance of a nutrition professional. It is important to calculate, educate, and monitor patients for appropriate dietary protein intake.

Dietary Supplements and Chronic Kidney Disease

What are supplements?

More than half of American adults, ages 20 years and older, use dietary supplements with the usage and amount increasing with age.[23] A dietary supplement is a substance used to add nutrients to a diet, lower health risks, and/or improve on a health condition. Dietary supplements contain one or more ingredients—vitamins, minerals, herbs, proteins, and/or enzymes—and are consumed in a variety of forms—pills, gummies, powders, as well as drinks and bars.[23,24] Diet patterns that include a variety of healthful foods (ie, fruits, vegetables, whole grains, and protein) are the best way to get sufficient nutrients. However, people living with certain health conditions may have difficulty meeting nutritional requirements through diet alone and may need to use a nutritional supplement to meet their dietary needs.

Why Do People With Chronic Kidney Disease Need a Supplement?

There are several plausible reasons people with CKD need to take supplements. First, late-stage CKD is often accompanied by a myriad of symptoms (ie, nausea, vomiting and/or decreased appetite), which may limit patients from consuming an adequate diet, thus supplementation may be needed to help meet their nutritional needs.

Although, dialysis is useful for removing waste buildup in the blood, it also removes water soluble vitamins: vitamin B1, B2, B6, B12, folic acid, and biotin. Therefore, patients on dialysis (all types), coupled with decreased dietary intake, are at increased risk for deficiency in these key vitamins.[25] Next, people with CKD may require following a special diet that may restrict key nutrients, thus making it difficult to meet daily nutrient needs; therefore, adding a single nutrient or multivitamin/mineral supplement may be helpful. Lastly, one important function of the kidneys is to convert the physiologically inactive form of vitamin D (calciferol) to the physiologically active form (calcitriol). Active vitamin D promotes intestinal absorption of calcium and maintains adequate calcium and phosphorus in the blood enabling bone mineralization.[26] However, due to the reduced ability to make active vitamin D, patients with CKD often suffer from vitamin D insufficiency.[27] Therefore, vitamin D supplementation maybe necessary.

Common Supplements in Chronic Kidney Disease

Because of the disturbances in nutrient balance and the adverse effects related to these imbalances, health care providers may recommend supplementation to people with kidney disease. Supplements often recommended or used by patients with CKD include vitamin D, B vitamins, protein, and/or fish oil.

Vitamin D

The prevalence of vitamin D deficiency is very high among people with CKD, ranging from 70% to 80% of the CKD population.[28] Observational studies among the CKD population suggest a significant link between vitamin D deficiency and poor outcomes, including secondary hyperparathyroidism, mineral bone disorders, cardiovascular disease, and mortality.[29–31] Evidence suggests that vitamin D supplementation in CKD may mitigate these adverse effects.[32] A double-blinded, randomized control trial examined the effects of vitamin D supplementation on vascular function among 120 adults with nondiabetic CKD stages 3 to 4.[33] The primary outcome was change in endothelium-dependent brachial artery flow dilation from baseline to 16 weeks compared with placebo. Researchers found that vitamin D supplementation significantly increased artery flow dilation at 16 weeks compared with placebo.[33] With the support of empirical evidence, the KDOQI and KDIGO guidelines recommend that patients with CKD and on dialysis receive vitamin D supplementation to increase arterial flow.[29]

B vitamins

Water-soluble vitamins are nutrients the body needs in small amounts to work and function properly. Unlike fat-soluble vitamins (vitamin A, D, E, and K) that are stored until needed, excess water-soluble vitamins are excreted through the urine. In the general population, megadoses of vitamins are often not warranted because there is no extra benefit to taking more than the recommended dose.[34] On the other hand, people with CKD may require supplementation of water-soluble B vitamins also known as vitamin B complex; B1, B2, B6, B12, folic acid, biotin, and pantothenic acid. These B vitamins play an important role in macronutrient (ie, carbohydrate, protein, and fat) metabolism, energy, and red blood cell production.[35] The patients with ESKD on dialysis are often prescribed a renal vitamin (a concentrated B vitamin) to replace water-soluble B lost during dialysis fluid removal. The patients with CKD with diabetes and long-term use of metformin (>5 years) are at higher risk for vitamin B-12 deficiency, as metformin alters gut absorption of vitamin B-12.[36] Vitamin B-12 deficiency limits the production of red blood cells, leading to pernicious anemia.[37] Therefore, vitamin B-12 or vitamins with B-12 may be prescribed to attenuate this effect among patients with diabetes and CKD. Currently, there is still debate on whether all patients treated with metformin should receive vitamin B-12 supplementation. At this time, the recommendation is to be aware of this risk and monitor B-12 levels in this group of patients.[38]

Protein supplements

Evidence on protein supplementation among patients with CKD has been mixed. It seems that protein supplementation is more beneficial in patients who are on HD and in those who are malnourished.[39] A systematic review of 22 randomized controlled trials examined the effect of oral-based protein supplementation among 1278 patients receiving kidney replacement therapy (KRT), with 80% on HD and 20% on PD. Researchers found oral-based protein supplementation led to higher serum albumin levels compared with controls. They also found that this effect was greater in patients receiving HD and patients who were malnourished (based on albumin and body mass index).[38] On the other hand, patients with CKD who are adequately nourished and/or not on KRT should avoid protein supplementation. As noted earlier, in people with CKD, protein supplements can worsen kidney function by increasing intraglomerular pressure and hyperfiltration of glomeruli, leading to a lower kidney filtration rate.[40] This adverse effect seems to be more prevalent among patients with CKD stage 3a/3b, the vast majority of CKD patients.[34]

Fish oil

In addition to vitamin D and protein supplements, fish oil or omega-3 fatty acids have been shown to improve kidney function.[41] Uremic pruritis (ie, itching) is associated with CKD and is a bothersome burden for patients with CKD reducing one's quality of life.[42] Literature demonstrates the efficacy of omega-3 fatty acid supplementation improving symptoms of uremic pruritis.[43] Fish oil supplementation is also believed to improve kidney function but evidence has been mixed. A systematic review to examine the effectiveness of common dietary supplements used in the CKD population found the effects of omega-3 fatty acids on the progression of kidney disease to ESKD seemed to be very low to moderate.[41]

Other Herbals and Botanicals

Medical cannabis and cannabidiol

For the past few years medical cannabis (marijuana) has gained popularity among health professionals and the public. The use of medical cannabis has significantly increased, especially among adults older than 50 years. By the end of 2021, 18 states, 2 territories, and the District of Columbia allowed recreational cannabis use, whereas 36 states and 4 territories established medical marijuana programs.[44] Tetrahydrocannabinol (THC) is one of the most prevalent derivatives of the cannabis plant with psychoactive and intoxication effects. THC has been shown to have medicinal properties including pain relief, antiemetic effects, and appetite stimulation.[45] The medication Marinol, which is a THC-based derivative, has been approved by Food and Drug Administration (FDA) to treat nausea and vomiting in patients with cancer receiving chemotherapy. It is also used to treat weight loss and poor appetite in patients with human immunodeficiency virus/AIDS.[45] The use of THC-based medication is often recommended after other treatments have been tried and failed. A nonhallucinogenic portion of the marijuana plant, cannabidiol (CBD) is found in the cannabis flower but with less, if any, intoxicating effect.[46] Recently, a CBD-based medication has been FDA approved for severe epilepsy in children.[47] However, CBD is widely used by the public for various reasons including as a pet supplement. CBD is legal in all states and available to order on the Internet.

Cannabis and chronic kidney disease

Unregulated, CBD-based products are widely available with health claims for treating a host of symptoms including insomnia, anxiety, and chronic pain.[48] Patients with CKD and receiving KRT experience many of these symptoms and may benefit from an alternative to opioids and nonsteroidal antiinflammatory drugs (NSAIDs). Patients using cannabis to treat symptoms related to CKD should be cautioned. Although generally recognized as safe, patients with CKD who use cannabis products may be at higher risk for adverse outcomes including progression of kidney disease and interference with kidney transplant listing.[48] CBD products that contain additives or other ingredients may interact with other medications and negatively affect kidney function.[47] Therefore, patients should be educated on the use of these products and be leery of false health claims and inaccurate labeling. What is more, studies involving cannabis and health benefits in humans are limited to association studies, thus inhibiting the ability to infer a cause and effect on many of these claims. Hence, clinical trials in humans are needed to prove these benefits.[46]

Choosing Supplements

Health care providers introduce or recommend dietary supplementation depending on a patient's need; however, a significant percent of patients choose to start supplements on their own.[49] Dietary supplements are regulated by the FDA as a food and not as drugs; therefore, many supplements do not require a prescription from a health care provider and are sold as over-the-counter drugs.[24] Although dietary supplements are generally recognized as safe, some may be harmful for people living with CKD. Certain ingredients may interact with other prescription medications or not be eliminated by the kidneys, thus accumulating in patients with CKD and leading to adverse outcomes; this has been described in star fruits (neurotoxins) and aristolochic acid (which was taken off the market but reappears online frequently). If supplements are not recommended by a provider but are a personal decision, it is important that health care providers know how to properly educate patients with CKD on choosing the right supplement. Equally important, health care providers should ask patients about cannabis, herbals, and over-the-counter preparations they use.

Choosing dietary supplements

According to the FDA, products sold as supplements must come with a *Supplemental Facts Label* that includes all the active ingredients, the serving amount, as well as other ingredients. Although, the manufacturer suggests serving size, health care providers might choose a different, more appropriate amount. Guidance is provided in chapter IV of the dietary supplement labeling guide (https://www.fda.gov/food/dietary-supplements-guidance-documents-regulatory-information/dietary-supplement-labeling-guide-chapter-iv-nutrition-labeling) on understanding a supplemental fact label allowing patients to make educated decisions.[50]

SUMMARY

Nonadherence to suggested diet and fluid recommendations can lead to rapid worsening CKD. Overall, there is not a one-size-fits-all solution to any dietary or supplement recommendations for patients living with kidney disease. To complicate issues more, the stage of kidney disease, medication regimens, and patient comorbidities can all significantly alter dietary recommendations to maintain a patient's overall health and improve prognosis. Even the type of dialysis a patient receives (HD, PD, home hemodialysis, or nocturnal HD) as well as residual kidney function, offer a multitude of different recommendations. Fortunately, dialysis patients have access to dietitians within their dialysis units; this is rarely true for the patient with CKD.

No matter what stage of kidney disease, patients need to modify their lifestyle to focus on diet and fluid intake, as their prognosis largely depends on adherence to recommended nutritional regimes.[51] Socioeconomic status, age, social support, and self-efficacy are all associated with patterns of dietary adherence.[52] Many tools, including the *Nutrition and Supplemental Fact* labels, are available to assist patients in making better choices to prolong kidney health. In this tech savvy age, patients lean on the Internet to fill in the missing pieces of education for making healthier choices. However, without the proper direction or diet education, patients may adhere to information completely opposite to their actual individualized personal plan of care. KIDGO recommends individuals living with CKD receive expert dietary advice and information in the context of an educational program. The education program should be tailored to the severity of CKD and the need to intervene on certain nutrients such as sodium, phosphorus, potassium, and protein intake where indicated.

It is important to note if a patient's insurance will cover a referral to a nutrition professional. Keep in mind, Medicare reimburses for medical nutrition therapy, *"for diagnoses of diabetes, non-dialysis kidney disease, and 36 months post kidney transplant when a Medicare beneficiary has been referred by a physician, and when provided by an RD/ Nutritionist, who is enrolled as a Medicare Provider."*[53] The Academy of Nutrition and Dietetics (AND) (www.eatright.org/) has a quick and easy "Find an Expert" link to assist in locating a local nutrition professional. AND has developed a nutrition care process for assessing individual patients. Medical Nutrition Therapy (MNT) is used for nutritional diagnostic, therapy, and counseling services for the purpose of disease management furnished by RDs or nutrition professionals. MNT is a specific application in a clinical setting focused on disease management and involves an in-depth, individualized nutrition assessment using the Nutrition Care Process to manage disease. Dietetic professionals also use education to reinforce essential nutrition-related knowledge.[54]

While awaiting a referral to a nephrologist or an RD, health care providers can use behavior change techniques to set achievable goals with patients. Printable, reliable, and free online handouts, including some in Spanish, are available through the AND, the NKF, the National Institute of Health, and/or the FDA. As research has shown Americans eat far more sodium than the dietary guidelines recommend; this may be a good place to start, no matter what the diagnosis.

CLINICS CARE POINTS

- Consuming too much sodium puts patients at risk for developing serious medical conditions including HTN, heart disease, and stroke; using educational materials and teaching food label reading to reduce sodium intake can benefit most patients.

- High-protein and fad diets may accelerate progression of kidney disease; therefore, calculate, educate, and monitor for appropriate protein intake.

- Diet plays a key role in guiding patients to manage their kidney disease; consider a Registered Dietitian referral for Medical Nutrition Therapy

- Management of hydration status in both CKD and ESRD is diverse; consider all aspects of the patient's lifestyle, stage of kidney disease, medications, residual kidney function, and multiple other factors to determine acceptable fluid intake recommendations.

- Dietary supplements should be used with caution in patients with kidney disease. For example, protein supplements can worsen kidney function by increasing intraglomerular pressure and hyperfiltration of glomeruli leading to a lower kidney filtration rate among patients with CKD stage 3a/3b. Therefore, in addition to evaluating need for

> supplementation, consider educating patients with kidney disease about potential risks before use.

DISCLOSURE

The authors have nothing to disclose.

REFERENCES

1. Hruby A, Hu FB. The epidemiology of obesity: a big picture. Pharmacoeconomics 2015;33(7):673–89.
2. National Institute of Health. Overweight and obesity. National Heart, Lung, and Blood Institute, Bethesda (MD). Available at: www.nhlbi.nih.gov/health-topics/overweight-and-obesity. Assessed April 1, 2021.
3. National Institute of Diabetes and Digestive and Kidney Diseases. Kidney disease statistics for the United States. Health statistics. Available at: https://www.niddk.nih.gov/health-information/health-statistics/kidney-disease. Assessed April 1, 2021.
4. National Kidney Foundation. Estimated glomerular filtration rate. National Kidney Foundation; 2020. Available at: www.kidney.org/atoz/content/gfr. Assessed July 12, 2021.
5. Okrent AM, Howard E, Park T, et al. Measuring the value of the U.S. Food System: Revisions to the Food Expenditure Series, TB-1948. U.S. Department of Agriculture, Economic Research Service; 2018.
6. American Heart Association. Food labeling survey. International Food Information Council Foundation. Available at: https://foodinsight.org/wp-content/uploads/2019/01/IFIC-FDN-AHA-Report.pdf. Assessed May 1, 2021.
7. United States Department of Agriculture. Changes to the nutrition facts label. Food and Drug Administration. Available at: https://www.fda.gov/food/food-labeling-nutrition/changes-nutrition-facts-label. Assessed May 1, 2021.
8. United States Department of Agriculture. Nutrition Facts Labels for Download. Food and Drug Administration. Available at: www.fda.gov/food/food-labeling-nutrition/nutrition-facts-label-images-download https://nam11.safelinks.protection.outlook.com/?url=http%3A%2F%2Fwww.fda.gov%2Ffood%2Ffood-labeling-nutrition%2Fnutrition-facts-label-images-download&data=04%7C01%7CE.Bennitta%40elsevier.com%7C753b6bffa82c4e947dac08d9ca10d8ba%7C9274ee3f94254109a27f9fb15c10675d. Assessed May 1, 2021.
9. Centers for Disease Control and Prevention. Get the facts: sodium and the dietary guidelines. Centers for Disease Control and Prevention. Available at: https://www.cdc.gov/salt/pdfs/sodium_dietary_guidelines.pdf. Assessed May 15, 2021.
10. Cheung AK, Chang TI, Cushman WC, et al. Executive summary of the KDIGO 2021 clinical practice guideline for the management of blood pressure in Chronic Kidney Disease. Kidney Int 2021;99(3):559–69.
11. Centers for Disease Control and Prevention. Salt. Centers for Disease Control and Prevention. Available at: https://www.cdc.gov/salt/reduce_sodium_tips.htm. Assessed June 1, 2021.
12. Langston C. Managing fluid and electrolyte disorders in Kidney Disease. Vet Clin North Am Small Anim Pract 2017;47(2):471–90.
13. Chuang CL. Fluid management in acute kidney injury. Contrib Nephrol 2016;187:84–93.

14. Chebib FT, Torres VE. Recent advances in the management of Autosomal Dominant Polycystic Kidney Disease. Clin J Am Soc Nephrol 2018;13(11):1765–76.
15. Kodner C. Diagnosis and management of nephrotic syndrome in adults. Am Fam Physician 2016;93(6):479–85.
16. National Kidney Foundation. Fluid overload in a dialysis patient. Available at: https://www.kidney.org/atoz/content/fluid-overload-dialysis-patient.   Assessed August 11, 2021.
17. National Institute of Diabetes and Digestive and Kidney Diseases. Kidney failure. US Department of Health and Human Services National Institutes of Health. Available   at: https://www.niddk.nih.gov/health-information/kidney-disease/kidney-failure. Assessed July 1, 2021.
18. Paquette IM, Solan P, Rafferty JF, et al. Readmission for dehydration or renal failure after ileostomy creation. Dis Colon Rectum 2013;56(8):974–9.
19. Gluba-Brzózka A, Franczyk B, Rysz J. Vegetarian diet in Chronic Kidney Disease- A Friend or Foe. Nutrients 2017;9(4):374.
20. Inker LA, Astor BC, Fox CH, et al. KDOQI US commentary on the 2012 KDIGO clinical practice guideline for the evaluation and management of CKD. Am J Kidney Dis 2014;63(5):713–35.
21. National Institutes of Health Office of Dietary Supplements. Nutrient recommendations: dietary reference intakes. US Department of Health and Human Services National Institutes of Health. Available at: https://ods.od.nih.gov/HealthInformation/ Dietary_Reference_Intakes.asp. Assessed July 1, 2021.
22. Ikizler TA, Burrowes JD, Byham-Gray LD, et al. KDOQI Clinical Practice Guideline for Nutrition in CKD: 2020 Update. Am J Kidney Dis 2020;76(3 Suppl 1):S1–107 [Erratum appears in Am J Kidney Dis. 2021 Feb;77(2):308].
23. Mishra S, Stierman B, Gahche JJ, et al. Dietary supplement use among adults: United States, 2017–2018. NCHS Data Brief, no 399. Hyattsville (MD): National Center for Health Statistics; 2021. https://doi.org/10.15620/cdc:101131external icon.
24. U.S. Department of Health and Human Services, National Institutes of Health. Should you take dietary supplements?. 2013. Available at: https://newsinhealth. nih.gov/2013/08/should-you-take-dietary-supplements. Accessed June 12, 2021.
25. Clase CM, Ki V, Holden RM. Water-soluble vitamins in people with low glomerular filtration rate or on dialysis: a review. Semin Dial 2013;26(5):546–67.
26. U.S. Department of Health and Human Services, National Institute of Health. Vitamin D fact sheet for health professionals. 2021. Available at: https://ods.od. nih.gov/factsheets/VitaminD-HealthProfessional/.
27. Williams S, Malatesta K, Norris K. Vitamin D and chronic kidney disease. Ethn Dis 2009;19(4 Suppl 5):S5–11.
28. Kandula P, Dobre M, Schold JD, et al. Vitamin D supplementation in chronic kidney disease: a systematic review and meta-analysis of observational studies and randomized controlled trials. Clin J Am Soc Nephrol 2011;6(1):50–62.
29. Jean G, Souberbielle JC, Chazot C. Vitamin D in Chronic Kidney Disease and Dialysis Patients. Nutrients 2017;9(4):328.
30. Capelli I, Cianciolo G, Gasperoni L, et al. Nutritional vitamin D in CKD: Should we measure? Should we treat? Clin Chim Acta 2020;501:186–97.
31. Kurani S, Hickson LJ, Thorsteinsdottir B, et al. Supplement use by US Adults With CKD: A Population-Based Study. Am J Kidney Dis 2019;74(6):862–5.
32. Lips P, Goldsmith D, de Jongh R. Vitamin D and osteoporosis in Chronic Kidney Disease. J Nephrol 2017;30(5):671–5.

33. Kumar V, Yadav AK, Lal A, et al. A Randomized Trial of Vitamin D Supplementation on Vascular Function in CKD. J Am Soc Nephrol 2017;28(10):3100–8.

34. National Research Council (US) Committee on diet and health. Diet and health: implications for reducing chronic disease risk. 12, Water-Soluble Vitamins. Washington (DC): National Academies Press (US); 1989. Available at: https://www.ncbi.nlm.nih.gov/books/NBK218756. Accessed June 12, 2021.

35. National Kidney Foundation. Vitamin and minerals IN chronic kidney disease. 2019. Available at: https://www.kidney.org/atoz/content/vitamineral.

36. Aroda VR, Edelstein SL, Goldberg RB, et al. Long-term Metformin Use and Vitamin B12 Deficiency in the Diabetes Prevention Program Outcomes Study. J Clin Endocrinol Metab 2016;101(4):1754–61.

37. National Institute of Health. National heart, lung, and blood institute (UNK). Pernicious anemia. Available at: https://www.nhlbi.nih.gov/health-topics/pernicious-anemia#. Accessed June 12, 2021.

38. Kim J, Ahn CW, Fang S, et al. Association between metformin dose and vitamin B12 deficiency in patients with type 2 diabetes. Medicine (Baltimore) 2019; 98(46):e17918.

39. Mah JY, Choy SW, Roberts MA, et al. Oral protein-based supplements versus placebo or no treatment for people with chronic kidney disease requiring dialysis. Cochrane Database Syst Rev 2020;5(5):CD012616.

40. Ko GJ, Obi Y, Tortorici AR, et al. Dietary protein intake and chronic kidney disease. Curr Opin Clin Nutr Metab Care 2017;20(1):77–85.

41. Lin PC, Chou CL, Ou SH, et al. Systematic Review of Nutrition Supplements in Chronic Kidney Diseases: A GRADE Approach. Nutrients 2021;13(2):469.

42. Mettang T, Kremer AE. Uremic pruritus. Kidney Int 2015;87(4):685–91.

43. Panahi Y, Dashti-Khavidaki S, Farnood F, et al. Therapeutic Effects of Omega-3 Fatty Acids on Chronic Kidney Disease-Associated Pruritus: a literature review. Adv Pharm Bull 2016;6(4):509–14.

44. National Conference of State Legislatures, state medical marijuana laws. Available at: https://www.ncsl.org/research/health/state-medical-marijuana-laws.aspx. Accessed August 13, 2021.

45. National Institute on Drug Abuse. Is marijuana safe and effective as medicine?. 2021. Available at: https://www.drugabuse.gov/publications/research-reports/marijuana/marijuana-safe-effective-medicine on 2021. Accessed June 19, 2021.

46. Grinspoon P. Medical marijuana. 2020. Available at: https://www.health.harvard.edu/blog/medical-marijuana-2018011513085. Accessed June 19, 2021.

47. FDA. What you need to know (and what we're working to find out) about products containing cannabis or cannabis-derived compounds, Including CBD. 2020. Available at: https://www.fda.gov/consumers/consumer-updates/what-you-need-know-and-what-were-working-find-out-about-products-containing-cannabis-or-cannabis.

48. Rein JL. The nephrologist's guide to cannabis and cannabinoids. Curr Opin Nephrol Hypertens 2020;29(2):248–57.

49. Jakimowicz-Tylicka M, Chmielewski M, Kuźmiuk-Glembin I, et al. Dietary supplement use among patients with chronic kidney disease. Acta Biochim Pol 2018; 65(2):319–24.

50. U.S. Food and Drug Administration. Dietary supplement labeling guide: chapter IV. Nutrition labeling. 2005. Available at: https://www.fda.gov/food/dietary-supplements-guidance-documents-regulatory-information/dietary-supplement-labeling-guide-chapter-iv-nutrition-labeling. Accessed June 19, 2021.

51. Beerendrakumar N, Ramamoorthy L, Haridasan S. Dietary and Fluid Regime Adherence in Chronic Kidney Disease Patients. J Caring Sci 2018;7(1):17–20.
52. Lambert K, Mullan J, Mansfield K. An integrative review of the methodology and findings regarding dietary adherence in end stage kidney disease. BMC Nephrol 2017;18(1):318.
53. Medicare Part B, Nutrition therapy services. Available at: https://www.medicare.gov/coverage/nutrition-therapy-services. Accessed August 13, 2021.
54. Academy of Nutrition and Dietetics. MNT versus nutrition education. Academy of Nutrition and Dietetics. Available at: https://www.eatrightpro.org/payment/coding-and-billing/mnt-vs-nutrition-education#lnd. Assessed July 1, 2021.

The Secret Side of the Military and the Kidney

Kim Zuber, PAC, MS[a],*, Rodney Ho, PhD, MPH, PA-C, Psychiatry-CAQ[b]

KEYWORDS

• Nephrology • Military medicine • PA • Berry Plan • Willem Kolff • Thomas Starzl

KEY POINTS

• Military training of physicians led to better outcomes for the US civilian population.
• Military medicine is responsible for many of the treatments used in nephrology.
• The Berry Plan introduced PAs to an entire generation of physicians.
• The GI Bill led directly to the incorporation of nephrology as a board-certified specialty.

Audio content accompanies this article at https://www.physicianassistant. theclinics.com.

The relationship between the military and kidney disease has been a long and fruitful partnership, one which continues today. Medical training has always included rotations in military medicine, but the collaboration is much more than that. Young, healthy patients with horrific injuries (crush injuries, major trauma, gunshot wounds) and world-class medical care (often at the site of the trauma) have combined to negate or decrease many unfortunate sequalae. Battlefield medicine allows for innovation in a way unavailable to controlled trials. Within the Veterans Administration (VA) and military medical systems, researchers are able obtain detailed data from large cohorts of patients, which translates into "large data" analysis. This large data analysis allows researchers to identify even very small risk factors or treatments that can change outcomes for everyone.

If not for the military, nephrology would not have many of the common treatments we take for granted today: erythropoietin, tourniquets to decrease blood loss (previously, blood loss could send a patient into shock and acute kidney injury [AKI]), point-of-care blood transfusions, ubiquitous use of penicillin and sulfanilamide to decrease sepsis and AKI, blood vessel ligation/repair techniques leading to dialysis access development, ambulance transport to medical care decreasing incidence of AKI, paracentesis with sodium hypochlorite to decrease sepsis and death (the first

[a] American Academy of Nephrology PAs, 131 31st Avenue North, St Petersburg, FL 33704, USA;
[b] University of West Florida, 2614 Brad Clemmons Drive, JBSA–Lackland, 78236, USA
* Corresponding author.
E-mail address: aanpa1@yahoo.com

Physician Assist Clin 7 (2022) 347–356
https://doi.org/10.1016/j.cpha.2021.11.012
2405-7991/22/© 2021 Elsevier Inc. All rights reserved.

incident of solute and peritoneal absorption), plastic surgery techniques leading to organ transplantation, anesthesia advances, decreased surgical times to lower the risk of AKI, portable radiograph facilities, and nursing care.[1-3] Mary Merritt Crawford, the only woman doctor at the American Hospital during World War I (WWI), stated: *"A war benefits medicine more than it benefits anybody else. It's terrible, of course, but it does."*[1]

Although "The Military" is often considered the 5 services (Air Force, Army, Navy, Marines, and Space Force), military medicine includes significantly more. The government has multiple medical divisions spread out among departments (ie, The Department of Homeland Security and Department of the Interior). The Public Health Service includes Commissioned Officers who are activated and sent to disaster zones as part of a Federal Emergency Management Agency response when medical assistance is needed following disasters, such as hurricanes, earthquakes, floods, fires, pandemics. The Bureau of Indian Affairs, part of the Interior Department, relies on the medical experts at the National Institutes of Health (NIH), including the nephrology section, for medical care on Indian lands. NIH itself operates a hospital on its campus that includes active, retired, and civilian medical staff with supplementation from Walter Reed Medical Center (WRMC) staff. Active-duty medical staff (including physician assistants [PAs]) are on site at the White House to care for the President, Vice-President, the Secret Service, and all workers on the White House campus. The VA system is responsible for the retired military members (veterans).

Military medical treatment facilities are found around the world and are often the first stop for US citizens in need of medical care before returning to the United States. The largest US overseas hospital is Landstuhl Regional Medical Center in Germany, which serves nonmilitary patients when critical care is needed, as happened for the embassy staff from Benghazi, Libya after an attack in 2012 or after release of the hostages from the 1979 Iranian hostage crisis.[4]

HISTORICAL

Although the history of medical care and the military reaches back to the Romans, the intersection with nephrology did not occur until the twentieth century. During WWI, the practice of surgical debridement and "flushing" of wounds with copious fluid was introduced. This in turn led to the development of plastic surgical techniques and rehabilitation for patients who survived their original injuries.[3] Marie Curie, awarded the Nobel Prize in 1911 for her discovery of radium and polonium, developed and trained a corps of female radiological technicians who drove converted cars to the battlefield, allowing surgeons to see inside the human body: the first "portable X-ray."[5] These radiographs allowed physicians to open chest cavities to find bullets or shrapnel. These thoracotomy procedures would later be used in the first heart and lung transplants.

Between the World Wars, biochemistry and the concepts of electrolyte imbalance were studied and discussed. Survival on the battlefield was dependent on both blood and fluid, and the best minds of the generation worked to solve the first "nephrology-dominated" fluid and metabolic issue in military medicine.

Although blood types (A, B, O) were discovered in 1901 by Karl Landsteiner (winner of the 1930 Nobel Prize), transfusions during WWI were vein-to-vein transfer.[6] The addition of sodium citrate in 1935 as an antiagglutinant allowed the blood to be transfused slowly and via a drip method.[3] Citate is still the anticoagulant of choice in the intensive care unit of the twenty-first century.

As World War II (WWII) began, anesthesia was coming into its own along with antibiotic treatment. Penicillin and sulfonamides were responsible for the decrease in deaths owing to wound infections. With anesthesia, including the development of curare for paralysis and pentothal for a safer "sleep," surgeons were able to remove bullets from chambers of the heart, lungs, and abdomen, along with the extremities.[3] This led to the development of a group of surgeons who would later go on to develop transplant procedures.

AFTER THE WORLD WARS

Acute renal failure (ARF) from crush injury was first described at the Battle of Britain in 1941.[7] It was acknowledged that crush injuries would lead to a severe, long, and protracted recovery period. Building on experiments done in the early twentieth century by Abel and Haas, in 1945, Willem Kolff developed a rotating drum kidney to be used in ARF.[8] This kidney used membranous tubes developed from a cellulose tissue used in sausage casing.[9,10] An electrolyte solution, dubbed dialysate, surrounded the tubes, and through diffusion, the uremic toxins were removed (**Fig. 1**).[11]

Kolff left the Netherlands for the United States in the years after the Nazis invaded his country and brought his rotating drum technology with him. It was later modified and adopted for use in the Korean War (**Fig. 2**).[11]

The Kolff rotating drum was initially used for hyperkalemia, which developed from massive blood transfusions but was soon used in ARF because of crush injuries. These initial hemodialysis procedures were done slowly (100 mL/h), with both physicians and nurses attending, and lasted 6 hours.[11]

TRANSPLANT

In the gap between the Korean and Vietnam wars, Joseph Murray,[12] Army-trained plastic surgeon, pioneered the first successful kidney transplant between identical twins. Murray developed many of his techniques during the 3-year stint he served as an Army physician in Pennsylvania treating patients with burn injuries from WWII.

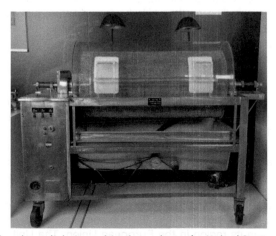

Fig. 1. Kolff rotating drum dialysis machine brought to the United States and later modified in Boston. Hoffman Collection (OHA 192.5), National Museum of Health and Medicine. The original is on exhibit at the WRMC Museum, used with permission, National Museum of Health and Medicine, Washington DC (Note: This image has been cropped to emphasize the subject; photo by Matthew Breitbart). (*From* Hoffman Collection (OHA 192.5), National Museum of Health and Medicine.)

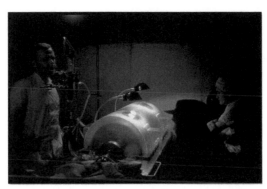

Fig. 2. Kolff rotating drum dialysis machine in use by Dr Irwin Hoffman during the Korean War while serving with the 11th Evacuation Hospital. This was the only Kolff dialysis machine in Korea. (Used with permission, National Museum of Health and Medicine, Washington, DC.)

Colonel James Brown, the military chief surgeon at the Pennsylvania military hospital, and Murray often discussed the anomalies of rejection and the concept of genetic compatibility. After leaving the military, Murray was appointed to the surgical service at Brigham and Women's Hospital in Boston. The chief of surgery at Brigham, Dr Francis Moore, was a longtime researcher in fluid loss and metabolism for burn injuries.[13] Moore and Murray transplanted kidney patients at Brigham, leading surgeons all over the United States to consider if other organs could be transplanted too. Dr Moore, after defining fluid metabolism in surgery at Brigham's, spent years as a consultant to WRMC.[13] This bidirectional medicine expertise was to continue throughout the twentieth century.

Dr Thomas Starzl,[14,15] considered the father of transplantation, was a Navy physician who trained in Chicago, Illinois at the VA Hospital before becoming chief of surgery at the VA in Denver, Colorado. He performed his first liver transplant in 1963 at the University of Colorado calling on the skills he learned from his training in Chicago, where he perfected his vascular surgery technique.[15] He then transferred to the Pittsburgh VA Medical Center in 1981 and was considered the most experienced liver transplant surgeon on the East Coast, transplanting both adults and children.[15] In what could only be called a fortuitous event, an electrician in the White House (Stu Thomas) had a 3-year-old daughter, Candi, who was dying of biliary atresia. There were no child livers available. Starzl called his previous chief in Chicago, Dr Lowell Davis, who called his daughter, Nancy Reagan, who told her husband to ask for liver donations (Audio 1).[16] After President Reagan's Saturday morning address in 1983, liver donations increased, allowing Starzl to transplant 13 children in 12 days. These children are still referred to as "*Ronnie's kids*," and Candi Thomas was among the transplants performed (**Figs. 3** and **4**). An Air Force jet flew Candi and her mom to Pittsburgh and returned them to the White House for a thank you.

The military continues to be on the cutting edge of transplant. Landstuhl, the military hospital and evacuation theater for all of Europe and Asia, is one of the top hospitals for organ donations in its region in the European Union. The United States allowed American troops who died of wounds sustained in Iraq or Afghanistan to donate their organs. Roughly half of the troops who died at Landstuhl from combat injuries from 2005 through 2010 were organ donors. From the 34 troops that donated organs, a total of 142 organs were obtained, according to the German organ transplant

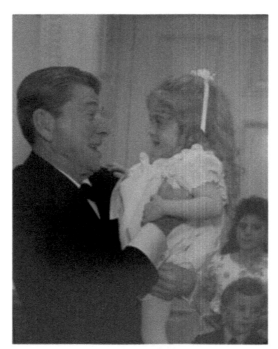

Fig. 3. President Ronald Reagan with Candi Thomas after her liver transplant, 1984. (Used with permission of the Thomas Family.)

organization, *Deutsche Stiftung Organ Transplantation*. In 2010, 10 of the 12 American service members who died at Landstuhl were donors, giving 45 organs.[17]

VIETNAM

Before introduction of the "Berry Plan" in 1954, a doctor's military draft would pull young doctors, in the midst of their training, to supplement military doctors in the battle theaters. Although the argument that the battle surgical experience was invaluable was valid, the randomness of the doctor's draft made it difficult for the physicians, hospitals, and training programs to plan residencies.[18] Dr Frank Berry, Army physician, put together a 3-point plan to accommodate the men (and they were all men at this time), the hospitals, and the military. All physicians would join the military (a particular service could be requested but it was not guaranteed) immediately after residency or after 1 year of fellowship or after completing residency.[18] By identifying when a physician would leave civilian service for military service, the hospitals and residency programs could plan multiple years in advance. This influx of trained physicians into the military continued until 1974 at which time the Vietnam War and the general draft were ending.[18]

Although the ability to do full "field" surgical medicine was popular with the surgeons, the development of the medic who would become the stateside PA was occurring on the battlefield too. Physicians learned to trust both medical care and procedures to these medics. The original cohort of PAs trained at Duke University were all retired military medics. Thus, it is not stretching the truth to say PAs would not exist today if not for the military. When the Berry Plan physicians worked with PAs after the war in their private practices and hospital systems, many of them were quite comfortable with the PA concept. PAs were also found at stateside military

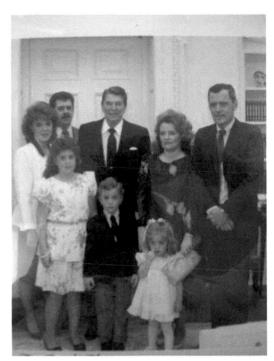

Fig. 4. A 1984 White House reception for Candi Thomas (*front*), President Ronald Reagan (*back*), Dr Thomas Starzl (*right*), Stu Thomas (White House electrician; *back left*), Janet Thomas (mother; *blue dress*). (Used with permission of the Thomas Family.)

centers with one nephrologist noting that although the first time he worked with PAs was on active duty, it certainly was not his last time.[19] The Berry Plan may have sped up the physician acceptance of PAs.

As part of the Berry Plan, several new physicians were used to "back fill" at the military hospitals stateside. The most prestigious and coveted nonsurgical positions were in Washington, DC at the WRMC (Army) or Bethesda, Maryland (Navy).[20] Although the roots of the NIH can be traced to 1887 as a public health initiative, the entity that presently occupies the Bethesda campus was developed in the 1950s and 1960s.[21] As these Berry Plan physicians arrived at NIH, Bethesda, and WRMC, they were able to learn from the best physicians and researchers in the United States.[2] Many well-known academic physicians who served both during and after the Vietnam War all rotated through the Walter Reed Army Institute of Research on the WRMC campus. This research institute was responsible for the development of war dialysis, and all physicians were trained on the dialysis machines at the institute. The Armed Forces Institute of Pathology, which is the repository of rare diseases and pathology, was also on the WRMC campus and taught both the civilian and the military physicians across the East Coast.[20,22] Experts on systemic lupus erythematosus, sickle cell, glomerulonephritis, bacterial and viral diseases along with public health, medication, and drug development were all on campus. *FEDMED* seminars, open to anyone (military, private practice, or trainees) who wished to attend, allowed interaction between world experts and the physicians who would treat the next generation of patients. The new hospital, opened in 1979, had the latest of everything, and many of the Berry Plan trainees were able to learn the newest techniques on the latest equipment before returning to civilian life with the expertise for their patients.[20]

The intersection of military and civilian medicine led to the introduction of the first nephrology boards in 1972.[23] Before this, nephrology was not an identified specialty, and thus, physicians were not eligible for the Government Issue (GI) Bill to pay for schooling/training. After the Medicare bill passed Congress in 1972 with a section referred to as the "end-stage renal disease (ESRD)" program, physicians who specialized in nephrology were needed. Training was offered, but the cost would not be covered by the GI Bill without a board-specialty examination. The American Society of Nephrology helped to push for "*Board Certification*," and the specialty of nephrology was born with the GI Bill covering training of these specialists.[23]

COMFORT

The military is sent to war zones but also to mass casualty zones. Techniques in treatment of crush injuries that were developed by the militaries in all countries have been adapted for civilian disasters. Often hyperkalemia and rhabdomyolysis sustained during earthquakes, tsunamis, volcanos, fires, and mudslides can result in deaths after the initial trauma.[24]

As medical care became more complicated and required more technical support, the concept of a floating hospital was developed. The *USNS Comfort* is a US Navy military ship equipped for any type of emergency from war to earthquakes to hurricanes to pandemics. Dialysis is available on the ship, and it is often used as an outreach of American medicine to victims of natural disasters.[24]

MEDICAL EDUCATION

After WWII, there was a shortage of military physicians, while at the same time, there was an overflow of veterans needing medical care. In 1945, General Omar Bradley pushed through Congress the "VA Department of Medicine and Surgery" bill, which allowed the VA system to run or manage their hospitals, while US medical schools were to supply medical staff, teaching staff, and students.[25] The agreement includes acute care hospitals, ambulatory care clinics, and long-term care sites.

The advantage to the medical school is a supply of patients, whereas the advantage for the VA was the ability to attract the best and the brightest of medical staff. The VA/medical school contract allows practitioners to be dually certified as both VA and medical school staff. As the VA system allows the student to follow the patient both in-clinic and in-house, the teaching aspects are significant for the students. The military was one of the first large organizations to integrate, and thus, veterans are of all races, genders, and backgrounds, allowing for a well-rounded student teaching experience. At the present time, every nephrology fellowship in the United States is affiliated with a VA hospital.

RESEARCH

As the United States does not have a centralized health care system and thus is unable to follow patients longitudinally, the VA has filled the gap for many researchers. Without the VA databases, many commonly used medications and procedures could not be tested, not to mention the 8 Nobel Prizes won by VA researchers.[26]

These researchers have developed erythropoietin and its methods of administration.[27] Organ transplant was developed at the VA. In 2008, researchers at the Pittsburgh VA determined that high-intensity renal replacement therapy is no better than less-acute care in the critically ill patient.[28] This same research group has trained nephrology PAs, published more than 200 articles on critical care nephrology, been responsible for the Up-to-Date nephrology section, and the chief of nephrology at the Pittsburgh VA, Paul Palevsky, MD, was the 2021 president of the National Kidney Foundation.[29,30]

By using big data, VA researchers have found that the patients with chronic kidney disease (CKD) are more likely to have other diseases: vascular, diabetes, hypertension, and cancer.[31] VA researchers in Vermont developed a predictive tool to determine who would develop AKI after angiograms.[32] The identification of AKI leading to CKD was identified by VA researchers.[33] The VA Nephropathy in Diabetes Trial (VA-NEPHRON-D) trial found the increase in ESRD can be traced to poor blood pressure control.[34] VA researchers found that veterans with restless leg syndrome were more likely to have CKD.[35] VA researchers in Palo Alto found that veterans who participated in kidney disease education had a lower mortality than those who did not participate.[36] The massive database trials, NEPHRON-D and PRESERVE, would not be possible without the researchers at the VA. We have gained new insights into hypertension and diabetic control, in progression of CKD/AKI, folic acid, and vitamin B supplementation of patients with CKD and dangers of combining ACEi and ARBs. In 2016, data from the VA showed sodium phosphate bowel preparations for colonoscopies increased kidney damage, leading to phosphate bowels preparations being taken off the market.[37] Without the big data available to the VA researchers, this rare complication would not have been seen except in anecdotal stories. In 2019, using data from more than three-fourths of a million active-duty military personnel, researchers were able to show that nonsteroid medications (ie, ibuprofen or naproxen) did cause AKI in a direct dose-related fashion.[38] The most recent VA publications are regarding the use of new diabetes medications and kidney care.[39]

Although these articles highlight the work of VA researchers, many more medical professors and part-time VA physicians are involved in US and international trials. The entire US population owes a debt of gratitude to the VA researchers and the veterans they serve. Without their publications, treatment of our patients would be less scientifically based and more regional.

SUMMARY

The PA profession has its roots in the military. In the same way, the recognition of nephrology as a specialty is also linked to the military. With their interlinked history, there is every expectation that the productive pairing will continue to improve and enhance medical care for years to come.

DISCLOSURE

K. Zuber: Nothing to disclose. R. Ho: The views and written materials expressed in this publication do not necessarily represent the views of the US Air Force, Department of Defense, and/or the US Government.

SUPPLEMENTARY DATA

Supplementary data related to this article can be found online at https://doi.org/10.1016/j.cpha.2021.11.012.

REFERENCES

1. Available at: https://www.statnews.com/2017/11/10/medical-innovations-war. Accessed January 9, 2021.

2. Available at: https://www.theatlantic.com/health/archive/2017/02/world-war-i-medicine/517656/. Accessed January 9, 2021.
3. Available at: https://www.britannica.com/science/history-of-medicine/Organ-transplantation. Accessed January 9, 2021.
4. Available at: https://www.stripes.com/news/officials-break-ground-on-hospital-to-replace-landstuhl-1.310376#:~:text=Expected%20to%20open%20in%202022%2C%20the%20new%20facility,cost%20millions%20of%20dollars%20a%20year%20to%20maintain. Accessed January 10, 2021.
5. Jorgensen TJ, editor. How Marie Curie brought X-ray machines to the battlefield. Washington, DC: The Conversation, Smithsonian Magazine; 2018. Available at: https://www.smithsonianmag.com/history/how-marie-curie-brought-x-ray-machines-to-battlefield-180965240. Accessed January 9, 2021.
6. Rosendaal FR, Reitsma PH. Karl Landsteiner. J Thromb Haemost 2018;16(6):1023.
7. Welch PG. Deployment dialysis in the U.S. Army: history and future challenges. Mil Med 2000;165(10):737.
8. Benedum J. Die Frühgeschichte der künstlichen Niere [The early history of the artificial kidney]. Anasthesiol Intensivmed Notfallmed Schmerzther 2003;38(11):681–8. German.
9. Fresenius medical care, the history of dialysis: historical basis of hemodialysis. Available at: file:///C:/Users/zuber/OneDrive/Desktop/PA%20Clinics%20%20Kidney%202022/12%20The%20military-Kim,%20Rodney/The%20history%20of%20dialysis%C2%A0-%C2%A0Fresenius%20Medical%20Care.pdf. Accessed January 9, 2021.
10. Henderson LW. A Tribute to Willem Johan Kolff, M.D., 1912–2009. Sorbent Therapeutics, Inc., South Kent, Connecticut. J Am Soc Nephrol 2009;20:923–4.
11. The Kolff rotating drum dialysis machine, Walter Reed Medical Library, photos and brochure.
12. Murray J. Interview with Dr Joseph Murray (by Francis L Delmonico). Am J Transplant 2002;2(9):803–6.
13. New York Times Obituary. Francis Daniels Moore dies at 88. 2001. Available at: https://www.nytimes.com/2001/11/29/us/dr-francis-moore-88-dies-innovative-leader-in-surgery.html. Accessed January 9, 2021.
14. Available at: https://blogs.va.gov/VAntage/35887/va-secretary-a-debt-of-gratitude-to-organ-transplant-pioneer-dr-thomas-e-starzl/. Accessed February 23, 2021.
15. Starzl T. A conversation with Thomas Starzl. Interview by Ushma S. Neill. J Clin Invest 2012;122(12):4304–5.
16. Available at: https://www.reaganlibrary.gov/archives/speech/radio-address-nation-international-monetary-fund-and-organ-donorship. Accessed March 9, 2021.
17. Jones M. Available at: https://pulitzercenter.org/reporting/soldiers-death-gives-life-another-man. Accessed January 10, 2021.
18. Berry Article.
19. Interview Steve Goldberger.
20. Interview Andrew Howard.
21. Available at: https://www.nih.gov/about-nih/who-we-are/history#:~:text=The%20Roots%20of%20NIH%20The%20National%20Institutes%20of,provide%20for%20the%20medical%20care%20of%20merchant%20seamen. Accessed March 6, 2021.
22. Available at: https://history.nih.gov/display/history/WWII%20Research%20and%20the%20Grants%20Program. Accessed March 6, 2021.

23. Bennett WM. The American Society of Nephrology at 50: a personal perspective. Clin J Am Soc Nephrol 2016;11(3):369–71.
24. Department of Defense. USN Comfort. Frequently asked questions. 2020. Available at: https://media.defense.gov/2020/May/18/2002302024/-1/1/1/FAQ_USNSCOMFORT_V6.PDF. Accessed January 9, 2021.
25. Hollingsworth JW, Bondy PK. The role of Veterans Affairs hospitals in the health care system. N Engl J Med 1990;322(26):1851–7.
26. Available at: https://www.research.va.gov/about/awards/awardee.cfm?award=53357. Accessed March 5, 2021.
27. Hynes DM, Stroupe KT, Greer JW, et al. Potential cost savings of erythropoietin administration in end-stage renal disease. Am J Med 2002;112(3):169–75.
28. VA/NIH Acute Renal Failure Trial Network, Palevsky PM, Zhang JH, O'Connor TZ, et al. Intensity of renal support in critically ill patients with acute kidney injury. N Engl J Med 2008;359(1):7–20.
29. Paul Palevsky discussion 2008
30. NKF. Available at: https://www.kidney.org/news/national-kidney-foundation-announces-appointment-university-pittsburgh-nephrologist-dr-paul-m. Accessed March 9, 2021.
31. Patel N, Golzy M, Nainani N, et al. Prevalence of various comorbidities among veterans with chronic kidney disease and its comparison with other datasets. Ren Fail 2016;38(2):204–8.
32. Brown JR, MacKenzie TA, Maddox TM, et al. Acute kidney injury risk prediction in patients undergoing coronary angiography in a national Veterans Health Administration cohort with external validation. J Am Heart Assoc 2015;4(12):e002136.
33. Heung M, Steffick DE, Zivin K, et al, Centers for Disease Control and Prevention CKD Surveillance Team. Acute Kidney injury recovery pattern and subsequent risk of CKD: an analysis of veterans health administration data. Am J Kidney Dis 2016;67(5):742–52.
34. Leehey DJ, Zhang JH, Emanuele NV, et al, VA NEPHRON-D Study Group. BP and renal outcomes in diabetic kidney disease: the Veterans Affairs Nephropathy in Diabetes Trial. Clin J Am Soc Nephrol 2015;10(12):2159–69.
35. Molnar MZ, Lu JL, Kalantar-Zadeh K, et al. Association of incident restless legs syndrome with outcomes in a large cohort of US veterans. J Sleep Res 2016; 25(1):47–56.
36. Kurella Tamura M, Li S, Chen SC, et al. Educational programs improve the preparation for dialysis and survival of patients with chronic kidney disease. Kidney Int 2014;85(3):686–92.
37. Schaefer M, Littrell E, Khan A, et al. Estimated GFR decline following sodium phosphate enemas versus polyethylene glycol for screening colonoscopy: a retrospective cohort study. Am J Kidney Dis 2016;67(4):609–16.
38. Nelson DA, Marks ES, Deuster PA, et al. Association of nonsteroidal anti-inflammatory drug prescriptions with kidney disease among active young and middle-aged adults. JAMA Netw Open 2019;2(2):e187896.
39. Xie Y, Bowe B, Gibson AK, et al. Comparative effectiveness of SGLT2 inhibitors, GLP-1 receptor agonists, DPP-4 inhibitors, and sulfonylureas on risk of kidney outcomes: emulation of a target trial using health care databases. Diabetes Care 2020;43(11):2859–69.

It's Not All Even
Health Disparities in Kidney Disease

Claretha Lyas, MD

KEYWORDS

• Chronic kidney disease • Disparities • LGBTQ+

KEY POINTS

• Populations of color have a disproportionate burden of chronic kidney disease and end-stage kidney disease.
• Minority groups are less likely to receive therapies shown to slow the progression of kidney disease, and they are less likely to receive kidney transplantation.
• The LGBTQ+ population shares similar kidney-related disparities as populations of color.

Health disparities have been present in the United States for generations. A nationalized system for recording health data originated in 1902 when the US Bureau of the Census was established as a permanent federal agency and began publishing vital statistics.[1] During this time, only a handful of states were participating, and much of the information reported involved birth and death statistics. Later, in 1960, the National Center for Health Statistics was established, leading the way for accurate, reliable health data to be published.[1] Since the 1960s, national health data have been reported annually on a variety of illnesses and health conditions. Not surprisingly, having a national system for reporting health data uncovered a disturbing trend of health disparities, particularly among individuals in minority groups. In the late 1990s, the infant mortality was 7.2/1000 live births overall; however, the rate for white infants was 6.0/1000 live births, whereas the rate for African American infants was 14.3/1000 live births.[1] In addition, health disparities in chronic illnesses became more apparent. For instance, the prevalence of obesity has been rapidly growing since the mid to late twentieth century. Since the 1980s, the highest rates have been among African Americans.[2] This has proven to be important given the well-established evidence that obesity is a predisposition for other chronic conditions, such as hypertension (HTN), cardiovascular disease (CVD), and type 2 diabetes (DM).

The prevalence of these 3 chronic illnesses has been increasing over time. A patient with HTN and/or DM has a higher risk of developing chronic kidney disease (CKD).

Division of Nephrology, Chronic Kidney Disease Clinic, University of Alabama at Birmingham, 624 Zeigler Research Building, 1720 2nd Avenue South, Birmingham, AL 35294-0005, USA
E-mail address: clyas@uabmc.edu

Physician Assist Clin 7 (2022) 357–365
https://doi.org/10.1016/j.cpha.2021.11.006
2405-7991/22/© 2021 Elsevier Inc. All rights reserved.
physicianassistant.theclinics.com

Many studies have shown that disparities exist in both the prevalence and the health outcomes among patients with these chronic conditions. Mokdad and colleagues[3] reported that in the year 2000, African Americans had the highest rate of DM in the United States among all racial groups. These data have been consistent across several other studies as shown by Voeks and colleagues,[4] Miech and colleagues,[5] and Bancks and colleagues.[6] Many studies have sought to understand why these disparities exist, including investigation of differences in health care resource allocation, health care utilization, quality of DM care, dietary habits, physical activity, perceived self-efficacy, and genetics. However, despite this work, the disparity in DM remains.

Similar trends are documented for HTN. There are numerous studies published over the past several decades that show an increased prevalence of HTN among African Americans along with an increasing trend of HTN-related complications, including CVD and stroke.[7–10] There are reports of increasing rates of uncontrolled HTN among African Americans.[11]

These trends have been disturbing and contribute to the increased risk of African Americans developing CKD and progressing to end-stage kidney disease (ESKD). In 2020, the US Renal Data System, a program designed to report annual data on ESKD and CKD in the United States, reported prevalence of CKD and ESKD based on data from the National Health and Nutrition Examination Survey (NHANES). NHANES is a program of studies designed to assess the health and nutritional status of adults and children in the United States and is a major program of the National Center for Health Statistics. This report showed that although the overall prevalence of CKD among African Americans and white Americans was similar, the prevalence of ESKD was 3.4 times higher in African Americans compared with whites; thus, highlighting the disparity that African Americans are more likely to experience progressive kidney dysfunction.[12]

Numerous other reports have highlighted similar disparities. Muntner and colleagues[13] showed that young African American individuals who participated in the community-based Coronary Artery Risk Development in Young Adults study, a prospective cohort study sponsored by the National Heart, Lung, and Blood Institute, had a 20-year higher CKD incidence compared with whites. In addition, Peralta and colleagues[14] showed that African Americans had a significantly higher rate of kidney function decline compared with whites, and this rate of decline occurred approximately 1 decade earlier in African Americans compared with whites. This same study also showed that Mexicans, South Americans, and other Hispanics had higher rates of kidney function decline compared with whites.[14]

There have been many other disparities reported within the realm of kidney disease, including inequities in medication management, specialty referral, transplantation, assessment of kidney function, and most recently, inequities surrounding the coronavirus pandemic.

Disparities have been reported in the medication-prescribing patterns of drug therapies known to slow the progression of kidney disease. It has been well established that angiotensin-converting enzyme inhibitors (ACE-i) or angiotensin receptor blockers (ARB) reduce albuminuria and help mitigate the risk of progressive CKD. In the 1980s through the early 2000s, it was thought that African Americans did not benefit from ACE-i/ARB medications because of differences in the renin-angiotensin-aldosterone axis and poorer cardiovascular outcomes (higher rates of acute myocardial infarction, stroke, and congestive heart failure).[15] As a result, many African Americans were preferentially treated with calcium channel blockers, whereas white Americans were treated with ACE-i/ARBs.[15] It was not until the publication of the African American Study of Kidney Disease and Hypertension (AASK) study in 2002 that this paradigm was questioned.[10] The AASK study was a randomized controlled trial that compared the effects of blood pressure control and antihypertensive medication classes on the rate of kidney function decline among African American hypertensive patients with kidney disease in the United States.[10] AASK showed that African American participants treated with an ACE-i had a decreased risk of the following endpoints: kidney function decline by 50% or more, ESKD, or death.[10]

Recently, there have been disparities reported in the prescribing patterns of sodium-glucose cotransporter 2 (SGLT2) inhibitors, medications designed to decrease kidney glucose reabsorption and increase urinary glucose excretion. In the landmark trial published by Heerspink and colleagues,[16] the SGLT2 inhibitor, dapagliflozin, reduced the risk of sustained decline in kidney function, ESKD, and death in patients with and without diabetes. Consequently, SGLT2 inhibitors have become the latest member in the CKD management repertoire. Unfortunately, in a study published by Eberly and colleagues[17] on SGLT2 inhibitor use among adult US patients with DM, including those with heart failure, atherosclerotic CVD, and CKD, African Americans were less likely to receive this beneficial therapy.

In addition to variations in medication-prescribing patterns, African Americans, as well as other minority groups, are more likely to experience delays in nephrology referral. Kinchen and colleagues[18] showed that in a national prospective cohort study of 81 dialysis facilities in the United States that African American men were more likely than white men to receive a late referral to a nephrologist, defined as less than 4 months from the time to initiation of dialysis. This later referral to nephrology was associated with a greater risk of death.[18]

Similarly, African Americans are less likely to receive a kidney transplant. A study published by Alexander and Sehgal[19] in 1998 demonstrated this finding. In this study, more than 7000 patients with ESKD on dialysis were followed to determine ability to complete the necessary steps for kidney transplantation. Steps were defined as follows19:

- Being medically suitable, possibly interested in transplant
- Definitely interested in transplant
- Completing the pretransplant workup
- Placed on the waiting list, with movement up the list and transplantation

The percentage of African Americans who were successfully able to complete all 4 steps and be successfully transplanted was substantially lower compared with whites.[19] Each step of the transplantation process showed a wider disparity gap between the 2 racial groups.[19] In the first step, being medically suitable and possibly interested in transplant, there were about 50% whites and 48% African Americans, with a difference of about 2%.[19] However, for the last step, which was moving up the transplant list and receiving a transplant, there were about 51% whites compared with 36% African Americans, or a difference of about 15%.[19]

There have been many variables reported to account for this disparity in transplantation. First, it has been described that whites are more likely to be referred to transplantation before initiation of dialysis compared with African Americans, in part because of greater access to care and bias from providers.[20] Also, it has been described that African Americans are less likely to identify potential living donors compared with whites. Those African Americans who are able to identify living donors have a greater likelihood of not receiving the living donor organ because of the donor having undiagnosed underlying HTN and glucose intolerance.[20]

Even after kidney transplantation, there are disparities in allograft survival. The review article by Young and Gaston[20] describes socioeconomic factors as a key variable in kidney allograft survival. It has been described by other investigators that patients without insurance before kidney transplantation, most often being African Americans, are more likely to have allograft loss. Butkus and colleagues[21] studied 100 cadaveric kidney allograft recipients at least 1 year after transplantation to evaluate variables associated with allograft loss. After controlling for other variables, such as immunosuppression regimen, age less than 30, and degree of immunologic mismatch between the donor and recipient, not having private insurance was associated with greater allograft loss, which was more apparent in African Americans compared with whites.[21] This decreased likelihood of having private insurance is a marker of African Americans' disparity in socioeconomic status, leading to poorer health outcomes.

In addition to disparities in transplantation, there has been widespread debate over the disparities caused in the assessment of kidney function. Glomerular filtration rate (GFR) equations, which estimate kidney function, have been in widespread use since the late 1970s. These equations use endogenous filtration markers, such as metabolites like creatinine, and the more recently recognized filtration markers like pseudouridine, acetylthreonine, myoinositol, phenylacetylglutamine, and tryptophan, and low-molecular-weight proteins, such as cystatin C, beta-2 microglobulin, and beta-trace protein, as a substitute for direct measurement.[22] These endogenous filtration markers are inversely related to GFR and directly related to other non-GFR determinants, including filtration marker generation, handling of the filtration marker by the kidney tubule, and extrarenal elimination of the marker.[22] These determinants are difficult to measure directly and often use surrogates for indirect measurement: age, sex, race, height and/or weight, or any combination of these. After the initial Cockcroft-Gault estimating equation was published in 1976, there was published research in 1999 by the National Institute of Diabetes and Digestive and Kidney Diseases and later by Levey and colleagues[22] that showed serum creatinine concentrations were higher among African Americans compared with whites.[23] The reason for this finding is often attributed to the presumption that African Americans have greater muscle mass compared with whites.[23] However, the validity of this assumption remains inconclusive, in part because of the challenges of reliably and noninvasively measuring lean body mass.[23] The subsequent GFR estimating equations (modification of diet in renal disease [MDRD] in 1999 and chronic kidney disease epidemiologic collaboration [CKD-EPI] in 2009) used race as one of the coefficients in the GFR equation.[24,25] In MDRD, the coefficient was equal to 1.20, which reflected a 20% higher measured GFR in African Americans compared with whites.[24] In CKD-EPI, the coefficient was 1.16, or a 16% higher measured GFR in African Americans.[25]

These estimating equations have since been scrutinized for contributing to disparities in kidney disease. The use of race in GFR-estimating equations reports a higher estimated glomerular filtration rate (eGFR), and resultant better kidney function, for African Americans compared with non-African Americans with the same serum creatinine. Consequently, this leads to delays in recognition of kidney disease, in referral to nephrologists and in referrals for transplantation.[26] In an effort to address these disparities caused by the existing CKD-EPI 2009 GFR equation, a task force created by the National Kidney Foundation and American Society of Nephrology adopted a new equation released in 2021 that refits the CKD-EPI equation without the race variable. This new equation is now more equitable for African Americans as it is designed to identify CKD earlier, thereby increasing the likelihood of nephrology referral and transplantation evaluation for African Americans.[27]

In addition to the systemic injustices contributing to kidney disease disparities in African Americans, there are also genetic variations recently described as playing a role. It has been shown that variations in the Apolipoprotein L1 (APOL1) gene contribute to the high burden of kidney disease in African Americans and individuals of African ancestry compared with white individuals.[28–31] The APOL1 gene is located on chromosome 22, and it encodes for the ApoL1 protein.[28] Circulating ApoL1 protein protects from *Trypanosoma brucei*, the parasite carried by the tsetse fly that causes African sleeping sickness.[28] Subspecies of *T brucei* have evolved resistance to the lytic effects of ApoL1 and can cause African sleeping sickness characterized initially by fevers and headaches, and later, by encephalopathy, ataxia, and insomnia. Individuals with the variant APOL1 gene (referred to as G1 and G2) are protected against *T brucei*, potentially conferring a selection advantage.[28,29] Studies over the past decade have shown that these gene variants (G1 and G2) confer an increased risk of kidney disease among nondiabetics, particularly in patients identified to have HIV-associated nephropathy (HIVAN), focal segmental glomerulosclerosis (FSGS), and HTN-associated ESKD.[29] One copy of the APOL1 gene is inherited from each parent. Individuals with 2 gene variants, one on each chromosome, have the greatest increased risk of kidney disease, whereas those inheriting only 1 high-risk gene variant have less of an increase in risk.[29] It is reported that about 13% of African Americans in the United States carry the high-risk genotype.[29] These gene variants carry an increased risk of kidney-related diseases. Studies have shown a 7- to 10-fold increased risk of HTN-associated ESKD, a 17-fold increased risk of FSGS, and a 29-fold increased risk of HIVAN in these individuals.[29]

These high-risk APOL1 gene alleles have also been found in Hispanic populations.[32] Hispanics have a diverse ancestral background encompassing African, Native American, and European ethnic groups. Hispanic individuals with the greatest proportion of African ancestry are found in the Caribbean, particularly Puerto Rico, Dominican Republic, and Cuba.[32] These groups have an increased risk of CKD.[32] A study by Kramer and colleagues[33] showed that Hispanics living in the Caribbean have a higher frequency of the 2 high-risk APOL1 gene variants, and this was associated with an increased risk of albuminuria and CKD.

Other kidney-related disparities are evident in the Latinx population, where there is a higher burden of CKD and progression to ESKD compared with non-Latinx white individuals. As in the African American patient population, Latinx individuals have a similar prevalence of CKD, especially in early stages of CKD, compared with white individuals.[32] However, progression to kidney failure is more rapid among both Latinx and African American individuals compared with whites.[32] Similar to African American individuals, Latinx populations suffer from similar socioeconomic disparities with decreased access to health care being the main contributing factor.[32] Pereira and Cervantes[34] report that 40% of Latinx individuals have either no health insurance or large copays that limit access to provider's visit and diagnostic test and procedures. Similar results were noted in a study by Hall and colleagues.[35] This study went further to examine use of medications known to slow the prevention of CKD. They showed that uninsured populations who historically have been predominantly Latinx and African American groups were less likely to be treated for HTN and less likely to be receiving an ACE-i or ARBs, both well known to slow the progression of CKD.[35]

In a review by Desai and colleagues,[32] it is noted that Hispanics have a greater than 50% chance of developing DM in their lifetime, and like other ethnic groups, DM is the most common cause of ESKD in Hispanic populations. Similarly, the progression to ESKD owing to diabetic nephropathy is higher in Hispanics, just as it is in African Americans, as compared with white individuals.[32]

As noted previously, Hispanics in the United States are more likely to have decreased access to care compared with non-Hispanic whites. Desai and colleagues[32] report that more than 25% of US Hispanics do not regularly see a health care provider. This disparity is thought to be related to socioeconomic factors: education, language barrier, or decreased likelihood of having health insurance.[32] In addition, Hispanics in the United States are less likely to receive a kidney transplant and are less likely to have a living kidney donor. The lack of living donors is attributed to decreased awareness about living donor kidney transplants and fear of the financial and health-related consequences of living kidney donation.[32]

Many minority groups have also been disproportionally affected by the coronavirus pandemic, and this has also contributed to kidney-related disparities. In the United States, the African American population carries the heaviest burden of COVID morbidity and mortality. Some estimates report that African Americans make up more than 25% of the coronavirus deaths even though African Americans comprise only 12% of the US population.[36] This disparity in mortality has been linked to the overrepresentation of black Americans in low-wage, service-related jobs that have been deemed "essential work."[36] Not only do African Americans suffer a disproportionately high rate of death from coronavirus but also they experience a high rate of kidney-related morbidity. Hirsch and colleagues[37] published findings of more than 5000 patients hospitalized with coronavirus in the New York metropolitan area from March 1, 2020 until April 15, 2020 and found that among the variables studied black race was associated with an increased risk of developing acute kidney injury. In addition, certain groups of African Americans, particularly those of recent African ancestry, may be more likely to have acute kidney injury along with high-grade proteinuria and hematuria from coronavirus as a result of possessing high-risk APOL1 gene alleles.[38]

There are also reports of fewer coronavirus vaccinations among African Americans compared with other racial groups. One report asserts that half of the states in the United States, only about 5% of coronavirus vaccines have gone to African Americans, whereas 2 to 3 times this number have gone to white Americans.[39] Increasing the rate of vaccination among African Americans will help mitigate the disparities in coronavirus and its kidney-associated morbidity.

Kidney-related disparities exist in LGBTQ+ individuals. However, adequate and accurate characterization of these disparities is lacking because of a lack of standardized methods of collecting data on sexual orientation and gender identity in large-scale research studies.[40] Stigmatization, medical mistrust, and decreased rate of health insurance also play a role in the limited amount of data known on disparities in LGBTQ+ individuals. In the few studies that are available, Dragon and colleagues[41] use Medicare claims data to describe aspects of the transgender population. They describe transgender individuals as having a high burden of chronic diseases, including CKD, with rates of CKD higher compared with their non-transgender, or cis-gender, counterparts.[41]

In addition to the high burden of CKD experienced by transgender individuals, there are also challenges in the management of CKD as it pertains to eGFR calculations. As discussed already, the currently available equations that estimate kidney function rely on endogenous biomarkers, with creatinine being the most common, as well as nonglomerular filtration determinants of kidney function, such as gender, age, and race. Transgender individuals may have variations in muscle mass owing to gender-affirming hormone therapy, leading to possible alterations in creatinine values.[42] This could in turn lead to bias and inaccuracy in estimating GFR. In a study reported by Collister and colleagues,[42] case reports of transgender men revealed an increase in serum creatinine after initiation of testosterone therapy, which later resulted in inaccuracies in both widely used GFR estimating equations. Such inaccuracies may prove consequential in clinical decision making for CKD in transgender individuals.

These and other disparities have been longstanding and pervasive across the spectrum of kidney disease. Recently, efforts have been instituted to address these disparities. The American Society of Nephrology and the National Kidney Foundation are working to provide recommendations to address race in the assessment of GFR.[26] There are numerous research efforts underway to address the morbidity associated with the high-risk APOL1 gene variants. These and other research efforts will go a long way in finding a cure for disparities in kidney disease.

CLINICS CARE POINTS

- It is important to recognize while managing patients with kidney disease that many disparities exist among minority populations.
- Understanding these disparities is important when developing minority patients plans of care.

DISCLOSURE

None.

REFERENCES

1. Guyer B, Freedman MA, Strobino DM, et al. Annual summary of vital statistics: trends in the health of Americans during the 20th century. Pediatrics 2000; 106(6):1307–17.
2. Mokdad AH, Serdula MK, Dietz WH, et al. The spread of the obesity epidemic in the United States, 1991-1998. J Am Med Assoc 1999;282(16):1519–22.
3. Mokdad AH, Bowman BA, Ford ES, et al. The continuing epidemics of obesity and diabetes in the United States. J Am Med Assoc 2001;286(10):1195–200.
4. Voeks JH, McClure LA, Go RC, et al. Regional differences in diabetes as a possible contributor to the geographic disparity in stroke mortality: the Reasons for Geographic and Racial Differences in Stroke Study. Stroke 2008;39(6): 1675–80.
5. Miech RA, Kim J, McConnell C, et al. A growing disparity in diabetes-related mortality U.S. trends, 1989-2005. Am J Prev Med 2009;36(2):126–32.
6. Bancks MP, Kershaw K, Carson AP, et al. Association of modifiable risk factors in young adulthood with racial disparity in incident type 2 diabetes during middle adulthood. J Am Med Assoc 2017;318(24):2457–65.
7. Wyatt SB, Akylbekova EL, Wofford MR, et al. Prevalence, awareness, treatment, and control of hypertension in the Jackson Heart Study. Hypertens 2008;51(3): 650–6.
8. Douglas JG, Agodoa L. ACE inhibition is effective and renoprotective in hypertensive nephrosclerosis: the African American Study of Kidney Disease and Hypertension (AASK) trial. Kidney Int Suppl 2003;(83):S74–6.
9. Lackland DT. Racial differences in hypertension: implications for high blood pressure management. Am J Med Sci 2014;348(2):135–8.
10. Wright JT Jr, Bakris G, Greene T, et al, for the African American Study of Kidney Disease and Hypertension Study Group. Effect of blood pressure lowering and antihypertensive drug class on progression of hypertensive kidney disease: results from the AASK trial. J Am Med Assoc 2002;288(19):2421–31.
11. Saeed, A et al. Racial disparities in hypertension prevalence and management: a crisis control? American College of Cardiology. American College of Cardiology

(acc.org). 2020. Available at: https://www.acc.org/latest-in-cardiology/articles/2020/04/06/08/53/racial-disparities-in-hypertension-prevalence-and-management. Accessed August 10, 2021.

12. United States Renal Data System. 2020 USRDS annual data report: epidemiology of kidney disease in the United States. Bethesda, MD: National Institutes of Health, National Institute of Diabetes and Digestive and Kidney Diseases; 2020.

13. Muntner P, Newsome B, Kramer H, et al. Racial differences in the incidence of chronic kidney disease. Clin J Am Soc Nephrol 2012;7(1):101–7.

14. Peralta CA, Katz R, DeBoer I, et al. Racial and ethnic differences in kidney function decline among persons without chronic kidney disease. J Am Soc Nephrol 2011;22(7):1327–34.

15. Norton JM, Moxey-Mims MM, Eggers PW, et al. Social determinants of racial disparities in CKD. J Am Soc Nephrol 2016;27(9):2576–95.

16. Heerspink HJL, Stefánsson BV, Correa-Rotter R, et al, for the DAPA-CKD Trial Committees and Investigators. Dapagliflozin in patients with chronic kidney disease. N Engl J Med 2020;383(15):1436–46.

17. Eberly LA, Yang L, Eneanya ND, et al. Association of race/ethnicity, gender, and socioeconomic status with sodium-glucose cotransporter 2 inhibitor use among patients with diabetes in the US. JAMA Netw Open 2021;4(4):e216139.

18. Kinchen KS, Sadler J, Fink N, et al. The timing of specialist evaluation in chronic kidney disease and mortality. Ann Intern Med 2002;137(6):479–86.

19. Alexander GC, Sehgal AR. Barriers to cadaveric renal transplantation among blacks, women, and the poor. J Am Med Assoc 1998;280(13):1148–52.

20. Young CJ, Gaston RS. Renal transplantation in black Americans. N Engl J Med 2000;343(21):1545–52.

21. Butkus DE, Meydrech EF, Raju SS. Racial differences in the survival of cadaveric renal allografts. Overriding effects of HLA matching and socioeconomic factors. N Engl J Med 1992;327(12):840–5.

22. Levey AS, Titan SM, Powe NR, et al. Kidney disease, race, and GFR estimation. Clin J Am Soc Nephrol 2020;15(8):1203–12.

23. Hsu J, Johansen KL, Hsu CY, et al. Higher serum creatinine concentrations in black patients with chronic kidney disease: beyond nutritional status and body composition. Clin J Am Soc Nephrol 2008;3(4):992–7.

24. Levey AS, Bosch JP, Lewis JB, et al. A more accurate method to estimate glomerular filtration rate from serum creatinine: a new prediction equation. Modification of Diet in Renal Disease Study Group. Ann Intern Med 1999;130(6):461–70.

25. Levey AS, Stevens LA, Schmid CH, et al, for the CKD-EPI (Chronic Kidney Disease Epidemiology Collaboration). A new equation to estimate glomerular filtration rate. Ann Intern Med 2009;150(9):604–12.

26. Delgado C, Baweja M, Burrows NR, et al. Reassessing the inclusion of race in diagnosing kidney diseases: an interim report from the NKF-ASN Task Force. Am J Kidney Dis 2021;78(1):103–15.

27. Delgado C, Baweja M, Crews DC, et al. A Unifying Approach for GFR Estimation: Recommendations of the NKF-ASN Task Force on Reassessing the Inclusion of Race in Diagnosing Kidney Disease. Am J Kidney Dis 2022;79(2):268–288.e1. https://doi.org/10.1053/j.ajkd.2021.08.003.

28. Pollak MR, Genovese G, Friedman DJ. APOL1 and kidney disease. Curr Opin Nephrol Hypertens 2012;21(2):179–82.

29. Friedman DJ, Pollak MR. APOL1 nephropathy: from genetics to clinical applications. Clin J Am Soc Nephrol 2021;16(2):294–303.

30. Freedman BI, Limou S, Ma L, et al. APOL1-associated nephropathy: a key contributor to racial disparities in CKD. Am J Kidney Dis 2018;72(5 Suppl 1): S8–16.
31. Umeukeje EM, Young BA. Genetics and ESKD disparities in African Americans. Am J Kidney Dis 2019;74(6):811–21.
32. Desai N, Lora CM, Lash JP, et al. CKD and ESRD in US Hispanics. Am J Kidney Dis 2019;73(1):102–11.
33. Kramer HJ, Stilp AM, Laurie CC, et al. African ancestry-specific alleles and kidney disease risk in Hispanics/Latinos. J Am Soc Nephrol 2017;28(3):915–22.
34. Pereira RI, Cervantes L. Reducing the burden of CKD among Latinx: a community-based approach. Clin J Am Soc Nephrol 2021;16(5):812–4.
35. Hall YN, Rodriguez RA, Boyko EJ, et al. Characteristics of uninsured Americans with chronic kidney disease. J Gen Intern Med 2009;24(8):917–22.
36. Crews DC, Purnell TS. COVID-19, racism, and racial disparities in kidney disease: galvanizing the kidney community response. J Am Soc Nephrol 2020; 31(8):1–3.
37. Hirsch JS, Ng JH, Ross DW, et al, for Northwell Nephrology COVID-19 Research Consortium. Acute kidney injury in patients hospitalized with COVID-19. Kidney Int 2020;98(1):209–18.
38. Shetty AA, Tawhari I, Safar-Boueri L, et al. COVID-19-associated glomerular disease. J Am Soc Nephrol 2021;32(1):33–40.
39. Newman AM. Institutional problems, individual solutions - the burden on black physicians. N Engl J Med 2021;384(22):2076–8.
40. Mohottige D, Lunn MR. Advancing equity in nephrology: enhancing care for LGBTQ+ patients and our workforce. Clin J Am Soc Nephrol 2019;14(7):1094–6.
41. Dragon CN, Guerino P, Ewald E, et al. Transgender Medicare beneficiaries and chronic conditions: exploring fee-for-service claims data. LGBT Health 2017; 4(6):404–11.
42. Collister D, Saad N, Christie E, et al. Providing care for transgender persons with kidney disease: a narrative review. Can J Kidney Health Dis 2021;8. 2054358120985379.

The Chromosomes and the Kidney
Genomics in the 21st Century

Nguyen H. Park, MS, PA-C

KEYWORDS

- Genetics • Genomics • Gene therapy • Molecular diagnosis

KEY POINTS

- Advances in genetic testing and molecular imaging reveal more genetic bases for kidney disease.
- As molecular diagnoses are established, novel targets for treatment and therapy will allow clinicians to prevent and slow the progression of CKD.
- Clinicians will require more familiarity with genetic testing and ethical issues surrounding testing in the treatment of kidney disease.

INTRODUCTION

Kidney disease affects more than 20 million people in the United States alone and more than 850 million people globally.[1] A family history of nephropathy is noted in almost one in three cases of chronic kidney disease (CKD); thus, a genetic cause of kidney disease should be on the differential diagnosis of every clinician.[1,2] Viewing kidney disease through the lens of genetics and genomics, implicated are not only cancer, congenital kidney diseases, and syndromes affecting the kidney, but also diseases thought previously to have primarily acquired causes (ie, diabetic kidney disease). Conditions previously were described by clinical characteristics (ie, Alport syndrome [AS]); however, medicine is rapidly moving toward a molecular analysis for the pathogenesis of disease. Learning a molecular diagnosis can have implications for changes in monitoring, testing, treatment, and familial testing. This article examines the current state of what is known about genetic and genomic mechanisms of a few of the most well-known and most common kidney diseases. It looks at basic genetic and genomic concepts including types of inheritance and mutations, and details some of the most recent discoveries regarding the molecular underpinnings of kidney disease. These discoveries offer windows into new treatments for diseases that

National Institutes of Health/NHGRI/ACMG, 9000 Rockville Pike, Clinical Research Center Building 10, Bethesda, MD 20892, USA
E-mail address: PAGeneSig@gmail.com

Physician Assist Clin 7 (2022) 367–375
https://doi.org/10.1016/j.cpha.2021.11.007
2405-7991/22/Published by Elsevier Inc.
physicianassistant.theclinics.com

previously could only be managed. Ethical, legal, and social implications (ELSI) surrounding genetics/genomics, testing, and access to care are explored, as are the challenges that accompany the influence of genetics/genomics on the care of patients with kidney disease across varying populations.

RENAL CELL CARCINOMA

Renal cell carcinoma (RCC) is one of the top 10 most common cancers in the United States and comprises approximately 90% of kidney cancer cases.[3] The clear cell RCC subtype comprises approximately 70% of cases of RCC. The rest of the RCC cases fall into the category of non–clear cell RCC, which includes papillary RCC, the second most common subtype of RCC, and other rare subtypes including chromophobe RCC. Numerous syndromes are associated with an increased risk of all types of kidney cancer (ie, von Hippel-Lindau syndrome, chromosome 3 translocations).[4] Strides in oncology continue to improve survival rates for patients with RCC with the most recent advances in treatment involving combinations of antiangiogenic therapies plus immune checkpoint inhibitors. This treatment combination is a logical progression because each medication used as monotherapy in advanced RCC is clinically efficacious.[5] Large randomized phase III trials are ongoing with vascular endothelial growth factor or vascular endothelial growth factor receptor inhibitors plus immune checkpoint inhibitors targeting the cancer. Preliminary results are promising, with increased median progression-free survival rates.[6–8]

NEPHROTIC SYNDROME

Nephrotic syndrome (NS), a condition characterized by phenotypes that are monogenic and polygenic, is the most common glomerular disease among children. There are several subtypes:

- Secondary NS
- Congenital
- Infantile
- Idiopathic
  - Steroid sensitive
  - Steroid resistant

Histologic classifications of NS noted on renal biopsy include focal segmental glomerulosclerosis (FSGS) and minimal change disease. These classifications are important, because when minimal change disease is noted, patients are more likely to respond to steroid therapy than patients with FSGS lesions. When FSGS is noted, NS frequently progresses to CKD and ultimately end-stage kidney disease (ESKD), with recurrence frequently noted on kidney transplant; thus, swift diagnosis and treatment can delay this onset.[9] Complicating FSGS diagnosis, as with many kidney diseases requiring histopathologic diagnosis, is the difficulty inherent with kidney biopsy missing the FSGS lesion. This can lead to underdiagnosis, especially in children. Investigations for the molecular basis for NS continue to reveal new mutations involved in monogenic forms of FSGS. Currently, next-generation sequencing has found more than 50 genes associated with steroid-resistant NS.[10] Because monogenic FSGS is usually steroid-resistant, a molecular diagnosis would enable providers to avoid the risks inherent with kidney biopsy, steroid exposure, the chance of a missed biopsy, and the side effects concomitant with immunosuppressive regimens.

FABRY DISEASE

Fabry disease (FD) is another example of how advances in novel therapies and the understanding of the genetic basis for the disease can change how a well-known disorder affecting kidneys is treated. FD is a metabolic disorder and results from a buildup of a glycosphingolipid called globotriaosylceramide (Gb3). This buildup is secondary to deficient production of the enzyme α-galactosidase A (α-gal A).[11] FD is characterized by multisystemic effects from the accumulation of Gb3 causing cellular and microvascular dysfunction throughout the body. In terms of kidney function, many patients progress to kidney failure, dialysis, and/or kidney transplant. FD is an X-linked lysosomal storage disorder; thus, males with a pathogenic variant on the *GLA* gene are affected because they have only one X chromosome. Similar symptoms are seen in heterozygous females, of a lesser severity and later onset, and kidney failure is rare.[12] Males with the pathogenic variant pass the pathogenic variant to their daughters, but not to their sons because of the X-linked method of transmission. Offspring of heterozygous females have a 50% chance of having the variant. Symptoms usually begin in childhood and misdiagnosis is not uncommon. Diagnosis in females requires GLA gene sequencing. α-gal A enzyme assays are confirmatory for males suspected of having FD, but follow-up GLA gene sequencing is recommended with a positive assay. Although FD was first described in 1898, the mutation of the *GLA* gene found at loci Xq 22.1 was not discovered until the 1970s. The mechanism of disease was discovered in the 1960s; however, no therapies were available until 2001. An enzyme replacement is the mainstay of therapy.[13] Gene therapy, introducing a working *GLA* gene to provide instructions to the cells to produce α-gal A, is in phase I/II pilot studies and demonstrates promising results. Patients have been responsive to the LV-mediated gene therapy at some level, showing plasma and leukocyte α-gal A–specific activity greater than or within the reference range, and reductions in Gb3 and lysosomal Gb3 levels.[14] Another recent study reports discovery of a novel *GLA* splicing mutation, which causes a remarkable increase in the alternatively spliced *GLA* transcript and, consequently, results in the kidney phenotype of FD.[15]

ALPORT SYNDROME

The incidence of AS is 1 in 5000 to 10,000 people; however, this prevalence may be revealed to be higher as more targeted genetic testing of patients occurs.[16] AS has multiple patterns of inheritance:

- X-linked AS
- Autosomal-recessive AS
- Autosomal-dominant AS

In AS, electron microscopic findings demonstrate irregular thickening and thinning of the glomerular basement membrane, lamellation and splitting of the lamina densa; however, because significant histopathologic variation is seen in AS depending on stage or inheritance pattern, AS is frequently mistaken for other syndromes. Targeted next-generation genetic testing can lead to in-depth genotype-phenotype correlations, and allow for first-line diagnosis of AS to be made without kidney biopsy. For example, patients with X-linked AS with wide deletions, nonsense mutations, or frameshift mutations were almost twice as likely to progress to ESKD by age 30 in comparison with patients with missense mutations. When definitive diagnosis of AS is made quickly, commencement of angiotensin-converting enzyme inhibitors (ACEi) is initiated when appropriate thereby significantly increasing the time until the onset of ESKD.[17]

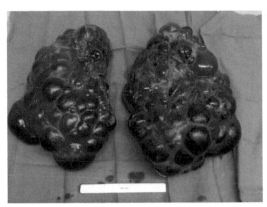

Fig. 1. Bilateral ADPKD kidneys. (Used with permission from Kim Zuber, PAC, 2021.)

AUTOSOMAL-DOMINANT POLYCYSTIC KIDNEY DISEASE

Autosomal-dominant polycystic disease (ADPKD) is another condition where genetic testing can lead to early diagnosis and therapy that can delay the onset of ESKD. ADPKD is caused by mutations in the polycystin genes: *PKD1* (80% of cases) or *PKD2* (15% of cases). ADPKD is the most common hereditary kidney disease occurring in 1 in every 400 to 1000 births, and in the United States, is one of the top five leading causes of ESKD.[18] In autosomal-dominant inheritance only one copy of the gene with the pathogenic variant is necessary to cause disease; thus, each child of a parent with the pathogenic gene has a 50% chance of developing ADPKD. Progression is marked by development and expansion of kidney cysts and progressive kidney enlargement, measured by total kidney volume. Total kidney volume can progress for years before a patient develops CKD (**Fig. 1**).

Systemic manifestations include hypertension, pain syndrome, hematuria, cystic infection, hemorrhage, and/or nephrolithiasis. Severity can range from mild cases managed with medications to more severe cases characterized by kidney failure, dialysis, and the need for kidney transplant. Disease-modifying therapies have been developed that target cystogenesis and suppress intracellular levels of cAMP.[19] Although the genes involved in ADPKD have been known for more than 20 years, a recent study using newly developed cilia electrophysiology and high-resolution microscopic imaging determined the exact molecular changes wrought by *PKD2* mutations, which may lead to additional therapies. *PKD2* is found in the primary cilia on the surface of cells involved in forming ion channels where ions move in and out of a cell. Mutations on *PKD2* destabilized ion channel structure in the cilia of kidney cells leading to impaired proper channel opening. With this discovery, investigation into therapy that targets the specific gene variant to restore function of the ion channels can begin.[20]

CHRONIC KIDNEY DISEASE

CKD affects more than 1 in 10 people worldwide and has significant associated morbidity and mortality.[21] Diabetic kidney disease, which develops in about 40% of patients with diabetes, is thought to be the most common cause of ESKD, although causes of CKD are often attributed by clinical correlation as opposed to histopathologic confirmation. Clinical correlation occurs because in the early stages of CKD, patients are often asymptomatic, and thus CKD may be missed. Once patients are in advanced stages of CKD, kidney biopsy may be contraindicated or inconclusive. For more than 10% of patients, the cause of CKD is unknown. Genetic kidney disease has typically been found in higher rates among pediatric CKD patients; a review of recent studies suggests 1 in 10 in adult patients with ESKD may have an identifiable genetic kidney disease contrasted with one in three pediatric patients. In one study of patients with CKD, discovery of a genetic diagnosis in up to 75% of cases led to changes in diagnosis, prognosis, risk stratification, and treatment.[2] Studies that identify modifier genes that may predispose patients to CKD or diabetic kidney disease are ongoing and are especially helpful in the cohort of patients with diabetes (type 1 and type 2). In one study, researchers analyzed data from greater than 1000 patients with type 2 diabetes, in which they prospectively followed nephrologic complications. Patients were randomized to ascertain the effect of the ACEi trandolapril on new-onset microalbuminuria. A new variant in the complement factor H gene that confers an increased risk of microalbuminuria was followed and cardiovascular complications. A decreased likelihood of benefit from ACEi therapy was noted for those patients who carried the factor H haplotype.[22] In another study, the benefits of widening investigations into diverse and multiethnic populations demonstrated a new genome-wide associated locus for mild to moderate CKD.[23] Investigators had studied multiethnic data on more than 40,000 participants in the Population Architecture using Genomics and Epidemiology (PAGE) study, which included African Americans, Hispanics/Latinos, East Asian, Native Hawaiian, and Native Americans.[23]

Findings in CKD incidence and progression among specific subgroups are undergoing even further scrutiny, with novel targets for therapy revealed as studies reveal the pathologic mechanisms of mutation. African Americans suffer disparately more kidney disease when compared with the entire population of patients with CKD, with kidney failure occurring at four to five times the rate of Americans of European ancestry. African American patients make up more than a third of dialysis patients despite representing only 13% of the overall US population. It is estimated that by 2030, globally almost three-quarters of patients with ESKD will be in low and lower-middle income countries including African countries.[24] Even accounting for known health disparities related to income disparity, African Americans not only have increased rates of CKD, but also have faster progression to kidney failure, independent of socioeconomic status or the presence of traditional clinical risk factors.[25] One known genetic risk factor identified in causing high rates of kidney disease in this population is the pathogenic variants in the Apolipoprotein L1 (APOL1) gene. Two alleles within the APOL1 gene, termed G1 and G2, encode the APOL1 protein.[26] In most instances, one APOL1 risk allele has no effect or, at most, a small effect on the incidence of kidney disease, whereas those carrying the two high-risk alleles have a 20% risk of developing CKD. Seventy percent of African American patients with FSGS or HIV-associated nephropathy carry the two APOL1 risk alleles. The APOL1 protein isoform lacks a signal peptide and is retained within cells leading to kidney injury, including arterionephrosclerosis, FSGS, and collapsing glomerulopathy.[26] Because recent studies have revealed pathophysiologic mechanisms of APOL1-associated CKD, targeted gene therapies are being developed, including an APOL1 antisense drug. This targeted APOL1 medication has been shown to ameliorate proteinuria in animal models.[27] All studies continue to demonstrate genetic and environmental causes of CKD and highlight the need for further investigation into mechanisms surrounding CKD.

ETHICAL, LEGAL, AND SOCIAL IMPLICATIONS

Although the advances in genetic testing are allowing clinicians to diagnose and treat more patients, the ELSI considerations that arise add an additional layer of complexity to the practice of medicine. One unique aspect of diagnosing conditions with a genetic/genomic cause is the potential for diagnosing family members. Although expanding the locus of benefit from patients to their extended family may be gratifying for providers, it also highlights some of the ethical concerns that accompany the practice of medicine in the genomic era. Issues of privacy, confidentiality, and informed consent require discussion before testing. Patients may not be cognizant of the ramifications of testing on their family members regarding not only the primary condition for which testing is ordered, but also any incidental findings.[28] Referral to genetic counselors, other genetics professionals, and to support groups is key to balanced and nuanced care of patients with genetic conditions. When the patient is a child or the patient's family includes children younger than the age of 18, further ELSI considerations arise. Genetic testing of children for conditions that have onset in adult years and without need for medical actions to be taken in childhood to prevent or ameliorate disease was generally not recommended until recently.[29] There is also the concern of obtaining health insurance with a known genetic defect. In 2008, Congress passed the Genetic Information Nondisclosure Act (GINA) which bars the use of genetic information in health insurance and employment.[30] GINA forbids group health plans and health insurers from denying coverage to a healthy individual or charging that person higher premiums based solely on a genetic predisposition to developing a disease. It also bars employers from using individuals' genetic information when making hiring, firing, job placement, or promotion decisions.[30]

With new therapeutic options developing, new consensus guidelines have recently been published by the American College of Medical Genetics and Genomics. These guidelines have changed recommendations for testing in the case of congenital anomalies, developmental delay, and intellectual disability. In those particular cases, systematic review has demonstrated the clinical utility of exome/genome sequencing.[31]

Challenges to integrating genetic/genomic data into the care of patients are manifold and have already started to change the practice of medicine. Patients are increasingly more familiar with genetic parlance with the rise of acceptability of direct-to-consumer genetic tests. In April 2017, the Food and Drug Administration granted approval for the first direct-to-consumer tests that provide genetic risk information for certain conditions, and in October 2018, *23andMe* received authorization to offer reports to customers on pharmacogenetics.[32,33] By 2019, more than 26 million people had purchased direct-to-consumer tests, with an estimated 100 million total by 2021.[34] Although the public perception of the utility of genetic/genomic data is largely positive, providers often feel unprepared to interpret genetic/genomic data for the diagnosis and treatment of their patients.[35] A study of family practice and specialty residents revealed that most of those surveyed felt unprepared to deal with genetic conditions despite believing that genetics is important.[36]

As testing choices have greatly expanded, from fluorescence in situ hybridization tests to next-generation sequencing to whole exome and whole genome sequencing, ordering the correct test is confusing. This is before taking into account which tests will be covered by the patient's insurance plan if at all. We are far from the science fiction fantasy of one machine that can determine a patient's condition with the touch of a button. Evaluation from clinicians regarding details of a patient's phenotype, carefully obtained family history, and other considerations (age, symptoms) are key factors to assist in choosing a test leading to a genetic diagnosis. The guidance of genetics professionals will continue to be germane.

Adding to the challenge of this ever-growing database of medical knowledge, is the continuing shortage of clinicians which impacts patients and their families at all stages of the diagnostic journey. Workforce studies forecast the acute lack of medical geneticists and other genetics professionals will continue as the current workforce ages and retires and demand outpaces availability. Access to primary care is already problematic in rural and remote communities, and access to genetic services is limited to primarily academic and large urban centers. Once the appropriate tests or referrals are made, the wait time to see genetics professionals is often months. After diagnosis, patients with genetic conditions often need a coordinated team of genetics professionals including occupational and physical therapists, social workers, and support groups for patients and their families. With all of these roadblocks, providers may feel overwhelmed. Concerted efforts in the genetics community are ongoing to educate providers, to increase workforce recruitment efforts including creating novel positions (genetics champions and genetics navigators), and to consolidate resources so efficient delivery of genetic care can occur. One positive change brought about by the COVID-19 pandemic was the exponential growth of telemedicine, with many genetics professionals now offering telegenetics visits, decreasing wait times and assisting families for whom long-distance travel is difficult.

SUMMARY

The promise of precision medicine is tantalizing to most physician assistants, with the goal of precise diagnosis leading to therapeutic interventions. The reality is that despite the start of mapping of the human genome occurring almost 30 years ago, the medical community does not yet have a complete understanding of all genetic/genomic causes of disease, let alone kidney disease. One effort to contribute to the understanding of kidney disease is the International Genetics & Translational Research in Transplantation Network (iGeneTRAiN), a multisite consortium that encompasses more than 45 genetic studies with genome-wide genotyping, including genome-wide data from greater than 30 kidney transplant cohorts. This program has already led to studies revealing details of disease etiologies in CKD and kidney transplantation.[37] As more secrets are unlocked, more and more frequently disease is noted to have a genetic basis, whether inherited or acquired. The challenge to all providers is in preparing for this revolution in how to care for patients with this mindset.[38] Physician assistants are uniquely poised to rise to this challenge with our focus on treating the whole patient; our broad, highly adaptable primary care training; and our team-based approach to caring for patients from birth through the end of life.[39]

DISCLOSURE

NHGRI/ACMG Genomic Medicine Program Management Fellow.

REFERENCES

1. Jager KJ, Kovesdy C, Langham R, et al. A single number for advocacy and communication-worldwide more than 850 million individuals have kidney diseases. Kidney Int 2019;96(5):1048–50.
2. Groopman EE, Marasa M, Cameron-Christie S, et al. Diagnostic utility of exome sequencing for kidney disease. N Engl J Med 2019;380(2):142–51.
3. Key statistics about kidney cancer, American Cancer Society. Available at: https://www.cancer.org/cancer/kidney-cancer/about/key-statistics.html. Accessed 31 July 2021.
4. Haas NB, Nathanson KL. Hereditary kidney cancer syndromes. Adv Chronic Kidney Dis 2014;21(1):81–90.

5. Gao X, McDermott DF, Michaelson MD. Enhancing antitumor immunity with anti-angiogenic therapy: a clinical model in renal cell carcinoma? Oncologist 2019; 24(6):725–7.

6. Lee WS, Yang H, Chon HJ, et al. Combination of anti-angiogenic therapy and immune checkpoint blockade normalizes vascular-immune crosstalk to potentiate cancer immunity. Exp Mol Med 2020;52:1475–85. https://doi.org/10.1038/s12276-020-00500-y.

7. Rini BI, Plimack ER, Stus V, et al. KEYNOTE-426 Investigators. Pembrolizumab plus axitinib versus sunitinib for advanced renal-cell carcinoma. N Engl J Med 2019;380(12):1116 27.

8. Motzer RJ, Penkov K, Haanen J, et al. Avelumab plus axitinib versus sunitinib for advanced renal-cell carcinoma. N Engl J Med 2019;380(12):1103–15.

9. Congenital Nephrotic Syndrome, Medline Plus. Available at: https://medlineplus.gov/genetics/condition/congenital-nephrotic-syndrome. Accessed 31 July 2021.

10. Bensimhon AR, Williams AE, Gbadegesin RA. Treatment of steroid-resistant nephrotic syndrome in the genomic era. Pediatr Nephrol 2019;34(11):2279–93.

11. American College of Medical Genetics, newborn screening ACT sheet, Fabry disease. Available at: https://www.acmg.net/PDFLibrary/Fabry.pdf. Accessed 31 July 2021.

12. Deegan PB, Bähner F, Barba M, et al. Fabry disease in females: clinical characteristics and effects of enzyme replacement therapy. In: Mehta A, Beck M, Sunder-Plassmann G, editors. Fabry disease: perspectives from 5 years of FOS. Oxford: Oxford PharmaGenesis; 2006. Chapter 30. Available at: https://www.ncbi.nlm.nih.gov/books/NBK11591. Accessed 31 July 2021.

13. Bartolotta C, Filogamo M, Colomba P, et al. History of Anderson-Fabray disease. Nephrol Dial Transplant 2015;30(Issue suppl_3). Page iii379, https://doi.org/10.1093/ndt/gfv186.08, Accessed 31 July 2021.

14. Khan A, Barber DL, Huang J, et al. Lentivirus-mediated gene therapy for Fabry disease. Nat Commun 2021;12(1):1178.

15. Li P, Zhang L, Zhao N, et al. A novel α-Galactosidase A splicing mutation predisposes to Fabry disease. Front Genet 2019;10:60.

16. Kashtan CE. Alport syndrome: achieving early diagnosis and treatment. Am J Kidney Dis 2021;77(2):272–9.

17. Nozu K, Nakanishi K, Abe Y, et al. A review of clinical characteristics and genetic backgrounds in Alport syndrome. Clin Exp Nephrol 2019;23(2):158–68.

18. Nobakht N, Hanna RM, Al-Baghdadi M, et al. Advances in autosomal dominant polycystic kidney disease: a clinical review. Kidney Med 2020;2(2):196–208.

19. Sussman CR, Wang X, Chebib FT, et al. Modulation of polycystic kidney disease by G-protein coupled receptors and cyclic AMP signaling. Cell Signal 2020;72:109649.

20. Vien TN, Wang J, Ng LCT, et al. Molecular dysregulation of ciliary polycystin-2 channels caused by variants in the TOP domain. Proc Natl Acad Sci U S A 2020;117(19):10329–38.

21. GBD 2015 DALYs and HALE Collaborators. Global, regional, and national disability-adjusted life-years (DALYs) for 315 diseases and injuries and healthy life expectancy (HALE), 1990-2015: a systematic analysis for the Global Burden of Disease Study 2015. Lancet 2016;388(10053):1603–58.

22. Valoti E, Noris M, Perna A, et al. Impact of a complement factor H gene variant on renal dysfunction, cardiovascular events, and response to ACE inhibitor therapy in type 2 diabetes. Front Genet 2019;10:681.

23. Lin BM, Nadkarni GN, Tao R, et al. Genetics of chronic kidney disease stages across ancestries: the PAGE study. Front Genet 2019;10:494.
24. Stanifer JW, Jing B, Tolan S, et al. The epidemiology of chronic kidney disease in sub-Saharan Africa: a systematic review and meta-analysis. Lancet Glob Health 2014;2(3):e174–81.
25. Aminu Abba Yusuf, Melanie A Govender, Jean-Tristan Brandenburg, Winkler Cheryl A. Kidney disease and APOL1. Hum Mol Genet 2021;30(Issue R1):R129–37. Available at: https://doi.org/10.1093/hmg/ddab024, Accessed 31 July 2021.
26. Friedman DJ, Pollak MR. APOL1 nephropathy: from genetics to clinical applications. Clin J Am Soc Nephrol 2021;16(2):294–303.
27. Aghajan M, Booten SL, Althage M, et al. Antisense oligonucleotide treatment ameliorates IFN-γ-induced proteinuria in APOL1-transgenic mice. JCI Insight 2019;4(12):e126124.
28. Miller DT, Lee K, Gordon AS, et al, for the ACMG Secondary Findings Working Group. Recommendations for reporting of secondary findings in clinical exome and genome sequencing, 2021 update: a policy statement of the American College of Medical Genetics and Genomics (ACMG). Genet Med 2021;23(8):1391–8.
29. Botkin JR. Ethical issues in pediatric genetic testing and screening. Curr Opin Pediatr 2016;28(6):700–4.
30. US Equal Employment Opportunity Commission, The Genetic Information Nondiscrimination Act of 2008. Available at: https://www.eeoc.gov/statutes/genetic-information-nondiscrimination-act-2008. Accessed 23 August 2021.
31. Manickam K, McClain MR, Demmer LA, et al. Exome and genome sequencing for pediatric patients with congenital anomalies or intellectual disability: an evidence-based clinical guideline of the American College of Medical Genetics and Genomics (ACMG). Genet Med 2021;23:2029–37. https://doi.org/10.1038/s41436-021-01242-6.
32. U.S. Food & Drug Administration. FDA allows marketing of first direct-to consumer tests that provide genetic risk information for certain conditions. 2017. Available at: https://www.fda.gov/news-events/press-announcements/fda-allows-marketing-first-direct-consumer-tests-provide-genetic-risk-information-certain-conditions. Accessed 31 July 2021.
33. 23andMe. 23andMe Granted The first and only FDA authorization for direct-to-consumer pharmacogenetics reports. Available at: https://blog.23andme.com/news/pharmacogenetics-report. Accessed July 31, 2021.
34. Regalado A. 2017 was the year consumer DNA testing blew up. Technology Review. 2018. Available at: https://www.technologyreview.com/s/610233/2017-was-the-year-consumer-dna-testing-blew-up. Accessed 31 July 2021.
35. Rubanovich C, Cheung C, Mandel J, et al. Physician preparedness for big genomic data: a review of genomic medicine education initiatives in the United States. Hum Mol Genet 2018;27(R2):R250–8.
36. Burke S, Stone A, Bedward J, et al. A "neglected part of the curriculum" or "of limited use"? Views on genetics training by nongenetics medical trainees and implications for delivery. Genet Med 2006;8(2):109–15.
37. Fishman CE, Mohebnasab M, van Setten J, et al. Genome-wide study updates in the International Genetics and Translational Research in Transplantation Network (iGeneTRAiN). Front Genet 2019;10:1084.
38. Campion M, Goldgar C, Hopkin RJ, et al. Genomic education for the next generation of health-care providers. Genet Med 2019;21(11):2422–30.
39. Hurst DJ. The future of precision medicine for physician assistants in family medicine. J Physician Assist Educ 2019;30(3):188–9.

The Kidney Goes to Congress

Troy Zimmerman, BA

KEYWORDS

- Chronic kidney disease legislation • Kidney disease advocacy
- National Kidney Foundation • Medicare kidney benefits

KEY POINTS

- Sixty years ago, nephrologists could offer few effective treatments for advanced kidney disease and kidney failure was quickly followed by death. Today, approximately 800,000 patients with kidney failure are alive because of dialysis or a kidney transplant.
- The first patient-oriented organization, the National Kidney Foundation, was founded in the 1960's. In the decades since, kidney advocacy organizations have educated Congress on the needs of kidney patients.
- Congress designated patients with kidney failure as Medicare-eligible regardless of age or Social Security disability status. This helped make dialysis available to everyone.
- Advocacy has led to the creation of other federal programs to increase CKD awareness and surveillance, increase the availability of kidney transplantation, and provide programs to help prolong kidney function or prepare for kidney replacement therapy.

INTRODUCTION

The Centers for Disease Control and Prevention (CDC) estimates that 37 million American adults have chronic kidney disease (CKD).[1] Approximately 90% of these patients are undiagnosed, resulting in countless lost opportunities for measures that can manage and slow disease progression, and in some instances, prevent end-stage kidney failure (ESKD).[2] Nearly 800,000 Americans have kidney failure, including 550,000 who require dialysis treatments and 250,000 who have a functioning kidney transplant.[3] ESKD incidence surpasses 130,000 patients annually and kidney disease was the nation's eighth leading cause of death in 2019.[1,3]

The toll of CKD on patients, families, and society through employment challenges and medical costs (including $130 billion in Medicare fee-for-service expenditures in 2019) is astounding.[3] Individuals with ESKD represent only 1% of Medicare beneficiaries but comprise 7% of Medicare expenditures.[4] Beyond a doubt, advocacy successes by the National Kidney Foundation (NKF) over six decades have resulted in tremendous strides for patients, yet much more remains to be done. NKF continues its wide-ranging efforts to address the tremendous impact of CKD and to meet the needs of patients, families, and caregivers.

Government Relations, National Kidney Foundation, 30 East 33rd Street, New York, NY 10016, USA
E-mail address: troyz@kidney.org

Physician Assist Clin 7 (2022) 377–384
https://doi.org/10.1016/j.cpha.2021.11.013
2405-7991/22/© 2021 Elsevier Inc. All rights reserved.

NATIONAL KIDNEY FOUNDATION: THE BEGINNING

More than 70 years ago in November 1950, Harry and Ada DeBold called the first meeting of the Committee for Nephrosis Research to order.[5] Subsequently, later that year, the National Nephrosis Foundation was created. The DeBold's infant son had been diagnosed with nephrosis and Mrs DeBold was determined to act. The DeBold's son died at age 4, but their resolve eventually became a life-saving event for millions of kidney patients.

A decade after the inaugural meeting of the DeBold's Committee for Nephrosis Research, the outlook for individuals diagnosed with kidney disease had not improved. Patients and families faced limited prospects to slow disease progression and a dramatically lower life expectancy was certain. Treatments for CKD were few and rudimentary dialysis was typically used only for acute kidney injury. Irreversible kidney failure meant imminent death for most patients because maintenance dialysis was available only to the select few. Kidney transplantation was in its infancy and extremely rare. The lack of successful treatments was especially impactful on families that experienced genetic kidney diseases, such as polycystic kidney disease. These families often witnessed relatives across multiple generations die years sooner than that of the average American.

Hope finally arrived with arguably the most significant development in the treatment of ESKD in 1960 when Dr Belding Scribner implanted the first arteriovenous shunt into a kidney patient at Seattle's University Hospital. Although death was no longer imminent for an individual with irreversible kidney failure, maintenance dialysis continued to be a reality only for few patients. The extremely limited availability of dialysis was powerfully illustrated in Alexander's[6] 1962 *Life Magazine* article. The author had access to the deliberations of a small committee, dubbed the "God Squad," which determined who would receive dialysis treatments, at the expense of those who would not.[6] The nation was shocked as it read about "Life or Death Committees" that decided who, candidly, was most worthy of this life-saving therapy. The seven-member Admissions and Policies Committee of the Seattle Artificial Kidney Center at Swedish Hospital was comprised of a surgeon and six other citizens who considered various factors and characteristics in their decision making including age, gender, marital status and dependents, income, net worth, emotional stability, educational background, occupation, past performance and future potential, and references. An interesting part of the deliberation gave more weight to males and to those who had more children. If readers were stunned in 1962, one can only begin to imagine the outcry that would occur today.

On September 21, 1964, the National Nephrosis Foundation officially became the NKF.[5]

MEDICARE COVERAGE OF KIDNEY FAILURE

As the 1960's progressed, dialysis became available in different areas of the nation, but the demand continued to outweigh the supply of machines. Further complicating the matter was how to pay for dialysis. Criteria, eligibility, and expenditures for maintenance dialysis differed depending on where one resided and if dialysis was even available in their community.

In 1964, NKF published *Proposal by The National Kidney Foundation for Kidney Programs under the Division of Chronic Diseases of the United States Public Health Service*.[5] The US Public Health Service covered no programs related to kidney disease at that time. The following year, NKF continued to urge Congress to support kidney programs, resulting in $6.4 million for kidney disease activities under the Department of

Health, Education and Welfare.[5] NKF advocacy to increase awareness of kidney disease programs continued for the remainder of the decade, often testifying before congressional committees. NKF's voice for kidney patients helped secure additional federal funding for kidney disease.

Federal examinations of the growing need for widely accessible and affordable care continued including the landmark 1967 report from the Committee on Chronic Renal Disease (Gottschalk Committee) presented to the US Bureau of the Budget.[7] The report recommended the establishment of a national program for the treatment of patients with kidney failure. NKF continued to mobilize efforts before Congress. Dr George Schreiner, a pioneer in dialysis at Georgetown University and then NKF President, was regularly present on Capitol Hill for meetings and testified more than two dozen times before Congress. Clearly, congressional interest in kidney disease, including irreversible kidney failure and dialysis, was growing.

NKF's advocacy efforts culminated in 1972 when Congress passed legislation (Public Law 92–603) that included an amendment that deemed patients with ESKD disabled and therefore eligible for Medicare, regardless of age or other qualification for Social Security disability.[5,7,8] This benefit applies even to patients who have group health insurance after a coordination period, after which Medicare becomes the primary payer for dialysis and/or transplant. The ESKD population has changed dramatically since passage of the Medicare benefit. A June 1975 House Ways and Means Committee hearing report (Background Information on Kidney Disease Benefits Under Medicare) noted more than one-third of dialysis patients in 1973 were on home dialysis, and only about 20,000 patients in the United States had chronic kidney failure.[5] This is quite different than the 800,000 Americans living with kidney failure in 2021. To this day, patients with ESKD are eligible for Medicare regardless of age and millions of lives have been saved by this unique Medicare benefit.

ORGAN DONATION AND TRANSPLANTATION

NKF has played a significant role in public policy surrounding organ donation and transplantation for more than 40 years, including its work on The National Organ Transplant Act (Public Law 98–507), which contained a prohibition on the sale or other valuable consideration of organs for transplantation.[9] To this day, the valuable consideration clause remains in federal law prohibiting the sale of organs and ensuring living and deceased organ donation is purely altruistic. In the 1980s, NKF conducted several donor blitzes with Members of Congress signing organ donor cards.[5] Shortly after the 1983 donor blitz, President Ronald Reagan met with NKF to highlight the importance of donation (see Audio 1 in The Secret Side of the Military and the Kidney).[10]

For more than three decades, a top priority for NKF and multiple other kidney focused organizations has been passing legislation to provide lifetime Medicare Part B coverage of immunosuppressive medications for organ transplant recipients. Although dialysis patients have indefinite Medicare eligibility as nonaged, nondisabled dialysis patients (Medicare end-stage kidney disease beneficiaries), transplant patients have Medicare for only for 36 months post-transplant.[11] Medicare paid for the kidney transplant (passed 1973) but did not cover immunosuppressive medications until 1986. Then, the eligibility was limited to 12 months post-transplant before Congress extended it to 36 months (2013).[5] Not surprisingly, many patients experienced significant difficulty affording medications that could cost $1000 or more per month or even opted out of transplant completely knowing they would not be able to afford the immunosuppressive drugs. Kidney organizations kept up the fight. In the Balanced Budget Act of 1997 (Public Law 105–33), Congress directed the Institute of Medicine to conduct an economic analysis of providing lifetime Medicare coverage of immunosuppressive drugs for kidney recipients.[12] The Institute of Medicine report determined that eliminating the 36-month limit would be cost effective although not cost neutral, which proved to be a barrier for legislative efforts for nearly two decades. Using that finding, NKF and partner organizations spearheaded the passage of legislation in 2000 to provide lifetime immunosuppressive coverage for Medicare-aged and disabled kidney recipients, who at that time faced the same 3-year immunosuppressive limit despite having lifetime Medicare eligibility for other health needs (the Medicare Part D prescription drug program was several years away from being established).[13]

With one exception, in every 2-year Congress afterward, legislation was introduced to address the immunosuppressive coverage gap. In 2020, after 20 additional years of advocacy, Congress passed legislation giving kidney recipients younger than age 65 and without other insurance indefinite Part B coverage for immunosuppressive drugs. This effort received a significant lift by the Trump Administration, which advocated for lifetime immunosuppressive coverage as part of its 2019 Advancing American Kidney Health initiative.[14] At a January 2020 hearing in the House, Dr Matthew Cooper, Director of Kidney and Pancreas Transplantation at Georgetown University's Medstar Transplant Institute and NKF National Board member, was the sole witness invited to testify on the legislation. Many other organizations submitted statements for the written record. Lifetime immunosuppressive coverage opens the door to transplantation for many patients who otherwise lacked permanent access to these life-saving medications. NKF was most grateful and appreciative for the tireless efforts and steadfast support from the immunosuppressive bill champions over the years, including Sen. Dick Durbin (D-IL) who helped lead the way for two decades. Joined by Sen. Bill Cassidy, MD (R-LA) and Reps. Ron Kind (D-WI) and Michael Burgess, MD (R-TX), these four champions were committed to closing the immunosuppressive coverage gap.

NKF advocacy, and that of other organizations, in support of organ donation, includes the Organ Donor Leave Act (Public Law 106–56), which provides federal civil servants who serve as a living organ donor with up to 30 days paid leave.[15] The leave is in addition to the donor's sick and annual leave. Multiple state and local governments have followed suit with a similar benefit for their employees and some private employers have done the same. The Charles W. Norwood Organ Donation Act (Public Law 110–144) clarified that paired kidney donation does not violate the National Organ Transplant Act (NOTA), opening the door to paired donations and kidney donor chains, making it possible for individuals who are medically incompatible with their intended recipient to donate to another patient.[16] In turn, their intended recipient receives a kidney from a different living donor. More than 1100 kidney transplants were made possible by paired donation in 2019.

NKF was the driving force behind a provision in the Organ Donation Recovery and Improvements Act (Public Law 108–216) that increased opportunities for living donation. The National Living Donor Assistance Center assists donors with unreimbursed expenses related to living donation.[17]

Working with Congress does not always mean getting a law passed or a provision included in legislation. Sometimes advocacy consists of preventing something that we believe would be detrimental to our patients and families. One such example is our opposition to a proposed legislation allowing for the creation of demonstration projects examining the potential impact of financial incentives to increase organ donation, thus waiving the "valuable consideration" clause. NKF's position was based on feedback from our professional and patient members that financial incentives could exploit the most vulnerable members of society (including those with low income) and would impact altruistic kidney donation.

In 2013, the American Society of Transplant Surgeons and the American Society of Transplantation spearheaded an effort that made it possible to use organs from an HIV-positive donor to an HIV-positive recipient. Multiple other organ transplant organizations collaborated to build bipartisan congressional support for the HIV Organ Policy Equity Act (HOPE Act) allowing scientists to carry out research into these organ donations. Resulting studies proved the feasibility, effectiveness, and safety of allowing transplantable organs from HIV-positive donors to be used for HIV-positive candidates.[18]

KIDNEY DISEASE AWARENESS AND DETECTION

NKF secured congressional support and funding to create two agency programs designed to increase awareness and surveillance of CKD funded through the annual appropriations bill for the Department of Health and Human Services. Beginning in 2000, Congress provided funding to the National Institutes of Health to promote evidence-based interventions to improve understanding, detection, and management of kidney disease.[19] Similarly, in 2006 Congress provided funding to establish a CKD program within the CDC.[20] The CDC CKD program promotes kidney health by preventing and controlling risk factors, raises awareness of CKD, and promotes early diagnosis and treatment. Key activities include the CKD Surveillance System to document CKD and its risk and monitor the progress of efforts to prevent, detect, and manage kidney disease. A significant amount of the data used to discuss kidney disease in every journal, oral and written presentations, and publications is because of these programs.

MEDICARE BENEFITS FOR KIDNEY DISEASE TREATMENT

President Lyndon Johnson signed legislation to create Medicare in 1965 and the Medicare end-stage renal disease program was added in 1972. As one would expect, enhancements and modifications for kidney patients have been made in the years since, as new needs and opportunities are brought forth.

The Medicare Nutrition Therapy benefit in 2000 (Public Law 106–554) provides Medicare reimbursement of nutritional counseling services by a dietitian or nutritional professional for patients with diabetes, late-stage kidney disease, or a functioning kidney transplant.[21] Utilization, however, has been less than anticipated, partly because only the physician is permitted to refer a patient for Medicare Nutrition Therapy services. Attempts to expand access by allowing nurse practitioners, physician assistants, clinical nurse specialists, and psychologists to refer patients has been introduced in Congress. The current legislation is championed by the Academy of Nutrition and Dietetics and is supported by NKF and other members of the kidney community. The bills also include attempts to increase medical diagnoses (ie, prediabetes, hypertension, high cholesterol, cardiovascular disease).

Because education of patients can slow progression of kidney disease and increase comfort of the patient, NKF was instrumental in the creation of the Medicare Kidney Disease Education Benefit.[19] This legislation created a Medicare program that provides up to six educational sessions for individuals with stage 4 CKD. Sessions include information on different modalities of dialysis, compassionate care conservative management, and kidney transplantation. Patients are overwhelmed when they reach kidney failure and most often select in-center dialysis as their treatment. Although this may truly be what the patient wants, all patients and their families should have information on modality choices.

IN THE FUTURE

Congressional support is needed for a CKD public awareness program to help educate Americans on the impact of CKD. Ninety percent of the nation's estimated 37 million adults with CKD are undiagnosed and 80 million more are at risk.[1] In 2019, NKF signed a Memorandum of Understanding with the Department of Health and Human Services to establish a public awareness program (the Are You the 33%). To further highlight that all politics is local, the kidney initiatives that were introduced during the Trump White House were strongly supported by Health and Human Services Secretary Azar, whose own father was a dialysis and transplant patient.[22,23]

NKF and other members of the transplant community continue to build bipartisan support for the Living Donor Protection Act to prohibit discrimination in the offering, pricing, and level of benefits for life, disability, and long-term care insurance for living donors. This act would codify that living organ donation is covered under the Family and Medical Leave Act, providing job protection for donors who take leave from work for surgery and recovery. Legislation to remove home dialysis barriers remains among NKF's initiatives.

Kidney disease is more common in patients affected by social determinants of health. The kidney community is working on legislation to address disparities in access to transplant, which may include a discretionary grant program to address social determinants of health barriers in underserved communities. More robust transparency and data reporting on the transplant process, with a special emphasis on racial and socioeconomic barriers that may hinder transplantation for certain patients, is needed. Every patient must be afforded equal access to early detection and appropriate treatment of CKD. The entire kidney community continues to support policy changes to increase organ availability and improve use of donor kidneys, including reducing kidney discards that are deemed suitable for use.

It is vital that research in kidney disease continue. To this end, NKF joined with the American Society of Nephrology to dramatically increase federal support of kidney disease research under the National Institutes of Health. Although treatments for CKD have seen some advances, the pace of innovation lags far behind that of other diseases and is insufficient to meet the growing burden kidney disease places on patients and the health system. Treatment options for kidney failure are the same as they were 40 years ago: dialysis, transplant, and/or palliative care and hospice. More federal support is needed to promote critical research that will expand knowledge on kidney health and disease, develop new and effective therapies, and reduce health disparities. KidneyX, one such program, brings together government and private organizations to jump-start innovation in the kidney space.[24]

During the COVID-19 pandemic, NKF worked for expanded access to telehealth services, access to personal protective equipment for dialysis workers, prioritizing kidney patients for early vaccine availability, and advocating for additional research on vaccine effectiveness for immunocompromised patients. Data were presented to Congress regarding COVID-19 disparities and the pandemic's impact on racial and ethnic populations.

NATIONAL KIDNEY FOUNDATION AND FRIENDS

For nearly 60 years, the dedication, diligence, and expertise of the NKF community has enabled the broader kidney community to collectively cultivate congressional champions to create, support, and fund numerous federal laws and programs to improve the lives of patients with kidney disease. However, this is never done alone and if not for the strong support of the American Society of Nephrology, the Renal Physicians Association, Dialysis Patient Citizens, the American Kidney Fund, the American Association of Kidney Patients, and countless other local and national patient and professional organization support groups, kidney disease legislation would not be where it is today. Advocacy is not possible without a strong patient component. The 150,000 patient and family members who lobby Congress are the most effective voices we have. No one can explain kidney disease better than someone who is going through it, whether as a patient or a caregiver. Advocacy comes in many forms, including meetings with members of Congress and their staffs by patient advocates and nephrology professionals. Kidney advocacy groups reach out to a congressional office on every given day, often multiple times. Just as important are written statements to committees, letters, emails, and telephone calls from patients and health professionals. Most importantly, advocacy requires time, patience, and the understanding that victories often are incremental. Being a successful advocate requires thorough preparation, straightforwardness, and much persistence. Ada DeBold would be pleased with what has been accomplished since the first meeting of the Committee for Nephrosis Research. Passion and determination live on in the kidney community as we continue to work toward improvements in the prevention, detection, and treatment of kidney disease.

DISCLOSURE

National Kidney Foundation Government Relations.

REFERENCES

1. Chronic Kidney Disease (CKD) Surveillance System. Centers for Disease Control and Prevention. Available at: https://nccd.cdc.gov/ckd/default.aspx. Accessed August 1 2021.
2. Szczech LA, Stewart RC, Su HL, et al. Primary care detection of chronic kidney disease in adults with type-2 diabetes: the ADD-CKD Study (awareness, detection and drug therapy in type 2 diabetes and chronic kidney disease). PLoS One 2014;9(11):e110535.
3. United States Renal Data System. 2020 USRDS annual data report: epidemiology of kidney disease in the United States. Bethesda, MD: National Institutes of Health, National Institute of Diabetes and Digestive and Kidney Diseases; 2020.
4. The Kidney Project, statistics. Available at: https://pharm.ucsf.edu/kidney/need/statistics. Accessed August 6 2021.
5. The National Kidney Foundation. In: Massry S, editor. The first 40 years. copyright: W.B. Saunders Company; 1990.
6. Alexander S. They decide who lives and who dies. Life Magazine, . '. Available at: http://www.nephjc.com/news/godpanel. Accessed 6 August 2021.
7. Rettig RA. Special treatment: the story of Medicare's ESRD entitlement. N Engl J Med 2011;364(7):596–8.
8. Fact Sheet, Medicare ESRD program. Available at: https://www.cms.gov/Medicare/End-Stage-Renal-Disease/ESRDNetworkOrganizations/Downloads/ESRDNWBackgrounder-Jun12.pdfgz. Accessed August 4 2021.
9. United States. National Organ Transplant Act: Public Law 98-507. US Statute Large 1984;98:2339–48.

10. Brown WW. History of the National Kidney Foundation. Am J Kidney Dis 2000; 35(4 Suppl 1):S3–18.
11. Immunosuppressive drug coverage, NKF. Available at: https://www.kidney.org/atoz/content/faq-expanded-medicare-coverage-immunosuppressive-drugs-kidney-transplant-recipients. Accessed August 4 2021.
12. H.R. 2015. Balanced Budget Act of 1997. Available at: https://www.congress.gov/bill/105th-congress/house-bill/2015. Accessed August 4 2015.
13. H.R.5661 - Medicare, Medicaid, and SCHIP Benefits Improvement and Protection Act of 2000. Available at: https://www.congress.gov/bill/106th-congress/house-bill/5661. Accessed August 6 2021.
14. Advancing American Kidney Health. Available at: https://www.federalregister.gov/documents/2019/07/15/2019-15159/advancing-american-kidney-health. Accessed August 4 2021.
15. H.R.457 - Organ Donor Leave Act. Available at: https://www.congress.gov/bill/106th-congress/house-bill/457. Accessed August 4 2021.
16. H.R.710 - Charlie W. Norwood Living Organ Donation Act. Available at: https://www.congress.gov/bill/110th-congress/house-bill/710. Accessed August 4 2021.
17. H.R.3926 - Organ Donation and Recovery Improvement Act. Available at: https://www.congress.gov/bill/108th-congress/house-bill/3926. Accessed August 4 2021.
18. Durand CM, Zhang W, Brown DM, et al. for the HOPE in Action Investigators. A prospective multicenter pilot study of HIV-positive deceased donor to HIV-positive recipient kidney transplantation: HOPE in action. Am J Transpl 2021; 21(5):1754–64.
19. About the CKD Initiative. Available at: https://www.cdc.gov/kidneydisease/about-the-ckd-initiative.html. Accessed August 4 2021.
20. Narva AS, Briggs M. The National Kidney Disease Education Program: improving understanding, detection, and management of CKD. Am J Kidney Dis 2009;53(3 Suppl 3):S115–20.
21. Public Law 106-554, Dec 21. 2000. Available at: https://www.congress.gov/106/plaws/publ554/PLAW-106publ554.pdf. Accessed August 4 2021.
22. Quote, Thomas P (Tip) O'Neill, 47th Speaker of the House of Representatives, 1935.
23. HHS Secretary Azar talks kidneys during Kidney Month. Available at: https://www.kidneyfund.org/advocacy-blog/hhs-secretary-azar-talks-kidneys.html. Accessed August 4 2021.
24. The next stage in the fight against kidney diseases, KidneyX innovation accelerator. Available at: https://www.kidneyx.org/. Accessed August 27 2021.

An Expectant Future for Patients with End-Stage Kidney Disease

Melanie T. Stapleton, MS-PAS, PA-C

KEYWORDS

- Advancing America Kidney Health Initiative • Re(building) kidney consortium
- KidneyX project • Wearable artificial kidney • Porcine kidney transplants

KEY POINTS

- Collaborative research efforts have expedited kidney research in all areas.
- Portable or implantable dialysis devices are in development to improve dialysis tolerance.
- Stem cells and xenotransplantation could provide healthy kidney tissue and more donor organs.
- Governmental support and funding are essential to advancing research to combat kidney diseases.

INTRODUCTION

Nearly 40 million Americans have some form of chronic kidney disease (CKD) and 90% have no knowledge of their condition.[1,2] Individuals with advanced CKD (defined as ≤30% kidney function) suffer from both physiologic and psychological impairments. These can include major cardiovascular disease, disability with loss of income, and emotional isolation.[2–4] The stratification of CKD in adults in the United States shows a concentration predominantly among those older than 65 years[5] (**Fig. 1**). Those who have end-stage kidney disease (ESKD) or kidney function so poor as to necessitate a replacement therapy such as dialysis or transplant have a mortality risk greater than 3 times of those who have early CKD.[6]

In 2019, the annual cost for treatment of CKD stage 2 was $17,000 per patient, whereas the cost for ESKD was $100,000/patient.[2] The Advancing America Kidney Health (AAKH) initiative, Executive Order No. 13,879 presented on July 10, 2019, was a public declaration of the United States of America commitment to win the battle against CKD for millions of patients and to end its exorbitant financial implications.[7] The AAKH's chief initiatives include the following:

- Reduce the risk of kidney failure
- Improve access to and quality of person-centered treatment options
- Increase access to kidney transplants

HealthPartners Nephrology, 205 Wabasha St S, Saint Paul, MN 55107-1805, USA
E-mail address: Melanie.T.Stapleton@HealthPartners.com

Physician Assist Clin 7 (2022) 385–395
https://doi.org/10.1016/j.cpha.2021.11.008
2405-7991/22/© 2021 Elsevier Inc. All rights reserved.

physicianassistant.theclinics.com

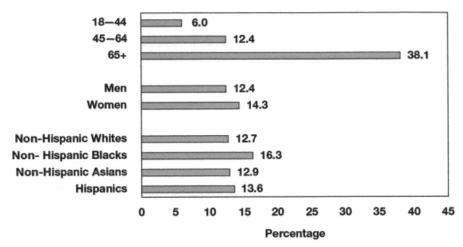

Fig. 1. Percentage of US adults aged 18 years or older with CKD. https://www.cdc.gov/kidneydisease/images/publications-resources/adults-with-CKD-cr-medium.png. (*Centers for Disease Control and Prevention. Chronic Kidney Disease in the United States, 2021, Atlanta, GA: US Department of Health and Human Services, Centers for Disease Control and Prevention; 2021.*)

Since the announcement, millions of dollars in dedicated CKD funding have been allotted to stimulate research supporting the use of stem cells to grow kidneys and for the development of a bioartificial kidney.[7] Other innovative, therapeutic strategies such as biomarkers for early CKD detection and specific gene targeting to interrupt CKD at its inception are independently in the works and are discussed here as well.

And finally, a myriad of natural disasters and the SARS-2 COVID-19 pandemic highlighted the urgent need for novel ESKD interventions to avoid congregate settings while promoting patient independence and protecting the health care workforce.[8–10] Toward that end, there is tremendous effort being made to find viable, animal donors for human kidney transplantation and biomarkers, and the long-awaited wearable kidney is on the way at last!

WHAT IS ON THE HORIZON?
Biomarkers

The first step in any battle is identifying the enemies. Increases in serum creatinine, urea, chloride, parathyroid hormone, phosphate, and urine protein (or albumin) to creatinine ratio (UPCR, UACR) are proved to indicate worsening kidney function.[11] The Chronic Renal Insufficiency trial, Modification of Diet in Renal Disease study, and African American Study of Kidney Disease and Hypertension study also correlated a positive improvement in serum bicarbonate levels, back to normal range, with slowing the progression of CKD.[12] An investigative study by Owens and colleagues based in Australia built on this knowledge by demonstrating that markers of inflammatory states and tissue injury also correlate to CKD progression, namely *"osteopontin, tissue factor, TNF-alpha receptors sTNFR-I and sTNFR-II as well stem cell factor and tryptase."*[12] Osteopontin, known as the *"bone bridge"* protein, is an extracellular matrix phosphoprotein whose overexpression is associated with cancerous tumors, cardiac fibrosis, and heart failure but also has positive associations to wound healing.[13] Although there is variability in the outcomes in studies performing complete knockout of osteopontin in mice models, a *reduction* in circulating osteopontin seems to be mostly favorable to decrease cardiac fibrosis.[13] Reducing levels of osteopontin, as well as the other biomarkers above which are associated with the induction of inflammatory processes leading to fibrosis, may also produce favorable results in CKD, if identified early in the course.[13]

Genetic Targets

Hepatocyte growth factor and cMet fibrosis

The endpoint of prolonged kidney injury is fibrosis, tissue that is no longer able to renew itself and has lost the ability to perform most of its cellular operations. Hepatocyte growth factor (HGF) is a protein made by mesenchymal cells and whose presence has been found to be critical for the growth, longevity, and renewal of multiple organs including the kidneys.[14,15] HGF is known to be upregulated as a defense mechanism during many disease processes.[14] The administration of anti-(HGF) antibody hastened tissue death in subject mice.[14] Kim and colleagues proposed that increasing cMet activity, a receptor for the (HGF) protein, could serve to ward off tissue fibrosis.[15] Identifying the cMet receptor as the potential target for manipulation rather than the HGF protein itself was a key turning point. Based on this research, cMet could provide an avenue to circumvent HGF's unpredictable inherent nature, a previous obstacle to its use as part of a manufactured drug therapy.[15]

Cubilin/albuminuria. Albuminuria is a known independent risk factor for CKD progression.[16] Albuminuria's origin has been found on the gene cubilin (CUBN).[16] Reznichenko and colleagues used the genetic alteration in CUBN to compare the presence of certain CUBN genotypes in transplanted kidneys: native kidneys and transplant donor kidneys.[16] There was more CUBN found in the ESKD transplant recipients at the time of transplant than in the donor organs.[16] Over the course of the life of the donated organ, there was an increase in the donor genotype of CUBN, correlating to the organ's declining function.[16] This increase provides a potential pathway for a new class of drug agent, perhaps an adjuvant immunosuppressive agent that would target albuminuria/proteinuria at the genetic level.

Sensors/noninvasive and real-time detection

Not to be left out, acute kidney injury (AKI) is getting some attention regarding the use of enhanced recognition technologies. Rhabdomyolysis can occur in athletes and otherwise healthy individuals after intense activities.[17] A small study conducted by Rojas-Valverde and colleagues sought to demonstrate that intense physical activities (contact and noncontact) contribute to internal trauma, resulting in transient AKI, which can be detected *during* the activity by using G force measuring devices.[18] Serum kidney injury markers and urine-specific gravity measurements before and after physical activity were evaluated in participants to measure volume depletion, a common confounding factor in AKI.[18] This trial found that in roughly 50% of the participants, including both low-intensity and high-intensity ranked runners, the corresponding levels of G force could account for the corresponding increase in serum creatinine.[18]

(Re)Building a Kidney: collaborative efforts in stem cell research. Joint kidney research efforts on the macro level combined with dedicated funding has proved to be an efficient and successful endeavor.[19] The (Re)Building a Kidney (RBK) consortium is a nationwide collaboration of cellular and molecular biologists, nephrologists, and surgeons established to further kidney research. Funded and founded in 2015 by the National Institute of Health's Kidney Disease Institute (NIH/NIDDK), RBK's chief initiative has been to make viable kidney cells and tissue that can be engrafted into humans to prevent and treat a myriad of kidney diseases.[19]

The key aspect of the RBK research is utilization of induced pluripotent stem cells (iPSCs) and renal progenitor cells.[19] These cells are intact, harvested, embryonic stem cells which can be isolated, protected, and nurtured while they form into kidney tissue in a controlled environment or as they are alternatively guided through a process of differentiation in culture to become distinct parts of the kidney organ or a complete kidney,[19,20] the idea being that these *kidney organoids* would then be in possession of all critical apparatuses that comprise and power the multitude of functional units of the kidney (**Figs. 2** and **3**).[19–21] The value of this research is not only in the finished product but also in observing the development of a kidney to determine where disease processes have their origin and to intervene using genetic and cellular strategies to alter the process.[19,20] Another ultimate goal of the iPSC research is for healthy kidneys or kidney tissue to be directly implanted into diseased kidneys to disrupt the disease and repair the organ.[19,20]

Multiple projects geared toward the goals as stated earlier have already been completed by RBK-funded researchers. The RBK Web site, www.rebuildingakidney. org, offers a complete listing of its research areas and current studies, which includes these 2 successfully completed projects:

Harvard University: construction of a perfused, 3-dimensional proximal tubule in a manufactured extracellular matrix.[19]

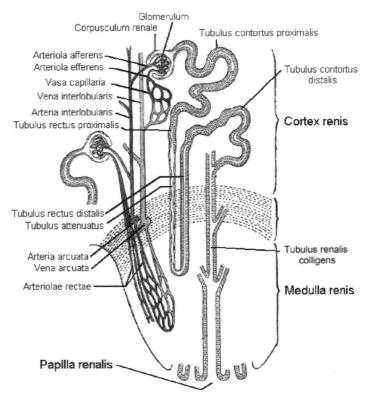

Fig. 2. Anatomy of the nephron, taken from Grays Anatomy, 1918. (Gray, Henry. Anatomy of the Human Body. Philadelphia: Lea & Febiger, 1918; Bartleby.com, 2000. www.bartleby.com/107/. [Date of Printout]. This work is in the public domain in the United States because it was published (or registered with the U.S. Copyright Office) before January 1, 1926.)

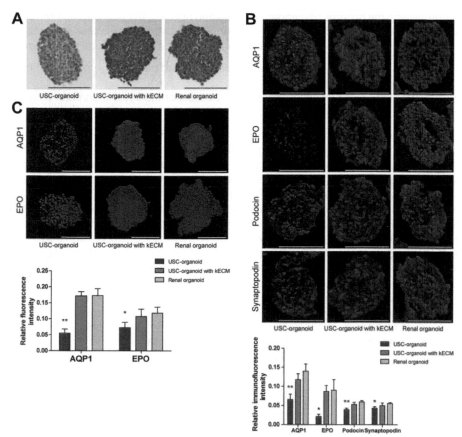

Fig. 3. (*A-C*) Kidney organoids, 3 dimensional histology (USC-organoids, USC-organoids with kECM, and renal organoids). (Image was taken directly from source without alteration. https://media.springernature.com/lw685/springer-static/image/art%3A10.1186%2Fs13287-020-01822-4/MediaObjects/13287_2020_1822_Fig4_HTML.png?as=webp; Sun, G., Ding, B., Wan, M. *et al.* Formation and optimization of three-dimensional organoids generated from urine-derived stem cells for renal function in vitro. *Stem Cell Res Ther* 11, 309 (2020). https://doi.org/10.1186/s13287-020-01822-4. http://creativecommons.org/licenses/by/4.0/. The Creative Commons Public Domain Dedication waiver (http://creativecommons.org/publicdomain/zero/1.0/))

University of Washington: an in-vitro study demonstrating the steps and setting that kidney iPSCs and parietal epithelial cells create and use to successfully renew glomeruli and reproduce podocytes, as well as valuable insight into where the process fails.[19]

KidneyX artificial kidney (innovation accelerator) project. The *KidneyX project*, similar to the RBK consortium, is an invitation and a challenge to researchers, developers, and biotech companies around the world who support the research and cure of kidney diseases to improve the quality of life of patients. The KidneyX project, a joint venture by the Health and Human Services department in league with the American Society of Nephrology (ASN), is a multimillion-dollar kidney research award established in 2019.[22] The artificial kidney prize portion of this project seeks to increase the number of functional kidneys that are readily available to patients with ESKD while circumventing the hazards of standard dialysis and avoiding the philosophic and logistical obstacles of kidney transplant.[22] The funding is distributed via tasked competitions divided into phases. The phases of the artificial kidney prize include the following:

1. Design of an artificial kidney that is reproducible and has high probability of both functionality and dependability
2. The actual production of an artificial kidney model or the innovation/enhancement of a preexisting artificial kidney model[22]

In the *Redesign Dialysis* competition, the title was itself the goal: to create a kidney replacement therapy or revolutionizing technology that could supplant the expensive, outdated, and life-limiting current options of peritoneal dialysis and hemodialysis. Among the list of winners is the Intracorporeal Hemodialysis System (iHEMO), a joint effort by *University of California-San Francisco*, led by Dr Shuvo Roy, *Vanderbilt University*, and Silicon Kidney.[23] iHEMO is a small device that houses the key components of a standard hemodialyzer, including a unique filter in a specialized membrane that is surgically placed and connected to the patient's central blood supply internally.[23] The iHEMO would theoretically eliminate the need for 3 to 5 times a week needle placement or external central venous catheter access, eliminating mortality risks associated with AV access failure, bleeding, catheter-associated clotting events, and blood stream infections.[22] However, the iHEMO device still requires an internal to external connection as well as in vivo placement of a foreign body, which could necessitate intermittent maintenance requiring invasive procedures.[22,23] The iHEMO is in the category of bioartificial kidneys and is still in the developmental phase.[23,24]

According to Wragg and colleagues, *renal assistive devices or RADs* (**Fig. 4**) offer internal dialysis while recreating the kidney's natural immunoprotective barrier by integrating proximal tubule cells with synthetic fibers to build this safety net. They also repair the function of the damaged kidney that houses it.[24] However, RAD production has suffered because of a limited supply of kidney host organs and could not demonstrate long-term or even intermediate reparative effects.[24]

The ambulatory kidney to improve vitality (AKTIV) by the *University of Washington* Center for Dialysis Innovation was another finalist in the *Redesign Dialysis* competition.[25] Although the specific design of the AKTIV is not presently available to the public, reportedly it is a compact replica of hemodialysis that provides portability, greatly conserves water (standard hemodialysis uses 18,000 L of treated water per patient each week or 100,000 L of water per person each year), decreases the need for large doses of anticlotting agents, and provides effective dialysis at a much more affordable price.[26,27] AKTIV differs from iHEMO in that it falls under the category of *wearable artificial kidneys* or WAKs, another frontrunner in innovative dialysis solutions.[24,25]

WAKs and wearable ultrafiltration units are devices housed in a garment, either around the waist or in a jacket type structure, which contains all components of a standard dialysis or ultrafiltration machine and is formatted to the patient with the intent to be a convenient, easily removable, battery powered device (see **Fig. 4**).[24] WAKS will still require connection to the patient's central blood supply through the superior vena cava or the subclavian vein. This design characteristic may still pose a significant risk for infection.[24]

In March 2021, Dr Victor Gura of the *University of California-Los Angeles* was issued the first US patent for his company's version of a WAK.[27] Per news media press releases, clinical trials of the device are hoped to be underway in the near future.

Porcine Kidney Transplants

Stem cell kidney organoid research and development of artificial kidney replacement devices may soon facilitate a major shift in the management of advanced CKD.

A *Renal Assistive Device*

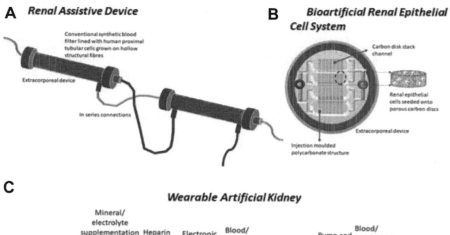

B *Bioartificial Renal Epithelial Cell System*

C *Wearable Artificial Kidney*

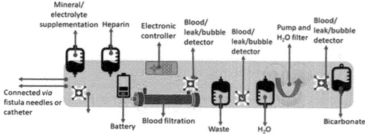

D *Wearable Ultrafiltration*

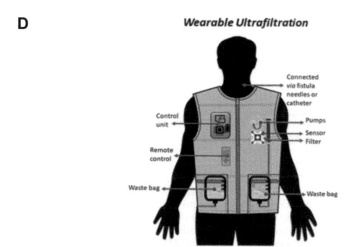

Fig. 4. (*A*) Renal assistive device, (*B*) bioartificial renal epithelial cell system, (*C*) wearable artificial kidney, (*D*) wearable ultrafiltration. https://media.springernature.com/lw685/springer-static/image/art%3A10.1186%2Fs41100-019-0218-7/MediaObjects/41100_2019_218_Fig1_HTML.png?as=webp (Wragg, N.M., Burke, L. & Wilson, S.L. A critical review of current progress in 3D kidney biomanufacturing: advances, challenges, and recommendations. *Ren Replace Ther* 5, 18 (2019). https://doi.org/10.1186/s41100-019-0218-7; Image was taken directly from source without alteration. (http://creativecommons.org/licenses/by/4.0/) (http://creativecommons.org/publicdomain/zero/1.0/))

However, the field of kidney transplantation is also evolving and broadening its scope to offer a potential solution to one of its lingering challenges: the incongruity between transplant listed ESKD patients and the number of transplantable kidneys.[28] In 2019, the waitlist for kidneys had grown to more than 110,000 individuals.[28] Yet, in 2018, less than 25,000 kidney transplants were done simply due to lack of available kidneys.[28] In more populous nations such as China, the divide is even greater, wherein only 5% of the 300,000 individuals on their active kidney transplant list receive kidney transplants.[28]

Table 1
Types of rejection and related factors in organ transplants from porcine donors

	Timing	Mechanisms	Solutions	Organ Survival
Hyperacute	Minutes	• Complement activation via xenoreactive antibodies in host immune system, for example. • Presence of Galα(1,3)Gal antigen on porcine epithelial cells. • Leads to membrane attack complexes (MACs) and ultimately cell death	• CRISPR/Cas9 knockout of GGTA1 in porcine donor, the catalyst for Galα(1,3)Gal antigen • Increase, modify CD46, CD55, & CD59 in porcine donors • Increased immunosuppression (CsA), splenectomy, B-cell depletion	∼3–8 mo
Delayed	Hours to days	• Immunoglobulin (IgG) and endothelial cell type II activation including: • Intravascular coagulation challenges/ variations in vWF, CD 39, & CD73 in porcine donors • Lack of binding between porcine TM and human thrombin • Porcine tissue factor pathway inhibitor (TFPI) problems	• Insert human CD39, CD73, and TM genes and inactivate vWF in porcine donors, • Knockout CD46 and use anti-CD 40 IS • Use of heme degradation products to fight apoptosis • TFPI overexpression in porcine donors	∼3–32 mo
Acute cellular	Days to months	• Cellular invasion->cell lysis by mononuclear cells by NK and T lymphocytes induction, macrophages • ULBP1 protein to NKG2D receptor	• HLA-E gene insertion into porcine cells Anti-ULBP1 polyclonal antibodies • uman CD47 into porcine cells	Markedly prolonged
Chronic	Months to years	Additive effect of aforementioned, minimal data. Possibly killer T lymphocytes, tissue factor activation->destruction of vasculature	Unknown	Unknown

This table was created using data including exact wording and phrases taken directly from Hryhorowicz M, Zeyland J, Słomski R, Lipiński D. Genetically Modified Pigs as Organ Donors for Xenotransplantation. Mol Biotechnol. 2017;59(9-10):435-444. doi:10.1007/s12033-017-0024-9. (http://creativecommons.org/licenses/by/4.0/)

Xenotransplantation or attempts to engraft animal tissue and organs into humans has been occurring for more than one hundred years.[28] Apes and monkeys, which are very similar to humans in genetic make-up, are considered to be workable option.[28] However, the successful use of these *nonhuman primates* has been halted due to donor to recipient size mismatch, probable transference of disease, and as well as the moral quandary of using primates purely for research or organ donation.[28] Instead, pig or porcine kidneys have recently emerged as the best option, given the potential ability to breed them in mass in various environments all around the world and allowing many options of kidney organ size, stage of development, and function. In addition, there is less potential for public or animal advocacy group resistance on the use of an animal, who is already categorized as farm stock, to be used for research and organ harvesting.[28]

Porcine organs have one major obstacle working against their use as organ donors for humans, *"molecular incompatibility between the donor and recipient, resulting from large phylogenetic distance, leading to xenograft rejection."*[28] Hryhorowicz and colleagues discussed the types, timing and mechanisms of porcine organ, transplant rejection, as well as the current solutions involving donor genetic editing for improved recipient immune system regulation and response.[28] Details of these mechanisms and the potential genetic and immunologic interventions are cited in **Table 1**.[28] Strategies applied thus far have improved organ graft survival (most data available describe pig heart to nonhuman primates transplant) through delayed graft rejection, up to 3 years in some instances.[28] In September 2021, multiple news media sources were notified and reported on the successful completion of a kidney transplant from a genetically modified pig donor to a brain dead, human recipient by a surgical team led by Dr Robert Montgomery of New York University-Langone. This achievement is a major first step in transcending the immunologic hurdle and paving a pathway for the future.

SUMMARY

CKD, particularly in later stages, has overwhelmed the US health care system for many years. Generally available, current therapies to manage advanced kidney disease (ie, hemodialysis and peritoneal dialysis) are noncurative, life-limiting, and costly. Kidney transplantation restores function and can improve quality of life, but the supply of organs is limited and requires an extensive selection process and the ability to tolerate both a major operation and the required immunosuppressive drugs. Thanks to a recent public/governmental coalition with matching funding programs, as well as a worldwide pandemic establishing a sense of urgency, CKD is now a major focus of research and innovation. Stem cells are on the path to eliminate kidney disease at their inception and restore healthy function to injured organs. Artificial kidneys, either internally placed or portable, may soon be a convenient reality to replace standard, stationary dialysis. Xenotransplantation, in particular pig kidneys to humans, may have many steps remaining before proving to be consistent and suitable source of donor organs, yet much progress is being made to combat rejection. Now that multiple solutions are on the way to prevent the development of CKD and improve treatment options. Those who suffer from the debilitating side effects of kidney failure can look toward the future with expectation rather than frustration.

DISCLOSURE

The author has no disclosures or conflicts of interest to report.

REFERENCES

1. Centers for Disease Control and Prevention. Chronic kidney disease in the United States, 2021. Atlanta, GA: US Department of Health and Human Services, Centers for Disease Control and Prevention; 2021. Available at: https://www.cdc.gov/kidneydisease/pdf/Chronic-Kidney-Disease-in-the-US-2021-h.pdf. Accessed July 1, 2021.
2. Elshahat S, Cockwell P, Maxwell AP, et al. The impact of chronic kidney disease on developed countries from a health economics perspective: a systematic scoping review. PLoS One 2020;15(3):e0230512.
3. Zha Y, Qian Q. Protein nutrition and malnutrition in CKD and ESRD. Nutrients 2017;9(3):208.
4. Podkowińska A, Formanowicz D. Chronic kidney disease as oxidative stress- and inflammatory-mediated cardiovascular disease. Antioxidants (Basel) 2020; 9(8):752.
5. Centers for Disease Control and Prevention. Chronic kidney disease in the United States, 2021. Atlanta, GA: US Department of Health and Human Services, Centers for Disease Control and Prevention; 2021. Available at: https://www.cdc.gov/kidneydisease/publications-resources/ckd-national-facts.html. Accessed July 1, 2021.
6. Centers for Disease Control and Prevention. All cause mortality rates by year and CKD stage, Veterans Affairs Health System. Available at: https://nccd.cdc.gov/ckd/detail.aspx?Qnum=Q185. Accessed July 1, 2021.
7. Federal Register, Exec. Order No 13,879, 84 Fed. Reg. 33817. 2019. Available at: https://www.federalregister.gov/documents/2019/07/15/2019-15159/advancing-american-kidney-health. Accessed July 1, 2021.
8. Verma A, Patel AB, Tio MC, et al. Caring for dialysis patients in a time of COVID-19. Kidney Med 2020. https://doi.org/10.1016/j.xkme.2020.07.006.
9. Lew SQ, Wallace EL, Srivatana V, et al. Telehealth for home dialysis in COVID-19 and beyond: a perspective from the American Society of Nephrology COVID-19 home dialysis subcommittee. Am J Kidney Dis 2021;77(1):142–8.
10. Truong T, Dittmar M, Ghaffari A, et al. Policy and pandemic: the changing practice of nephrology during the coronavirus disease-2019 outbreak. Adv Chronic Kidney Dis 2020;27(5):390–6.
11. Owens E, Tan KS, Ellis R, et al. Development of a biomarker panel to distinguish risk of progressive chronic kidney disease. Biomedicines 2020;8(12):606.
12. Adeva-Andany MM, Fernández-Fernández C, Mouriño-Bayolo D, et al. Sodium bicarbonate therapy in patients with metabolic acidosis. ScientificWorldJournal 2014;2014:627673.
13. Abdelaziz Mohamed I, Gadeau AP, Hasan A, et al. Osteopontin: a promising therapeutic target in cardiac fibrosis. Cells 2019;8(12):1558.
14. Nakamura T, Mizuno S. The discovery of hepatocyte growth factor (HGF) and its significance for cell biology, life sciences and clinical medicine. Proc Jpn Acad Scr B Phys Biol Sci 2010;86(6):588–610.
15. Kim YC, Lee J, An JN, et al. Renoprotective effects of a novel cMet agonistic antibody on kidney fibrosis. Sci Rep 2019;9(1):13495.
16. Reznichenko A, Snieder H, van den Born J, et al. for the REGaTTA (REnal GeneTics TrAnsplantation) Groningen group. CUBN as a novel locus for end-stage renal disease: insights from renal transplantation. PLoS One 2012;7(5): e36512.

17. Schlader ZJ, Hostler D, Parker MD, et al. The potential for renal injury elicited by physical work in the heat. Nutrients 2019;11(9):2087.
18. Rojas-Valverde D, Timón R, Sánchez-Ureña B, et al. Potential use of wearable sensors to assess cumulative kidney trauma in endurance off-road running. J Funct Morphol Kinesiol 2020;5(4):93.
19. Available at: https://www.rebuildingakidney.org/about/,Accessed July 1, 2021
20. Woolf AS. Growing a new human kidney. Kidney Int 2019;96(4):871–82.
21. Gray H. Anatomy of the human body. Philadelphia: Lea & Febiger; 1918. Bartleby.com, 2000. Available at: www.bartleby.com/107/.
22. KidneyX artificial kidney prize offers $10 million to accelerate artificial kidney development. Available at: https://www.hhs.gov/about/news/2020/10/30/kidneyx-artificial-kidney-prize-offers-10-million-accelerate-artificial-kidney-development.html. Accessed July 1, 2021.
23. Finalist: the ambulatory kidney to improve vitality (AKTIV), KidneyX innovation accelerator. Available at: https://www.kidneyx.org/PrizeCompetitions/RedesignDialysisPhaseII/KidneyProject. Accessed July 1, 2021.
24. Wragg MN, Burke L, Wilson SL. A critical review of current progress in 3D kidney biomanufacturing: advances, challenges, and recommendations. Ren Replace Ther 2019;5:18. Available at: https://doi.org/10.1186/s41100-019-0218-7. Accessed July 1, 2021.
25. Finalist: the Ambulatory Kidney to Improve Vitality (AKTIV). Available at: https://www.kidneyx.org/PrizeCompetitions/PastCompetitions/redesigndialysisphaseiproposal121.
26. Water use in dialysis, Center for Disease Control and Prevention, Atlanta, GA. Available at: https://www.cdc.gov/dialysis/guidelines/water-use.html. Accessed July 1, 2021.
27. US issues patent for wearable artificial kidney Artificial Kidney News. Available at: https://www.artificialkidneynews.com/log-in/us-issues-patent-for-wearable-artificial-kidney. Accessed July 1, 2021.
28. Hryhorowicz M, Zeyland J, Słomski R, et al. Genetically modified pigs as organ donors for xenotransplantation. Mol Biotechnol 2017;59(9–10):435–44.

Saying Goodbye

Lindsay Paige Penninger, PA-C*, Samantha Gwyn Collins, PA-C

KEYWORDS

• ESKD • CKD • End-of-life (EOL) care • Dialysis • Palliative care • Nephrology

KEY POINTS

- Chronic kidney disease (CKD) is often a comorbid disease leading to end-of-life (EOL) care.
- End-of-life care planning discussions with patients with CKD, acute kidney injury (AKI), and end-stage kidney disease (ESKD) should be done before the advanced stages of the disease.
- It is important to stress ethical considerations in end-of-life discussions.
- EOL discussions incorporate patient's wishes for supportive care versus kidney replacement therapy in ESKD.

A SHIFTING PATIENT POPULATION

The prevalence of CKD has risen steadily since the 1980s, in part due to a rise in diabetes, hypertension, and obesity in the US. The increased life expectancy has also led to more elderly patients on dialysis. When introduced in the 1940s, dialysis was considered a life-saving treatment. When the end stage kidney disease (ESKD) Medicare entitlement program was created in 1972, the goal of dialysis shifted from life-saving to rehabilitation as the dialysis population was predominantly young patients without multiple comorbidities.[1] In the 21st century, the ESKD patient population has again shifted. Currently, more than half of new start dialysis patients are over 60 years old.[1] Though the patient population has changed, the approach of the dialysis provider has largely remained the same: focused on quality metrics and life extension, rather than patient comfort and goals. As the kidney disease patient population grows and shifts toward older adults, the percentage of patients dying with a chronic kidney disease (CKD) diagnosis increases. It is important to address the management of CKD at end of life (EOL).

FACTORS IMPACTING MORBIDITY/MORTALITY

Mortality in CKD and ESKD is highly dependent on comorbid conditions. The most common comorbidities include diabetes and cardiovascular disease. Death rates in

Carolina Kidney Associates, 309 New Street, Greensboro, NC 27405, USA
* Corresponding author.
E-mail addresses: lpenninger@carolinakidney.com (L.P.P.); scollins@carolinakidney.com (S.G.C.)

Physician Assist Clin 7 (2022) 397–408
https://doi.org/10.1016/j.cpha.2021.11.009
2405-7991/22/© 2021 Elsevier Inc. All rights reserved.

CKD are predicted by several factors including age, cigarette smoking, troponin-T level, and/or N-terminal pro-brain natriuretic peptide.[2] Estimated glomerular filtration rate (eGFR) is also a predictive factor; for every 30% decrease in eGFR, there is a 1.3 times higher death rate.[2] Hospitalizations are common in patients with ESKD due to cardiovascular events, access-related complications, fluid overload, GI bleed, and sepsis.

CKD can also directly cause death, most frequently due to hyperkalemia, volume overload, access infections, or anemia. CKD increases morbidity through complications such as renal osteodystrophy and fluid-related hypertension and/or hypotension.

Ethical Considerations

Ethics play an important role in the management of patients with CKD especially when it comes to EOL. There are 9 principles of medical ethics for consideration when caring for patients (**Box 1**).

Respecting patient wishes, human dignity, and rights while providing competent, compassionate care in the best interest of the patient is of utmost importance while helping those who are making EOL decisions. This is what makes advance care planning (ACP) so essential, to ensure patients have had time to decide their wishes and convey these to their family and health care providers.

It is important for providers to continue to expand their scientific knowledge and provide relevant information to patients/families regarding their disease state and likely trajectory of progression. To make informed decisions, patients need to have as much education as possible regarding their state of health. The goal is an informed patient who can understand choices associated with disease progression, specifically

---

Box 1
American Medical Association Principles of Medical Ethics

1. Provide competent care with compassion and respect for human dignity and rights

2. Uphold the standards of professionalism, be honest in all professional interactions and strive to report physicians deficient in character or competence, or engaging in fraud or deception, to appropriate entities

3. Respect the law and recognize a responsibility to seek changes in those requirements which are contrary to the best interests of the patient

4. Respect the rights of patients, colleagues, and other health professionals and safeguard patient confidences and privacy within the constraints of the law

5. Continue to study, apply and advance scientific knowledge, maintain a commitment to medical education, make relevant information available to patients, colleagues, and the public, obtain consultation and use the talents of other health care professions when indicated

6. In the provision of appropriate patient care, except in emergencies, be free to choose whom to serve, with whom to associate, and the environment in which to provide medical care

7. Recognize a responsibility to participate in activities contributing to the improvement of the community and betterment of public health

8. Regard responsibility to the patient as paramount

9. Support access to medical care for all people

CKD, Chronic Kidney Disease; EOL, end-of-life; American Medical Association. AMA Principles of Medical Ethics.[3]

dialysis versus compassionate care. When patients choose compassionate care, palliative care services/hospice consults are imperative to provide the highest level of care. It is the health care provider's responsibility, if attainable, to make EOL as peaceful and asymptomatic as possible.

Caring for patients at EOL is one of the codes of medical ethics developed by the American Medical Association (AMA). This code incorporates 8 topics to be considered or addressed with every advanced CKD patient (**Table 1**).

Vulnerable Chronic Kidney Disease Populations

Specific CKD patient groups are considered vulnerable and require a more in-depth analysis and ethical deliberation. Davison and Holley specifically listed the following patient populations as requiring additional consideration when determining appropriate initiation or withdrawal of dialysis, transplantation and ACP.[11]

1. Elderly
2. Cognitively impaired
3. Cultural minorities or cultural backgrounds differing from the provider

Older age is considered a predictor of death along with increased number of comorbidities and nonambulatory status.[11] Survival on dialysis is affected by psychosocial factors, patient nutrition, and functional status.[11] All of these must be factored in when making decisions. Previously determined time-limited trials can provide an ethically sound way to initiate dialysis and determine whether it is beneficial and well-tolerated. At the end of the time trial, the patient and care team can determine if it would be the best interest of the patient to continue dialysis long term. As for transplantation in elderly populations, age is a consideration. It is often not considered the sole reason for denying patients to be listed for deceased donor transplant but it is a factor as "deceased donor kidneys are a scarce resource" and require criteria for exclusion.[11]

A patient's ability to provide informed consent is one of the basic ethical principles. With patients who are cognitively impaired and unable to understand what it is to initiate or withdrawal dialysis, special consideration must be taken in these decisions. This is an area whereby the clinical picture and advance directives can help to guide decision making.

Patients and practitioners do not always share the same cultural background and this must be considered when approaching EOL conversations. There are differences in thought on who should be making important medical decisions for a patient as well as different cultures' views on morals, religion, illness, and health care. Western cultures mostly hold the belief that all patients have the right to make their own decisions whereas many other cultures believe a family or society should help to make these decisions. In western culture, when dialysis becomes futile, the decision to withdrawal dialysis is deemed appropriate as it is no longer upholding ethical standards of beneficence and nonmaleficence.[11] Yet, in other cultures, this decision would not be morally acceptable. For example, "In Buddhist ethical framework, it is impossible to withdraw life-sustaining treatment with beneficial intent."[11] It is best that when a provider is unsure how a patient's cultural background will play a role in their care to ask the patient. This will help to establish the patient care team and guide future decision making.

Barriers to End-of-Life Discussions

Due to shifting patient demographics, more patients are dying with a diagnosis of CKD rather than progressing to dialysis. It is important for providers to discuss EOL and goals of care as part of the patient treatment plan. However, studies have shown

Table 1 Code of medical ethics: end of life care	
Advance Care Planning	• Allows patients to "express values they want to govern their care, articulate factors that are of importance to them for QOL and make clear preferences they have with respect to specific interventions"[4]
Advance Directives	• Can be oral or written • Valid and upheld across all health care settings • Reflects patients "values, goals of care and treatment preferences to guide future decisions about health care"[5] • Allows patient to name a health care proxy to make decisions on their behalf when they do not have the capacity to do so
Withhold or withdrawing life-sustaining treatment	• Patient with decision-making capacity has "the right to decline any medical intervention or ask that an intervention be stopped, even when that decision is expected to lead to his or her death and regardless of whether or not the individual is terminally ill"[6] • Health care proxy may make this decision if the patient lacks capacity • "When an intervention no longer helps to achieve the patient's goals for care or desired quality of life, it is ethically appropriate for physicians to withdraw it"[6]
Orders not to attempt resuscitation	• Apply across all care settings • Ethically important to follow to "respect autonomy and self-determination"[7]
Medically ineffective interventions	• Only recommend interventions that are medically appropriate "scientifically grounded"[8] • Not required to offer treatments that do not offer a clinical benefit or align with patient goals of care • "Futile" depends on the values and goals of a particular patient in specific clinical circumstance"[8]
Sedation to unconsciousness in EOL care	• "When a terminally ill patient experiences severe pain or other distressing clinical symptoms that do not respond to aggressive, symptom-specific palliation it can be appropriate to offer sedation to unconsciousness as an intervention of last resort"[9] • Must never be used to intentionally cause death
Physician-assisted suicide & Euthanasia	• "Fundamentally incompatible with the physician's role as healer, would be difficult or impossible to control, and would pose serious societal risks"[10] • "Physicians must aggressively respond to the needs of patients at the end of life"[10]

QOL, quality of life; American Medical Association. AMA. ETHICS. [4–10].

many patients with later-stage CKD are not aware of the actual state of their health. One meta-analysis found that many patients did not know their prognosis and did not recall being offered alternatives to dialysis, while another study showed that less than 10% of patients presenting for kidney replacement therapy (KRT) had a previous EOL discussion with their nephrologist.[12,13]

Patients may not be aware that they have treatment options other than KRT. Dialysis carries physical, emotional, and socioeconomic burdens, thus patients with CKD 5/ ESKD may opt to stop dialysis or forgo initiation of dialysis altogether. Though KRT is viewed as a life-sustaining treatment, studies have found a similar 1-year survival rate between elderly people receiving dialysis (73.0%), and those receiving supportive care (70.6%).[14] For elderly patients with multiple comorbidities and less than 1-year life expectancy, the socioeconomic burden and physical goal of dialysis may not be in line with the patients' care goals.[1]

There are also barriers to EOL discussions from a provider perspective. As outlined above, most patients with CKD have multiple comorbidities and will often die from a condition other than their kidney disease. This can make it challenging to know which provider should be having these conversations with the patients. There may not be time to form a patient-provider relationship in which the patient trusts the provider to have an open discussion about goals of care. In such situations, the nephrology provider may feel it is better for a different provider, such as a primary care provider, to initiate the conversation. Additionally, although the dialysis patient population has shifted, the metrics that providers are expected to meet for dialysis patients are largely unchanged and are focused on morbidity and mortality outcomes rather than a patient-centered approach. Well-controlled phosphorus and parathyroid hormone levels may not be a priority for older patients who primarily continue dialysis to increase their comfort, rather than their life expectancy. There are also some patients who present to nephrologists for the first time in the late stages of CKD. Time is also a factor, as providers are often expected to see a high volume of patients which limits the time to complete sensitive, complicated discussions with patients and their families. Finally, there is a lack of privacy in the dialysis treatment area, and neither patient or providers may not be comfortable approaching these topics when other patients are nearby.

Approach to Discussing the End-of-Life

One of the most difficult, but also rewarding tasks as a provider is to discuss EOL care with patients. As the progression of CKD ultimately leads to ESKD and death, it is imperative to have these discussions with patients to determine what type of disease management they would like to pursue. Ultimately there are 3 options:

1. KRT (hemodialysis or peritoneal dialysis)
2. Transplantation
3. Comfort or compassionate care

As stated previously it is very important to know what options patients would prefer to better plan and prepare for the patients' needs in the future. This conversation may be held multiple times and the patients should understand that they may change their minds.

Shared Decision Making

The Renal Physicians Association (RPA) developed recommendations regarding approaching these choices in individual patients (**Box 2**). Initially, a relationship must be developed with patients to establish shared decision making.[15] "*Shared*

> **Box 2**
> **RPA recommendations for adults shared decision making in the appropriate initiation and withdrawal from Dialysis[15]**
>
> 1. Develop a physician–patient relationship for shared decision making
>
> 2. Fully inform AKI, stage 4 and 5 CKD, and ESKD patients about their diagnosis, prognosis, and all treatment options
>
> 3. Give all patients with AKI, stage 5 CKD, or ESKD an estimate of prognosis specific to their overall condition
>
> 4. Institute advance care planning
>
> 5. If appropriate, forgo (withhold initiating or withdraw ongoing) dialysis for patients with AKI, CKD, or ESRD in certain well-defined situations
>
> 6. Consider forgoing dialysis for AKI, CKD, or ESRD patients who have a very poor prognosis or for whom dialysis cannot be provided safely
>
> 7. Consider a time-limited trial of dialysis for patients requiring dialysis, but who have an uncertain prognosis, or for whom a consensus cannot be reached about providing dialysis
>
> 8. Establish a systematic due process approach for conflict resolution if there is disagreement about what decision should be made with regard to dialysis
>
> 9. To improve patient-centered outcomes, offer palliative care services and interventions to all AKI, CKD, and ESKD patients who suffer from burdens of their disease
>
> 10. Use a systematic approach to communicate about diagnosis, prognosis, treatment options, and goals of care
>
> AKI, Acute Kidney Injury; CKD, chronic kidney disease; ESKD, end-stage kidney disease; Renal Physician Association. Shared Decision-Making in the Appropriate Initiation of and Withdrawal from Dialysis.[15].

decision making is a process of communication by which physicians and patient agree on specific course of action based on a common understanding of the patient's treatment goals, taking into account the benefits and harms of treatment options, and the likelihood of achieving the outcomes that are most important to individual patients."[15] Family members or friends are important to involve especially so a health care proxy can be determined for if the patient becomes incapable of making their own decisions.

It is important for providers to share information with patients and families regarding the diagnosis, expected prognosis specific to that diagnosis and all available treatment options.[15] Poor prognosis has been associated with specific patient populations with 2 or more characteristics (**Table 2**).

Those with a poor prognosis should be informed that pursuing dialysis may not provide improvement in quality of life (QOL) or *"functional status"*, as well as not increasing survival when compared with medical management without dialysis.[15] *"Research has shown that open, honest discussions with patients with advanced CKD about prognosis and end of life care promote self-reliance, alleviate fear and uncertainty, and reinforce both trust and hope."*[16]

With shared decision making, it is important to initiate advance care planning (ACP) to solidify patient care goals and ensure health care proxy is aware and agrees to patient's wishes to prepare for a situation whereby the patient may no longer have decision making capacity.[15] As stated by Davison, *"evidence supports ACP as a means of improving end of life care, decreasing inappropriate life sustaining treatment, increasing the use of hospice and supportive care, preventing hospitalizations and*

Table 2	
CKD patient with 2+ characteristics have poor outcomes[15]	
Characteristic	**Defined as**
Elderly	age 75+
High comorbidity scores	modified Charlson Comorbidity Index 8 or greater (19 comorbid conditions are given a weighted score then tallied to create CCI)[16]
Marked function impairment	Karnofsky Performance Status Scale score <40 (overall <40 defined as "*Unable to care for self; requires equivalent of institutional or hospital care; disease may be progressing rapidly, deceased*")[17]
Severe chronic malnutrition	Serum albumin <2.5

CCI, Charlson Comorbidity Index. Renal Physician Association. Shared Decision-Making in the Appropriate Initiation of and Withdrawal from Dialysis.[15–17].

increasing compliance with patient's end of life wishes."[18] As part of the ACP, the decision whether or not to initiate dialysis is of utmost importance. It is equally as important to readdress ACP for established dialysis patients to determine if they are continuing to benefit from dialysis and ensure their goals of care have not changed.

Withdrawal/Withhold Dialysis

RPA describes 4 situations whereby it is appropriate to withdraw ongoing dialysis or withhold initiating dialysis (**Box 3**).

Certain patient populations (**Table 3**), have a very poor prognosis or cannot be safely provided dialysis. With these patients, it is often not best to not initiate dialysis.[15]

One simple clinical tool which can be useful to help identify dialysis patients at risk for early mortality is *"The Surprise Question"* which asks *"would you be surprised if this patient were to die in the next 12 months?"*[18] If no, it is important to have an EOL discussion with this patient. Careful consideration must be taken, and in-depth conversations about expected outcomes, benefits, and burdens associated with dialysis to ensure the appropriate ethical decision are made regarding the patients' care.

Time-Limited Trials

As noted above, a time-limited trial of dialysis can be initiated for patients with ESKD with uncertain prognosis or uncertainty about whether or not dialysis should be

Box 3
Situations appropriate to withhold initiation or withdraw ongoing dialysis[15]
Patients with decision-making capacity, who being fully informed and making voluntary choices, refuse dialysis or request that dialysis be discontinued
Patient who no longer possess decision-making capacity who have previously indicated refusal of dialysis in an oral or written advance directive
Patients who no longer possess decision-making capacity and whose properly appointed legal agents/surrogates refuse or request that it be discontinued
Patients with irreversible, profound neurologic impairment such that they lack signs of thought, sensation, purposeful behavior, and awareness of self and environment
Renal Physician Association. Shared Decision-Making in the Appropriate Initiation of and Withdrawal from Dialysis.[15].

Table 3	
Categories of patients to consider forgoing dialysis[15]	
Category	**Examples**
Medical condition precludes the technical process of dialysis because patient unable to cooperate	Advanced dementia patient pulling out dialysis needles
Medical condition precludes the technical process of dialysis because condition is too unstable	Profound hypotension
Terminal illness from non-kidney causes	Metastatic cancer
Age >75 with 2+ criteria for very poor prognosis	Saying "No" to surprise question, high comorbidity score, significantly impaired functional status, and/or severe chronic malnutrition

Renal Physician Association. Shared Decision-Making in the Appropriate Initiation of and Withdrawal from Dialysis.[15].

initiated.[15] Often patients or families are uncertain about whether or not dialysis would be the right choice for them. A time-limited trial can help determine if the patient would tolerate treatment. Before beginning the time-limited trial, it is important to establish the length of time when a reevaluation will be done to determine whether or not the patient is benefitting from dialysis and if it should be continued. Providers, patients/medical proxy, and other health care providers do not always agree about decisions regarding dialysis. It is important to have a "*systematic due process approach*" to help resolve any conflicts in decision making that may arise.[15] Potential sources of conflict include:

1. Miscommunication or misunderstanding about prognosis
2. Intrapersonal or interpersonal issues
3. Special Values

Depending on the situation it may be beneficial for an ethical committee to review the decision.

Supportive Care

Palliative care and hospice care are both types of supportive care.[18] Palliative care helps patients with life-threatening illness cope with living and dying despite life expectancy. Hospice is EOL care that is implemented when patients are believed to be within months of death. Palliative care and hospice services are a helpful resource for patients with terminal conditions but are significantly underutilized in nephrology. According to a cohort study of 1226 patients on hemodialysis studied from 2001 to 2015, only 34% of patients who withdrew dialysis treatment received palliative care services, even though the median time to death after stopping dialysis was 7 days.[19] It is important to offer palliative care services to all patients with KRT and late-stage CKD patients who are symptomatic from their disease. These services help continue the discussion about patient's goals of care while also providing support to patient families including bereavement. Supportive care and symptom management are key in improving QOL as well as allowing patients the opportunity to die in the setting of their choice. Many patients in the hospital often say *"let me go home and die with dignity"* and they have the right to this choice.

Communication

Good communication and education are essential in providing patients with the highest quality patient care. These have been shown to *"improve patient's adjustment to illness, increase adherence to treatment, and results in higher patient and family satisfaction with care."*[15] Providers have to find a way to inform patients/families about the trajectory of their diagnosis and treatment options in a way that is well understood by all.

In both dialysis patients and CKD patients while continuing communication and discussing treatment options it is beneficial to complete a Medical Orders for Scope of Treatment (MOST) form. MOST allows patients to define their preference for life-sustaining treatments. The largest advantage of the MOST form is that these conversations have specific examples:

- If your heart were to stop do you want me to do CPR, perform compressions on your chest?
- If you were to stop breathing, would you want me to put a tube down your throat to help you to breathe?
- If it came down to it, would you agree to have a trach placed?
- Would you want medication to maintain your blood pressure, antibiotics, or nutrition?
- If you could no longer eat and needed a feeding tube, would you want to have one placed?
- What if you were unconscious, with no signs of waking, how long would you want to continue lifesaving interventions?
- Would you want to continue dialysis?
- If you were not able to go home, would you want to go to a nursing home?

Every patients answers are different and some wish to discuss it with their family before making a decision. It is important to inform the patients that their choices will be carried out but that they can amend the form at any time.

Communication skills in the area of conservative care, particularly in the past, have not been a large focus in nephrology provider education. Cohen noted that nephrology fellows reported *"limited teaching and comfort in performing"* primary palliative care skills.[20] One program which seeks to help improve these skills is *NephroTalk. a* multimodal conservative care curriculum developed to teach conservative care concepts and communication skills to nephrology fellows.[20] When this program was piloted, fellows felt it improved comfort and willingness in having these discussions.[20] Additional education in this area for providers is important to provide patients with the highest standard of care.

CASE STUDY

Ms Doe is an 83-year-old female with a history of diabetes, heart failure, hypertension, medication-induced angioedema, and breast cancer. She has had stable CKD for years with an eGFR of 20 for the last 3 years. She has the usual sequalae of CKD: lethargy, mild anemia, edema, and chronic vitamin D deficiency (resolved on weekly supplementation). Ms Doe's heart failure has been maintained on furosemide 20 mg BID and is relatively stable. She occasionally requires an extra 20 mg of furosemide for lower extremity edema. She has indicated repeatedly that she is not interested in transplant or dialysis.

Ms Doe presented to the clinic for an acute visit for increased lower extremity edema. She had no respiratory symptoms at that time. Her eGFR remained close to baseline at 19 mm/min but she was having increased albuminuria, a bad prognostic sign. Her history and physical examination showed an increase in her lower extremity edema to 2+ pitting to her knees and thus her furosemide was increased to 40 mg BID. An appointment was made for 2 weeks hence. At her follow-up visit, she reported feeling much worse. Her edema has increased to 3+ pitting edema and she had significant leg pain. Her potassium was unchanged but her eGFR dropped to 15 mm/min and her albuminuria continued to worsen. She began to have mild uremic symptoms including decreased appetite, fatigue, and difficulty sleeping. At this time, we revisited her goals of care. We discussed the risks and benefits of dialysis and discussed that she may not have much longer to live without KRT. She confirmed she would never agree to dialysis, even in an emergency situation. She expressed that she felt she lived a very happy and full life and was content with dying whenever that time came.

Ms Doe's goals were to reduce swelling in her legs to improve her comfort and live to see her children and grandchildren for Mother's Day in 4 weeks. We increased her furosemide to 80 mg BID and planned a 1-week follow-up while advising the patient to see her cardiologist evaluate for worsening heart failure.

Three days later, the patient presented to the hospital with shortness of breath. Her chest x-ray revealed stable cardiac enlargement and pulmonary edema. Her eGFR had worsened to 8 mm/min and her UA showed albuminuria/proteinuria but no other changes. She again declined dialysis and was treated with aggressive IV diuresis with moderate response. Diuretics were changed to torsemide with metolazone as needed. Her phosphorus was elevated at 6.2 mg/dL but she showed no signs of hyperphosphatemia (IE: itching) and declined to start a low phosphorus diet or phosphorus binders, as food was very important to her and she preferred to enjoy her meals without restrictions. She reported her leg pain improved and after a hospice/palliative care consult, she was discharged home with hospice. She continued to follow-up with our office periodically for diuretic dose adjustments. She lived to see her family for Mother's Day and passed away 2 days after that.

This case illustrates the importance of a patient's goals in medical decision making. Though her life likely could have been prolonged with dialysis, her current way of life was more important to her than longevity. She also had multiple comorbid conditions and may have been at risk for complications from both access surgery and dialysis treatments. Lowering her phosphorus was not as important to her as she enjoyed eating and she was not symptomatic from hyperphosphatemia. As medical providers, we were able to help her achieve her goals through medical management and hospice services.

CONCLUSION

While many practitioners may find EOL discussions difficult, they are common in kidney disease. Kidney disease patients have a higher morbidity rate than oncology patients but this is rarely acknowledged outside of the specialty. The chance to discuss EOL goals and plans, to participate in one of the most precious times of life and death is a gift not given to many. In nephrology, it is a very tough but also a very rewarding talk. Where else can you expound on philosophy, religion, bucket lists, intimate physical symptoms, and make a difference in a patient's life; and eventually their death.

DISCLOSURE

Authors have nothing to disclose.

CLINICS CARE POINTS

- ESKD populations have shifted with over half new start dialysis patients being over the age of 60.
- Important to establish practitioner - patient relationship for shared decision making to initiate ACP and determine goals of care.
- Communication is key. Important to have honest conversation regarding prognosis, treatment options and EOL care. These conversations may need to occur multiple times.
- Good communication results in "improved patient adjustment to illness, increased adherence to treatment and results in higher patient and family satisfaction with care."
- Remember ethical principles when approaching EOL discussion. Vulnerable CKD populations, such as elderly, cognitively impaired and cultural minorities require additional consideration and deliberation in these discussions.
- Time limited trials of dialysis should be considered in patient who require dialysis but have uncertain prognosis or for whom a consensus can not be reached about providing dialysis.
- Offer palliative care and hospice services to all patients who suffer from the burden of their disease or have chosen comfort care to support patients and help make end of life as comfortable as possible.

REFERENCES

1. Grubbs V, Moss AH, Cohen LM, et al. A Palliative Approach to Dialysis Care: A Patient-Centered Transition to the End of Life. Clin J Am Sco Nephrol 2014; 9(12):2203–9.
2. Landray MJ, Emberson JR, Blackwell L, et al. Prediction of ESRD and Death Among People With CKD: The Chronic Renal Impairment in Birmingham (CRIB) Prospective Cohort Study. Am J Kidney Dis 2010;56(6):1082–94.
3. American Medical Association. AMA Principles of Medical Ethics. AMA. AMA Principles of Medical Ethics | American Medical Association (ama-assn.org) 1995. Revised 2021.Available at: www.ama-assn.org/about/publications-newsletters/ama-principles-medical-ethics. Accessed April 24, 2021.
4. American Medical Association. ETHICS: Advance Care Planning. AMA. Advance Care Planning | American Medical Association (ama-assn.org)1995. Revised 2021. Available at: www.ama-assn.org/delivering-care/ethics/advance-care-planning. Accessed April 24, 2021.
5. American Medical Association. ETHICS: Advance Directive. AMA. Advance Directives | American Medical Association (ama-assn.org)1995. Revised 2021. Available at: www.ama-assn.org/delivering-care/ethics/advance-directives. Accessed April 24, 2021.
6. American Medical Association. ETHICS: Withholding or Withdrawing Life Sustaining Treatment. AMA. Withholding or Withdrawing Life-Sustaining Treatment | American Medical Association (ama-assn.org)1995. Revised 2021. Available at: www.ama-assn.org/delivering-care/ethics/withholding-or-withdrawing-life-sustaining-treatment. Accessed April 24, 2021.
7. American Medical Association. ETHICS: Orders Not to Attempt Resuscitation. AMA. Orders Not to Attempt Resuscitation (DNAR) | American Medical

Association (ama-assn.org)1995. Revised 2021. Available at: www.ama-assn. org/delivering-care/ethics/orders-not-attempt-resuscitation-dnar. Accessed April 24, 2021.

8. American Medical Association. ETHICS: Medically Ineffective Interventions. AMA. Medically Ineffective Interventions | American Medical Association (ama-assn.org)1995. Revised 2021. Available at: www.ama-assn.org/delivering-care/ethics/medically-ineffective-interventions. Accessed April 24, 2021.

9. American Medical Association. ETHICS: Sedation to unconsciousness in EOL care. AMA. Sedation to Unconsciousness in end-of-life care | American Medical Association (ama-assn.org)1995. Revised 2021. Available at: www.ama-assn. org/delivering-care/ethics/sedation-unconsciousness-end-life-care. Accessed April 24, 2021

10. American Medical Association. ETHICS: Physician Assisted Suicide. AMA. Physician-Assisted Suicide | American Medical Association (ama-assn.org)1995. Revised 2021. Available at: www.ama-assn.org/delivering-care/ethics/physician-assisted-suicide. Accessed April 24, 2021

11. Davison SN, Holley JL. Ethical issues in the care of vulnerable chronic kidney disease patients: the elderly, cognitively impaired, and those from different cultural backgrounds. Adv Chronic Kidney Dis 2008;15(2):177–85.

12. Thorsteinsdottir B, Swetz KM, Tilburt JC. Dialysis in the frail elderly–a current ethical problem, an impending ethical crisis. J Gen Intern Med 2013;28(11): 1511–6.

13. Davison SN. End-of-life care preferences and needs: Perceptions of patients with chronic kidney disease. Clin J Am Soc Nephrol 2010;5(2):195–204.

14. Foote C, Kotwal S, Gallagher M, et al. Survival outcomes of supportive care versus dialysis therapies for elderly patients with end-stage kidney disease: A systematic review and meta-analysis. Nephrol 2016;21(3):241–53.

15. Renal Physician Association. Shared decision-making in the appropriate initiation of and withdrawal from dialysis. 2nd ed. 2010. Rockville, Maryland.

16. National Palliative Care Research Center. Karnofsky Performance Scale Index. karnofsky_performance_scale.pdf (npcrc.org). Available at: www.npcrc.org/files/news/karnofsky_performance_scale.pdf. Accessed August 5, 2021.

17. Figueiredo, S. Editors: Zeltzer, L; Korner, N. Charlson Comorbidity Index: In depth Review. Charlson Comorbidity Index (CCI) – Strokengine, 2009. Available at: strokengine.ca/en/assessments/charlson-comorbidity-index-cci/. Accessed August 5, 2021

18. Davison SN, Levin A, Moss AH, et al, for KDIGO. Executive summary of the KDIGO Controversies Conference on Supportive Care in Chronic Kidney Disease: developing a roadmap to improving quality care. Kidney Int 2015;88(3): 447–59.

19. Chen JC-Y, Thorsteinsdottir B, Vaughan LE, et al. End of Life, Withdrawal, and Palliative Care Utilization among Patients Receiving Maintenance Hemodialysis Therapy. Clin J Am Soc Nephrol 2018;13(8):1172–9.

20. Cohen RA, Bursic A, Chan E, et al. NephroTalk multimodal conservative care curriculum for nephrology fellows. Clin J Am Soc Nephrol 2021;16(6):972–9.

Moving?

Make sure your subscription moves with you!

To notify us of your new address, find your **Clinics Account Number** (located on your mailing label above your name), and contact customer service at:

Email: journalscustomerservice-usa@elsevier.com

800-654-2452 (subscribers in the U.S. & Canada)
314-447-8871 (subscribers outside of the U.S. & Canada)

Fax number: 314-447-8029

Elsevier Health Sciences Division
Subscription Customer Service
3251 Riverport Lane
Maryland Heights, MO 63043

*To ensure uninterrupted delivery of your subscription, please notify us at least 4 weeks in advance of move.

9780323897341